Global Health Nursing

Michele J. Upvall, PhD, RN, CRNP, is a professor of nursing at Carlow University in Pittsburgh, Pennsylvania. Michele has taught and researched global health since the beginning of her nursing career. She has studied the collaborative practices of nursing with indigenous healers in southern Africa and with the Navajo Nation in southwestern United States. Other populations she has worked with include Somali refugee women and their families; nurses and other health care providers in Bhutan, Cambodia, and Botswana; and rural populations in Ghana.

Michele developed and coordinated the first baccalaureate nursing (BSN) program for Navajo and Hopi students in Ganado, Arizona, while on faculty at Northern Arizona University. During that time, she also received her postmaster's certification as a family nurse practitioner. Michele then traveled to the Aga Khan University School of Nursing in Karachi, Pakistan, where she served as director of the prelicensure BSN and RN-to-BSN programs. While in Pakistan, she implemented the first master's of nursing program in the nation.

After 5 years in Pakistan, Michele returned to her home in Pittsburgh and facilitated the growth of the nursing programs division at Carlow University into a school of nursing as associate dean and director. While serving in this role, Michele developed a state-of-the-art nursing skills laboratory, facilitated curriculum revision for both undergraduate and graduate nursing programs, and was instrumental in developing the doctor of nursing practice (DNP) program. She has published numerous research-based and project development articles in cooperation with global health nursing colleagues in peer-reviewed journals and has also contributed book chapters based upon her experiences in the United States and abroad.

In addition, Michele is a fellow of the American Association of Colleges of Nursing's (AACN's) Leadership for Academic Nursing programs and a recipient of the Cameo of Caring Nurse Educator Award and the Community Service Award from Sigma Theta Tau International Lambda Omicron chapter. She is active in the Pennsylvania State Nurses' Association and serves as a peer reviewer for a variety of nursing and other health care–related journals.

Jeanne M. Leffers, PhD, RN, is currently professor emerita of nursing at the University of Massachusetts–Dartmouth, where she has taught in the undergraduate and graduate programs in nursing, has been the graduate program director, and served the College of Nursing using her expertise in public health, environmental health, and global heath. At the university, she has been involved in programs to advance faculty development for diversity initiatives, strengthen the academic programs in sustainable development, and engage international students in global learning. She has taught collaborative courses in both sociology and sustainability disciplines and has been a faculty member at the University of Rhode Island's College of Nursing. A graduate of Simmons College School of Nursing, she completed her master's in nursing at the University of Rhode Island and her MA and PhD in sociology at Brown University. During her professional nursing career, she worked with women and children and held positions as a public health nurse in Tennessee and Virginia prior to her 30-year career in nursing education. She continues to teach at the University of Rhode Island and at the University of Massachusetts–Dartmouth.

Jeanne has published in the areas of public health nursing, environmental health, and global health, including coauthoring the book *Volunteering at Home and Abroad: The Essential Guide for Nurses* with Julia Plotnick, MPH, FAAN. She has also been instrumental in the development of the Alliance of Nurses for Healthy Environments' (ANHE) website (www.anhe.org), an online resource helping nurses learn essential knowledge for environmental health and helping nurses network with nurse colleagues to promote healthy environments.

Jeanne is an active member of nursing organizations devoted to public health nursing, the nursing profession, and nursing research, and has served in a number of related leadership roles. Currently, Jeanne serves on the steering committee of the ANHE and the Health Volunteers Overseas Nursing Education Steering Committee, an association with which she is the nurse coordinator for the nursing education program in Uganda. In addition, Jeanne is a member of the Environmental Protection Agency's Children's Health Protection Advisory Committee (CHPAC). Locally, she serves on the board of directors for the Greater New Bedford Community Health Center and the South Coast Visiting Nurse Association of Southeastern Massachusetts.

Jeanne is the recipient of the University of Massachusetts–Dartmouth Drum Major Award, the Simmons College Distinguished Alumna Award, the Genesis Award, and the Theta Kappa Chapter Leader Award.

Global Health Nursing

Building and Sustaining Partnerships

Michele J. Upvall, PhD, RN, CRNP
Jeanne M. Leffers, PhD, RN
Editors

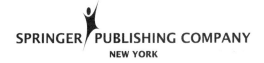

SPRINGER PUBLISHING COMPANY
NEW YORK

Springer Publishing Company, LLC
11 West 42nd Street
New York, NY 10036
www.springerpub.com

Acquisitions Editor: *Elizabeth Nieginski*
Composition: Amnet Systems

ISBN: 978-0-8261-1868-4
e-book ISBN: 978-0-8261-1869-1

14 15 16 17 / 5 4 3 2 1

The author and the publisher of this Work have made every effort to use sources believed to be reliable to provide information that is accurate and compatible with the standards generally accepted at the time of publication. The author and publisher shall not be liable for any special, consequential, or exemplary damages resulting, in whole or in part, from the readers' use of, or reliance on, the information contained in this book. The publisher has no responsibility for the persistence or accuracy of URLs for external or third-party Internet websites referred to in this publication and does not guarantee that any content on such websites is, or will remain, accurate or appropriate.

Library of Congress Cataloging-in-Publication Data

Global health nursing : building and sustaining partnerships / [edited by] Michele J. Upvall, Jeanne M. Leffers.
     p. ; cm.
  Includes bibliographical references and index.
  ISBN 978-0-8261-1868-4 (print : alk. paper) — ISBN 978-0-8261-1869-1 (e-book)
  I. Upvall, Michele J. (Michele Jean), editor of compilation. II. Leffers, Jeanne, 1947– editor of compilation.
  [DNLM: 1. Nursing. 2. Education, Nursing. 3. International Cooperation. 4. Nursing Research. 5. Public-Private Sector Partnerships. WY 16.1]
  RT42
  610.73—dc23
                                                                                          2013048451

Special discounts on bulk quantities of our books are available to corporations, professional associations, pharmaceutical companies, health care organizations, and other qualifying groups. If you are interested in a custom book, including chapters from more than one of our titles, we can provide that service as well.

For details, please contact:
Special Sales Department, Springer Publishing Company, LLC
11 West 42nd Street, 15th Floor, New York, NY 10036-8002
Phone: 877-687-7476 or 212-431-4370; Fax: 212-941-7842
E-mail: sales@springerpub.com

Printed in the United States of America by Courier.

Contents

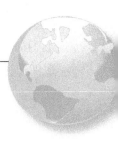

Contributors

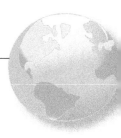

Sarah E. Abrams, PhD, RN
Associate Dean and Associate Professor
College of Nursing and Health Sciences
University of Vermont
Burlington, Vermont

Luisa Barton, NP-PHC, DNP
Faculty, MN-PHCNP Program
Ryerson University
Toronto, Canada

Linda Ciofu Baumann, PhD, APRN-C, FAAN
Professor Emerita
University of Wisconsin
Madison, Wisconsin

Debra Brady, PhD, RN
Associate Professor, Education Team Chair
College of Nursing
University of New Mexico
Albuquerque, New Mexico

Marion E. Broome, PhD, RN, FAAN
Dean and Distinguished Professor
Associate Vice President for Academic Affairs
IU Health School of Nursing, Indiana University
Indianapolis, Indiana

Alicia J. Curtin, PhD, GNP, RN
Associate Professor
College of Nursing
University of Rhode Island
Kingston, Rhode Island

Jill B. Derstine, EdD, RN, FAAN
Associate Clinical Professor
College of Nursing and Health Professions
Drexel University
Philadelphia, Pennsylvania

Jacqueline Maria Dias, RN, RM, BScN, MEd
Nurudin Jivraj Assistant Professor and Director
School of Nursing and Midwifery
Aga Khan University
Karachi, Pakistan

Myrna A. A. Doumit, PhD, MPH, BSN
Associate Professor and Assistant Dean
Alice Ramez Chagoury School of Nursing
Lebanese American University
Byblos, Lebanon

Elizabeth Downes, MPH, MSN, APRN, FAANP, DNP
Assistant Professor
Emory University
Atlanta, Georgia

Marie J. Driever, PhD, RN, FAAN
Clinical Practice and Research Consultant
Affiliate Assistant Professor
School of Nursing
University of Washington
Seattle, Washington

Nermine Elcokany, DNP, RN
Assistant Lecturer
Faculty of Nursing
Alexandria University
Alexandria, Egypt

Miguel Angel Estopinan, MS, RN
Universidad Nacional Autónoma de Nicaragua
Matagalpa, Nicaragua

Leah J. Hart, RN, MSN, MPH
Technical Development Officer
Jhpiego (An affiliate of Johns Hopkins University)
Baltimore, Maryland

Nancy Hoffart, PhD, RN
Founding Dean and Professor
Alice Ramez Chagoury School of Nursing
Lebanese American University
Byblos, Lebanon

Pamela Hoyt-Hudson, BSN, RN
Global Nursing Coordinator
Dreyfus Health Foundation
New York, New York

Gale Hull, Doctor of Humane Letters
President
Partners in Development
Ipswich, Massachusetts

Azza Hussein, DNS
Associate Professor and Department Head
Nursing Administration
Faculty of Nursing
Alexandria University
Alexandria, Egypt

Peter Johnson, CNM, PhD
Jhpiego (An affiliate of Johns Hopkins University)
Baltimore, Maryland

Nancy Kelly, MHS
Executive Director
Health Volunteers Overseas
Washington, DC

Jessica Larratt-Smith, NP-PHC
Ryerson University Graduate
Toronto, Canada

Janet L. Larson, PhD, RN, FAAN
Professor
School of Nursing
University of Michigan
Ann Arbor, Michigan

Alexis Lawton, BA
Haiti Project Director
School of Nursing and Health Professions
Regis College
Weston, Massachusetts

Jeanne M. Leffers, PhD, RN
Professor Emerita of Nursing
University of Massachusetts
Dartmouth, Massachusetts

Judy Liesveld, PhD, RN, PPCNP-BC
Associate Professor
College of Nursing
University of New Mexico
Albuquerque, New Mexico

Marilyn Lotas, PhD, RN, FAAN
Associate Professor
Frances Payne Bolton School of Nursing
Case Western Reserve University
Cleveland, Ohio

Cherlie Magny-Normilus, FNP-C, MSN, RN
Director of Policy and Advocacy, Haiti Project
School of Nursing, Science, and Health Professions
Regis College
Weston, Massachusetts

Barbara Mandleco, RN, PhD, ANEF
Professor Emerita
College of Nursing, Brigham Young University
Provo, Utah

Diane C. Martins, PhD, RN
Associate Professor
College of Nursing
University of Rhode Island
Kingston, Rhode Island

Speciosa M. Mbabali, MCommH, RNT, RM, RN
Department of Nursing
College of Health Sciences
Makerere University
Kampala, Uganda

Scovia Nalugo Mbalinda, MSc PRH, BSN
Department of Nursing
College of Health Sciences
Makerere University
Kampala, Uganda

Ruth McDermott-Levy, PhD, RN
Assistant Professor
College of Nursing
Villanova University
Villanova, Pennsylvania

Geoffrey Menego, MCHD
Jhpiego (An affiliate of Johns Hopkins University)
Kisumu, Kenya

Emma McKim Mitchell, PhD, RN
Assistant Professor
School of Nursing and Health Studies
University of Miami
Miami, Florida

Rose Chalo Nabirye, PhD, MPH, RN
Department of Nursing
College of Health Sciences
Makerere University
Kampala, Uganda

Marcia A. Petrini, PhD, RN, FAAN
Professor and Dean
HOPE School of Nursing
Wuhan University
Wuhan, Hubei Province, People's Republic of China

Julia Plotnick, MPH, RN, FAAN, RADM (retired), ScD (Hon)
Chief Nursing Officer
United States Public Health Service (retired)
Silver Spring, Maryland

Manila Prak, BSN, RN
Director of External Program Department
Angkor Hospital for Children
Siem Reap, Cambodia

Mary E. Riner, PhD, RN, FAAN
Associate Dean for Global Affairs
School of Nursing
Indiana University
Indianapolis, Indiana

Valentina Sarkisova, MSN, RN
President
Russian Nurses' Association
Saint Petersburg, Russia

Natalia Serebrennikova, PhD
International Relations Manager
Russian Nurses' Association
Saint Petersburg, Russia

Anne Sliney, BSN, RN, ACRN
Chief Nursing Officer
Clinton Health Access Initiative
Boston, Massachusetts

Michele J. Upvall, PhD, RN, CRNP
Professor of Nursing
Carlow University
Pittsburgh, Pennsylvania

Catherine Uwimana, RN, MSN
Acting Dean
Faculty of Nursing Sciences
Kigali Health Institute
Kigali, Rwanda

Jenny Vacek, MSN, RN
Senior Lecturer II
College of Nursing
University of New Mexico
Albuquerque, New Mexico

Judith Lupo Wold, PhD, RN
Distinguished Professor for Educational Leadership
Lillian Carter Center for Global Health and Social Responsibility
Nell Hodgson Woodruff School of Nursing, Emory University
Atlanta, Georgia

Foreword

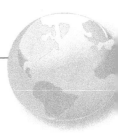

Global health, as a field of study, has undergone unprecedented transformation. As the world has evolved demographically, environmentally, and technologically, so too has the definition of global health. It has changed from being defined as infectious diseases, tropical medicine, or health care for developing nations to the health and well-being of populations in all nations. It is no longer just a field of study in which health care providers offer their knowledge and care, based on Western wisdom, to people less fortunate in faraway lands. It is now an area of study and investigation built on the premise that the health of the world is predicated on mutual respect among populations and reciprocal learning of best practices. It is also based on the transmission and receipt of knowledge from different corners of the world, collaborative practices, and partnered international teams working through volunteerism, nongovernmental organizations (NGOs), governments, academic institutions, and international organizations, all to keep populations well, prevent illness, and maximize health. Learning from others is also an ultimate overall goal of global health. It is through full collaboration, as well as a strong sense of accountability among all these sectors, that progress on improving health globally can be accelerated. Effective partnerships are essential to delivering equitable, high-quality, accessible global health care.

And while the complete engagement of these collaborations is essential to making the world healthier, it all starts with how we prepare the next generation of health care professionals to have the passion for making a difference. With the transformation of global health—or because of it—academic institutions have experienced unprecedented interest in learning about and partaking in global health experiences. As educators in health professional schools, we have committed ourselves to educating and graduating globally minded health care professionals who are ready to address worldwide issues and who are well equipped to translate research findings into policy and practice in the United States and globally. This yearning for being part of the world and expanding horizons to understand the different health contexts has resulted in a proliferation of student and faculty exchange programs as well as a need for clinicians whose experiences and learning are not bound by borders. With increases in population movements resulting in migration and immigration, and owing to the many wars that have driven people out of their countries seeking refuge, health care professionals have seen the necessity to understand the different sociocultural and ecological contexts for populations displaced for whatever reason.

Alongside the increase in interest, great strides in global health have been made that are partly owing to large-scale social and technological revolutions. For example, the decrease in infant mortality in 2012 has enabled more children than ever before to live to celebrate their fifth birthday (UNICEF, 2013). Antiretroviral drugs have increased the length and quality of life of those living with HIV. And unprecedented technological advances, such as telecommunications, mobile phone technology, the Internet, and broadband technology, have aided in bridging the gap between those who have access to health care information and those who don't, and while these advances are testaments to how far we've come, current global health issues and challenges serve as indications of how far we still have to go. The poliovirus, for example, is once again rearing its ugly head in Israel and parts of

Europe (Butler, 2013). With regard to the reduction of maternal mortality, progress remains slow. Every day, 800 women die from preventable causes related to pregnancy and childbirth because of a lack of access to a skilled health professional (doctor, nurse, midwife) to administer interventions that prevent and manage life-threatening conditions resulting from childbirth (WHO, 2012). Also, the impact of climate change and natural disasters on global health are being felt around the world. For example, the recent devastation and destruction of health care services in the Philippines as the result of supertyphoon Haiyan has put millions of survivors at risk of contracting life-threatening diseases.

All these happenings in global health support the timeliness of this book because of the absolute need for theories, evidence, and guidelines to support culturally competent and ethically sound global experiences. This book is built on a sound theoretical background that honors the principles of equity and justice, which should undergird and permeate all educational curricula, research, and evidence-based practice to advance global health and ensure health equity. The theoretical frameworks should stimulate productive research programs and the values of respect, civility, reciprocity, and collaboration that are manifested in the various chapters.

This book provides the readers, whether faculty members, clinicians, or students, with frameworks of prototypical experiences to prepare them for exchange and/or reciprocal work in other countries. The authors demonstrate how they prepared for their assignments, experiences, or missions by studying context, history, and sociocultural structure. There are examples of reciprocal exchanges of knowledge, ways by which goals were mutually modified, best practices of partnerships, and mutually agreed-upon goals and outcomes by host countries and the hosted clinician/faculty/student. Some of the authors also provide comparative data between countries. The volume also provides exemplars of courses, clinical experiences, reflective diaries, and final-outcome report writing. These and other pragmatic guidelines will be welcomed by those who provide the experiences and those who actually live through these experiences.

I commend the editors for their choice of chapters, and the authors for writing the chapters. This is a timely collection of chapters made very coherent by the editors' well-articulated, theoretical framework as well as by their conclusion. This book should be read by every person who is embarking on a global health experience or who is working or caring for immigrants and refugees. It will provide him or her with a context as well as with a framework for culturally competent and ethical practice.

Afaf I. Meleis, PhD, DrPS (hon), FAAN
Margaret Bond Simon Dean of Nursing
Professor of Nursing and Sociology
University of Pennsylvania School of Nursing
Director of the School's WHO Collaborating
Center for Nursing and Midwifery Leadership

REFERENCES

Butler, D. (2013). Polio risk looms over Europe. *Nature, 502,* 601–602.

UNICEF. (2013). *Levels and trends in child mortality: Report 2013.* New York, NY: United Nations Children's Fund.

World Health Organization (WHO). (2012). *Maternal mortality fact sheet.* Retrieved from http://www.who.int/mediacentre/factsheets/fs348/en/#

Preface

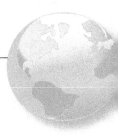

Nurses have shared stories of their global health experiences for decades, and many of these stories have significantly affected the nursing profession and the patients at the center of nursing care. Florence Nightingale and her efforts in the Crimea serve as a classic example of how nurses affect health globally. On a more contemporary note, organizations such as the American College of Nurse-Midwives (ACNM) have actively promoted the health of women and newborns globally over the past 30 years (Kennedy, Stalls, Kaplan, Grenier, & Fujoka, 2012). At an individual level, we see increased participation of nurses in volunteer organizations, nongovernmental organizations (NGOs), academic and research institutions, religious organizations, and governments to promote health worldwide. Even the tourism industry has aligned its profit motive with an appeal to good intentions through the rise of "voluntourism," whereby nurses can provide short-term care in local clinics, hospitals, or schools while also touring the local area or country.

Often in our efforts to help improve the health of the world's population we assume that our compassionate attitudes and good intentions will make a difference and are primary to facilitating health. But enthusiasm and compassion are not enough, regardless of practice setting, and the nurse who is a novice to global health may feel bewildered and confused when his or her efforts fail or are refused. We do not live or practice nursing in isolation, and our good intentions—though important—are not enough to guide practice anywhere in the world. We foster a collective sense of humanity by reflecting on our actions and asking how we individually, and as a profession, do good or do harm through our efforts in global health (McBride & Mlyn, 2012).

The premise of this book is one of connection and relationships. Globalization is a force through which we recognize our connections, promoting the concept of partnerships and shared responsibility. This book presents a framework for nursing to build and, ultimately, sustain partnerships. Exemplar case studies written by nurses working in global health follow each chapter to illustrate specific elements of a strong partnership. These nurses offer their stories from many different perspectives and backgrounds and include nurses working across national boundaries as well as those nurses effecting change within their own countries.

Our guiding principle for this book and its chapters is that partnerships are paramount in creating sustainable outcomes. Varying degrees of partnership integration can include coordination, cooperation, and close collaboration (Rosenberg, Hayes, McIntyre, & Neill, 2010). No matter their degree of partnership, nurses are ethically and morally obliged to be concerned with the world's suffering. We are connected: first through our humanity, then through our professional values and social responsibility as nurses. But we also recognize that many mistakes will be made by everyone along the global health road. Mistakes and challenges are learning opportunities; with kindness and forgiveness the outcomes of cultural humility should arise from them. And take courage: We may not always comprehend the full effect of our partnerships. By reflection we may identify an effect, but we must also appreciate the role of serendipity in our planning and be comfortable with varying degrees of ambiguity.

From our perspective, *global health nursing* can be defined as follows:

> Individual- and/or population-centered care addressing social determinants of health through a spirit of cultural humility, deliberation, and reflection in true partnership with communities and other health care providers.

Partnership is the central element of global nursing practice. Nurses must collaborate closely as an integrated team with host country partners to achieve optimum cross-cultural care reaching beyond disease management to build the capacity of partners and to avoid leaving holes in health care services upon departure. That partnerships occur both within a country's borders and across borders emphasizes the transnational component of global health. Through partnership we address health problems and their underlying social determinants, which affect all of us in varying degrees. Dichotomistic terminology such as "third world" and "first world" as well as "developing" versus "developed" nations distances partners and promotes an attitude of "us" and "them." Use of such labels conjures stereotypical images of people in the direst of circumstances as portrayed through media, which are not necessarily accurate. We use the terms *low resource* and *high resource* to encourage a less value-laden and more neutral perspective.

Although many international organizations promote a strong partnership model between host countries and visiting nurse volunteers or partners, the growth of unsustained short-term programs leaves ethical challenges and issues to be addressed (Crigger, 2008; Levi, 2009). Also, power imbalances persist among those receiving assistance and those providing it. Horton (2013) strongly, and correctly, condemns using the term *partner* in cases in which no partnership truly exists.

In our roles as global health nurse advocates and members of the Health Volunteers Overseas (HVO) Nursing Education Steering Committee, we have witnessed both strong, successful partnerships and partnerships that have faltered at various points. We believe that nurses seeking to develop or to enrich the global health partnerships they have already established will appreciate a model of partnership that includes practical considerations for ongoing development. Nurses serving in direct international clinical practice and nurse educators providing global learning opportunities for students, consultants, and researchers can also benefit from the theoretical foundation we provide and from the accompanying case studies. Reflective questions at the end of each case study can help stimulate critical and anticipatory thinking. We do not provide an extensive review of other readily available books that apply, more generally, to all health care providers. These books include global epidemiology of disease, international public health, infectious disease treatment, emerging infectious disease, and tropical medicine. Although such books are important as references for nurses who work globally, they do not focus specifically on nursing practice and the role of nurses in global health. We instead focus on the profession of nursing within the context of global health.

Michele J. Upvall
Jeanne M. Leffers

REFERENCES

Crigger, N. J. (2008). Towards a viable and just global nursing ethics. *Nursing Ethics, 15*(1), 17–27. doi: 10.1177/0969733007082121

Horton, R. (2013). Offline: The panjandrums of global health. *The Lancet, 382,* 112.

Kennedy, H. P., Stalls, S., Kaplan, L. K., Grenier, L., & Fujoka, A. (2012). Thirty years of global outreach by the American College of Nurse-Midwives. *Maternal Child Nursing, 37*(4), 290–295. doi: 10.1097/NMC.06013e318252ba71

Levi, A. (2009). The ethics of nursing student international clinical experiences. *Journal of Obstetrics, Gynecologic, and Neonatal Nursing, 38,* 94–99.

McBride, A. M., & Mlyn, E. (2012, January 25). International volunteer services: Good intentions are not enough. *Chronicle of Higher Education.* Retrieved from http://chronicle.com/article/International-Volunteer/130459/?sid=at&utm_source=at&utm

Rosenberg, M. L., Hayes, E. S., McIntyre, M. H., & Neill, N. (2010). *Real collaboration: What it takes for global health to succeed.* Los Angeles, CA: University of California Press.

Acknowledgments

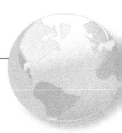

The global health context is a rich environment in which to meet and learn from others. Our own experiences in global health and the outstanding global health work done by nurses we encountered in global settings inspired this book. We acknowledge our partners worldwide who advance health for people across the globe. This book has provided numerous opportunities for us to network and learn about the work of those who have contributed to this book. We deeply appreciate their willingness to share their experiences as they truly live the partnership process in global health. As co-editors, we have learned from each other as well, and our friendship has deepened over these many months of work.

We are grateful to the members of the Health Volunteer Overseas (HVO) Nursing Education Steering Committee for supporting and encouraging this project. The idea for this book grew out of a discussion from this committee as we recounted both success stories and "not-so-successful" stories. We committed ourselves to creating a forum for these stories and to providing guidance to others through chapters explaining the theory behind the stories. We express our special thanks to Linda James, project manager, for her support of nursing education at HVO.

Our family and friends gave us the fortitude to keep reading, writing, and revising throughout the publication process. Our global health work would not have been possible without the support of our families over many years. Jeanne is deeply grateful to her husband, Jim, and to her children—Matt and his family, John, and Annie—for their loving support. Michele greatly appreciates the support, patience, and love of her husband, Richard, and of her children, Leah, Jonathan, and Rachel. Both our families have stood with us no matter where in the world we have found ourselves living.

In addition, we thank Dr. Afaf Meleis for generously contributing the Foreword for this book. As a world-renowned expert in global health and nursing, her contribution is unmatched, and we are sincerely grateful.

We could not have accomplished the work without the help of the editorial staff at Springer Publishing Company—in particular, Elizabeth Nieginski and Chris Teja, whose support and attention helped us in each phase of our work on this book.

We wish to thank those nurses and others dedicated to global health with whom we have had the privilege to work during our many years in global health nursing. There are too many for us to name individually, but without their partnership and friendship, our work would not have been collaborative, or so rewarding. We have learned more than we have shared.

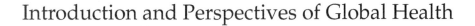

Introduction and Perspectives of Global Health

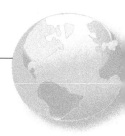

Michele J. Upvall
Jeanne M. Leffers
Emma McKim Mitchell

Globalization represents a paradigmatic shift in our relationships as individuals and as a nursing profession. We are now connected through the global economy, technology, and the larger sociopolitical environment across and within continents (www.globalization101.org). Globalization exemplifies our interdependence and requires a holistic view of our world. We are connected in myriad ways: culturally, economically, politically, psychologically, and spiritually (Crigger, 2008). Our understanding of health and the meaning of health for individuals and communities is also changing by the process of globalization. Health is no longer viewed as static, an either/or dichotomy with presence or absence of disease, but rather as dynamic and defined within the context of society. The World Health Organization (WHO) defines health as "a state of complete physical, mental and social well-being and not merely the absence of disease or infirmity" (WHO, 1948, p. 100). But how is global health defined? How is it similar to or different from international health or public health? Can these entities be combined? If so, what are their synergies? Exploring these questions while reviewing historical development and nursing perspectives of global health provides the foundation for understanding a conceptual model of partnership for global health embodied by social justice and equity.

INTERNATIONAL HEALTH, PUBLIC HEALTH, OR GLOBAL HEALTH

No clear consensus exists differentiating international and public health from global health, so various combinations of the terms have been developed, such as *international public health*, *global public health*, and *global health promotion* (Fried et al., 2010; Khubchandani & Simmons, 2012; Merson, Black, & Mills, 2006). Often the term *international health* is used synonymously with global health, but a closer look at each of the definitions (including that of public health) is important to clear communication among disciplines (Campbell, Pleic, & Connolly, 2012) and, ultimately, to evaluating health outcomes across professional and geographical boundaries (Dyar & deCosta, 2013).

International Health

Traditional definitions of international health represent a concrete and perhaps static view of health with providers from resource-rich countries crossing borders to countries with few resources. Sharma and Atri (2010) view international health as "the science and art of examining health problems in multiple countries, primarily those that are developing, and finding population-based solutions to their problems" (p. 6). Koplan et al. (2009) reviewed the concept of international health in their search for a comprehensive definition of global health and determined that international health efforts are targeted at low-income countries, and primarily at infectious diseases and maternal and child health issues.

These perspectives of international health illustrate what is referred to as a medical model approach to the world's health challenges. The focus is on diagnosis and treatment with the goal of curing the health problem or disease. While this approach has benefited the world in controlling communicable disease, it has not been totally successful, and in fact it represents what Frenk et al. (2010) designate as a form of professional tribalism—one profession operating either in isolation or in competition with other professions. For example, poliomyelitis is endemic in Pakistan and Afghanistan (Sultan & Khan, 2013) despite ongoing community campaigns to eradicate it. Efforts to control poliomyelitis may be more successful if both medical and public health professionals used a more collaborative approach to address this health challenge rather than working alone.

Public Health

Public health may be viewed as a subset of international health in which local and national governments are concerned with the health of communities. Winslow (1920) published one of the earliest definitions of public health:

> [T]he science and art of preventing disease, prolonging life, and promoting physical mental health and efficiency through organized community efforts toward a sanitary environment; the control of community infections; the education of the individual in principles of personal hygiene; the organization of medical and nursing service for the early diagnosis and treatment of disease, and the development of the social machinery to ensure to every individual in the community a standard of living adequate for the maintenance of health. (p. 30)

A more succinct definition from WHO (2013) is "all organized measures (whether public or private) to prevent disease, promote health, and prolong life among the population as a whole."

The American Public Health Association (APHA) defines public health from a disease prevention and health promotion perspective, inclusive of groups from small communities to nations. Policy and research are emphasized in order to understand and strategize priorities for health (www.apha.org/NR/rdonlyres/C57478B8-8682-4347-8DDF-A1E24E82B919/0/what_is_PH_May1_Final.pdf?gclid=CNqJ5trQ97cCFSxk7AodR2IA2A). Currently, the three priorities of the APHA (www.apha.org/advocacy/priorities) include:

- Building public health structure and capacity
- Ensuring the right to health and health care
- Creating health equity

These priorities, approached from a multidisciplinary perspective, are concerned with issues of social justice and distinguish public health from international health and a medical model. Again, health is more than absence of disease. All populations are entitled to health, including the alleviation of forces, such as poverty, that degrade health. Merson, Black, and Mills (2006) combined international and public health in their definition of international public health: "the application of principles of public health to health problems and challenges that affect low and middle income countries and to the complex array of global and local forces that influence them" (p. xiv). The confusion among terms continues with attempts at defining global health.

TABLE I.1 Definitions and Core Concepts of Global Health

Definition	Core concepts
". . . health problems, issues, and concerns that transcend national boundaries and may best be addressed by cooperative actions . . . goal of improving health for all people by reducing avoidable disease, disability, and deaths" (Institute of Medicine, 2009a, p. 5)	• Transcend boundaries • Cooperation • Health for all • Reduce disease, disability, death
"an area for study, research, and practice that places a priority on improving health and achieving equity in health for all people worldwide. Global health emphasizes transnational health issues, determinants, and solutions; involves many disciplines within and beyond the health sciences and promotes interdisciplinary collaboration; and is a synthesis of population-based prevention with individual-level care" (Koplan et al., 2009, p. 1995)	• Includes study, research, and practice • Improves health for all • Transnational • Determinants of health • Multidisciplinary • Interprofessional collaboration • Synthesis of individual care and population prevention
"collaborative trans-national research and action for promoting health for all" (Beaglehole & Bonita, 2010, p. 1)	• Collaboration • Transnational • Combines research with action • Provides health for all

Global Health

Attempts to distinguish public health from global health and provide a comprehensive definition of global health are ongoing. Fried et al. (2010) declare that there is no differentiation and cite principles of "global public health." Their core beliefs of global public health emphasize health for all with health seen as a public good that must be addressed using an interprofessional approach. Fried et al. (2010) note the interdependence of populations, such that by strengthening local populations the global health system will be stronger.

Other groups and individuals have also defined global health (see Table I.1). The definition of Koplan and colleagues (2009) has been widely accepted, but others view it as lengthy and unwieldy. Beaglehole and Bonita's (2010) simpler definition views global health as building on national public health efforts and action based on research to support policy based on evidence.

In an effort to determine Canada's strategic role in global health, the Canadian Academy of Health Sciences agreed on Koplan et al.'s definition of global health, but only after an inductive analysis of other definitions. Their analysis determined primary and secondary characteristics for any definition of global health. Primary characteristics included equity; a global conceptualization of health with the goal of health for all; causes or contextual factors of health such as the social, economic, and physical environment; means or methods for practicing global health; and solutions for addressing health issues. Secondary characteristics address the source of obligation for carrying out global health activities, typically resource-rich entities; a multidisciplinary approach defining the values and goals of the actors, or agents; and determining whether global health should be proactive or reactive or a combination of the two (Campbell, Pleic, & Connolly, 2012).

The definition and practice of global health is evolving despite lack of agreement on a single operational definition of global health (Khubchandani & Simmons, 2012). Rowson et al. (2012) frame the global health definition debates around three central aspects of a definition useful for educators of global health. In the first aspect, the object of knowledge, global health refers to the scope of problems and not just to geographical location. In addition, commonalities and differences need to be accounted for and are often related to context. For example, poverty occurs in all parts of the world, but knowing what causes poverty and how to address it requires knowledge of the local context.

The second aspect of any definition of global health should address types of knowledge. Multidisciplinary approaches are critical to understanding the underlying social, political, and economic determinants of health problems. Global health is more than having an intervention to cure a health problem. Rather, health is interconnected to social, political, and economic context and thus requires a multifaceted approach.

Finally, the purpose of knowledge for global health must be considered. It is not enough to approach global health from the perspective of how it is practiced—we must also ask *why* it is practiced. This approach goes beyond simple acceptance of equity as the primary value in global health to require critical thinking about power in relationships and to question all values related to global health. Developing partnerships in working toward mutually agreed-on global health goals promotes a sense of power *with* others as opposed to power *over* others.

A BRIEF HISTORY OF GLOBAL HEALTH

Concern about health and communicable disease dates back to the ancient civilizations of Mesopotamia, India, China, Egypt, and Greek and Roman civilizations. The Romans in particular contributed to public health with the development of sewer systems and aqueducts, as well as a system of military medicine (Sharma & Atri, 2010). While care of individuals and populations have always been of concern to society, examining historical antecedents of health promotes understanding of the shift from international to global health (Brown, Cueto, & Fee, 2006).

Present-day global health is rooted in the history of international health and colonization. European expansion brought disease and deaths to those who were subjugated by colonial forces, with public health viewed as a means of creating more wealth through expansion of power. Controlling disease enabled colonial forces to keep the workers healthy enough to extract resources and enrich the colonial powers (Unite for Sight, n.d.).

Nursing was not immune to the forces of colonialism, as Racine and Perron (2012) note in their discussion of professional imposition or imperialism. They relate the experiences of 19th-century British nurses in what is now Sri Lanka as an example of an exotic view of "the other," or cultural voyeurism. In their letters to the Overseas Nursing Association, these nurses wrote about the conditions of the hospital and their relationships with local providers. To be working in what was then known as Ceylon was an adventure, with the British nurses claiming superiority and emphasizing the difference between themselves and the locals. How different were these nurses from nurses and students of today who, without preparation in global health and cultural humility, perpetuate a similar attitude of distinction and superiority (Racine & Perron, 2012)?

WHO as a force for international health emerged from the precursor to the current United Nations, the League of Nations Health Committee; the United Nations Relief and Rehabilitation Administration; and the Paris-based L'Office Internationale d'Hygiene Publique in June 1948, the result of 3 years of meetings.

The Pan American Sanitary Bureau resisted integration into WHO and maintained its autonomy. Today, the Bureau is known as the Pan American Health Organization (PAHO) and is the WHO regional representative for the Americas. After being renamed in 1958, the agency focused its attention on controlling and eradicating infectious diseases such as smallpox, polio, and Chagas disease, developing research centers throughout Latin America to seek local solutions to local problems. More recently, PAHO has emphasized income inequity as a major problem affecting health (Fee & Brown, 2002).

Alma Ata Conference and Primary Health Care

During the 1960s, colonial powers ceded direct government control in many countries, with independence arising particularly throughout Africa. This new political environment affected WHO and the world of international health as well. The discord between control of infectious disease and recognition of socioeconomic forces influencing health forced a transformation of WHO. Mahler, who served as the director-general of the WHO from 1973 to 1988, convened the Alma Ata conference in Kazakhstan in 1978, in which the Declaration for Primary Health Care was passed by the delegates and "Health for all in the Year 2000" became the rallying cry (Brown, Cueto, & Fee, 2006).

The Alma Ata Declaration affirmed health as a human right, recognizing the inequality of health among those living in low-resource and resource-rich countries. Economic and social development was noted to be of basic importance to achievement for all, with people having the right and responsibility to participate in their own health care. Primary health care was to address health at the community level and existed within a referral system beginning with local clinics and continuing to comprehensive, tertiary care centers. Specific elements of primary health care included health education, nutrition, safe water and basic sanitation, maternal and child health care, immunizations, treatment of common diseases, provision of essential drugs, and family planning (WHO, n.d.).

The shift of thinking from international health to global health began with the Alma Ata Declaration, but as the World Bank and the field of health economics emerged, the WHO began to lose its power and the forces of neocolonialism became increasingly evident. Developing countries turned to international lending agencies, bankrupting themselves and setting the health of their populations back by decades (Ruger, 2005). The World Bank replaced the influence of the WHO, which from 1988 to 1998 was plagued by budget crises and accusations of corruption. In 1998, under the leadership of Gro Brundtland, a physician and former prime minister of Norway, the WHO embraced a new vision of global health and finance, aligning public–private partnerships such as the Bill & Melinda Gates Foundation with immunization programs and the Roll Back Malaria campaign (Brown, Cueto, & Fee, 2006).

Millennium Development Goals

In 2000, world leaders gathered at the United Nations in New York City to adopt the United Nations Millennium Declaration. The declaration, now known as the Millennium Development Goals (MDGs), offers an outline and specific targets for ending extreme poverty by 2015:

- Eradicating extreme hunger and poverty
- Achieving universal primary education
- Promoting gender equality and empowering women
- Reducing child mortality
- Improving maternal health
- Combating HIV/AIDS, malaria, and other diseases
- Ensuring environmental sustainability
- Creating global partnerships for development

Although these ambitious goals will not be realized in 2015, progress has been made. For example, as more than 90% of children in poorer countries of the world were enrolled in primary school, a demand for more secondary schools has been created. In addition, the number of deaths of children younger than age 5 has decreased from 12.4 million in 1990 to 6.9 million in 2011. Clearly, more progress is needed, especially in sub-Saharan African countries, but the effects of developing strong global partnerships to implement the MDGs have been positive (United Nations, n.d.a).

The question remains, what will happen after 2015? Countries with few resources are experiencing the double disease burden of both communicable and chronic problems such as cardiovascular disease and obesity. The Committee on the U.S. Commitment to Global

Health convened by the Institute of Medicine (IOM, 2009b) made the following recommendations for advancing global health in the future:

- Scale up existing interventions, with the United States demonstrating leadership in addressing chronic health problems
- Generate and share knowledge through expanding research and evaluation efforts
- Invest in capacity building with long-term partnerships between foundations and corporations with universities, research centers, and health care systems in low- and middle-income countries
- Increase U.S. financial commitments to global health
- Engage in respectful partnerships

The case studies offered in this book provide a glimpse into the future of how the MDGs will be addressed and which direction should be pursued based on failed attempts and success stories. As a result of work in respectful partnership, goals may need to be redefined and revised along with the strategies for achieving those goals.

GLOBAL HEALTH NURSING

The more than 35 million nurses in the world represent the largest pool of health care providers (WHO, 2007). Nursing is well positioned to meet the challenge of global health. Nurses are responsive to the transitions of individuals and groups, including refugees and immigrants (Schumaker & Meleis, 1994), and health promotion and disease prevention are central to the role of the nurse as demonstrated through the work of Pender and the development of the Health Promotion Model (Pender, Murdaugh, & Parsons, 2006). Recognition of the determinants of global health is a central part of nursing's holistic practice, and nursing students are taught to assess patients from a cultural, environmental, social, psychological, economic, and spiritual perspective. Nursing then is in an optimum position to face the challenges presented in global health according to the following definition of global health nursing:

> Individual- and/or population-centered care addressing social determinants of health with a spirit of cultural humility, deliberation, and reflection in true partnership with communities and other health care providers.

Merry (2012) suggests that priority roles for nurses in global health include "advocacy, healing and alleviating suffering through caring, and increasing nursing capacity globally" (p. 28). Nurses should be and are advocates for patients at all levels—for the individual seeking health care as well as at the national and international levels through policy development. The nurse as healer and alleviator of suffering directly relates to health promotion and the provision of primary health care. MDGs of reducing child mortality, improving maternal health, and combating HIV/AIDS and other diseases are within the realm of nursing care.

The role of nurse as diplomat (Hunter et al., 2013) and the potential for nursing to be a primary force in global health diplomacy can promote global partnership. According to Novotny and Adams (2007), health diplomacy "is a professional practice that should inform any group or individual with responsibility to conduct research, service, program, or direct international health assistance between donor and recipient institutions" (p. 2). Nurses working in any setting, whether as volunteers or as paid employees, have the potential to act as health diplomats and promote partnership. Nurse researchers are also health diplomats and particular attention to ethical issues regardless of research setting is crucial to the nursing research role.

Increasing the capacity of nursing is central to the mission of a number of nursing organizations, including the International Council of Nurses (ICN) and the American Academy of Nursing (AAN), and thus merits a chapter of its own (Chapter 8). Position statements from the ICN (1999) and WHO research on nursing mobility (2003) are reflected in the AAN's proposed actions for addressing the global nursing shortage. These actions include conferences with world leaders for further action as well as conferences on global nursing and health research, creating a database and inventory of existing faculty and student exchanges, soliciting models for addressing global recruitment and faculty exchanges, collaborating with other international organizations and agencies, encouraging countries to develop policies of self-sufficiency for all health care providers, supporting technology and distance education, and taking an active role in policy and legislation supporting research funding (Rosenkoetter & Nardi, 2007, p. 313).

Ethical Positioning for the Practice of Global Health Nursing

An overview of the history of global health discusses nursing from a colonialist perspective and asks about nursing's progress in an era of intense globalization. Nursing ethics have been taught in classrooms around the world, but do traditional ethical principles with their origins in deontology (i.e., following the rules and considering rights and duties) and teleology (or utilitarianism—considering the consequences and results of our actions) provide the guidance necessary in the context of global nursing partnerships? For example, what ethical guidelines are articulated when overseeing student and faculty exchanges? Virtue ethics applied to nursing seems to be a logical ethical stance for global health nurses. The desire to do good at home or across national boundaries is consistent with global health nursing. However, virtue ethics depends on context and the nurse must consider that what may be considered virtuous in one cultural setting may not be appropriate in another. Grace (2009) reminds us that there is no list of virtues that portrays a virtuous nurse and that "[c]ompassion for . . . suffering without knowledge of how to mitigate it and/or the motivation to alleviate is an empty virtue" (p. 80). Global health nursing must make progress in replacing the colonialist view of cultural voyeurism too often evident in global exchanges and clinical experiences with a more sustainable, inclusive perspective of global ethics (Crigger, 2008; Racine & Perron, 2012). Virtue ethics may offer some insight, but it is inadequate to address the reality of poverty and inequity in health care.

Davis and Tschudin (2008) remind us that "[w]hile it is extremely difficult for most individuals to have any impact on the development of globalization, it is possible for informed individuals working in groups and through various organizations to make a difference on specific aspects of this movement" (p. 6). How nurses make a positive difference in global health, beyond the position of "do no harm" and from the perspective of partnership, requires an understanding of human rights and social responsibility. Applying these concepts to global health nursing practice can facilitate the development of guidelines and best practices when working with students and health care providers in community to promote health.

Human Rights

The Universal Declaration of Human Rights adopted by the General Assembly of the United Nations in 1948 relates rights and health as follows (United Nations, n.d.b):

> 1. Everyone has the right to a standard of living adequate for the health and well-being of himself and of his family, including food, clothing, housing and medical care and necessary social services, and the right to security in the event of unemployment, sickness, disability, widowhood, old age or other lack of livelihood in circumstances beyond his control.

> 2. Motherhood and childhood are entitled to special care and assistance. All children, whether born in or out of wedlock, shall enjoy the same social protection. (Article 25)

Human rights and nursing's flexibility in conceptualizing human rights provide a foundation for a global nursing ethics. Crigger (2008) identifies five qualities for developing global nursing ethics, one of which is identified as an openness to new approaches in human rights. Crigger suggests that combining the approach of Sen's (2004) notions of freedoms with Nussbaum's theory of human flourishing (1998) may promote consensus in defining human rights. The central human functional capacities for human flourishing identified by Nussbaum include:

- Having a normal life span—that is, one which is not short or impacted by poor quality of life
- Having health, sufficient food, shelter, intimate relationships, and relocation; security against bodily and emotional harm
- Being able to avoid pain and experience pleasure
- Having the ability to imagine, think, reason, and be educated
- Loving and being loved; experiencing human emotion
- Planning one's own life . . . seeking work that is fulfilling and productive
- Being able to engage freely in social interactions
- Living in relation to animals and nature
- Playing and being able to experience recreation
- Leaving autonomously as one chooses with certain "guarantees" of non-interference (Crigger, 2008, p. 24)

Applying human rights to communities and population-based nursing care is the focus of rights-based public health nursing (Ivanov & Ode, 2013) and by extension, global health nursing. All actions of the nurse operating within a rights-based ethic of care should contribute to realization of human rights. Program development and policies in nursing must reflect understanding of the issues of health and social well-being with evaluation metrics providing assurance that human rights are not violated through nursing actions (Ivanov & Oden, 2013).

Social Responsibility

Nursing care is often focused at the individual level even in global health nursing. Shifting our thinking to the level of society must increase awareness of nursing's responsibility to society as a whole. Nursing does have "a social responsibility to address those issues affecting the health of the world's people, including concerns related to poverty, access to care in politically unstable climates, and environmental conditions affecting health" (Tyer-Viola et al., 2009, p. 110). The Nursing Social Policy Statement articulated by the American Nurses Association (ANA, 2010) also addresses the social responsibility of nursing by promoting quality health care for all individuals. At a macro level, concerns affecting the health of societies discussed by Tyer-Viola et al. (2009) include nursing migration and the global nursing shortage.

How nurses address the needs of society at a global level requires more attention and focus in nursing education. Service-learning activities are one way to promote awareness of social responsibility, but these types of projects must be designed *with* rather than *for* the community. Similarly, interest in providing global health experiences for nursing students has increased. However, we must ask who really benefits from these efforts. Some organizations such as the Consortium of Universities for Global Health (CUGH) directly address issues of equity and focus on long-term partnerships of mutual benefit to all (http://cugh .org/about-us). Other organizations have created best practice guidelines for developing and maintaining global health experiences (Crump & Sugarman, 2010). These efforts illustrate shared responsibility as the basis for creating partnerships (Dybul, Piot, & Frenk, 2012). Good intention is not enough in the practice of global health nursing. Global health nursing is not practiced in isolation but rather is realized only through partnership and mutual learning.

CONCEPTUAL MODEL FOR PARTNERSHIP AND SUSTAINABILITY

Nurses must ground their practice in scientific evidence to provide the most effective nursing care to individuals, families, and populations. When nursing practice extends to a global health focus, there is limited evidence to guide practice. Although some nursing research focuses on the health beliefs, health practices, and health outcomes of many population groups and diseases, the research has not examined the actual nursing role for effectiveness and ethics. The literature includes reports on the impact of global health experiences on the nurse or nursing student who works in a setting across national borders. However, these reports contain little measuring the impact on the host partner or the health outcomes (Bentley & Ellison, 2005; Casey & Murphy, 2008; Kulbok, Mitchell, Glick, & Greiner, 2012; Reising, Allen, & Hall, 2006). Central to all nursing practice is the relationship between the nurse and those cared for by the nurse. Due to the limited evidence to support global health nursing, we elected to use the Conceptual Model for Partnership and Sustainability in Global Health (Leffers & Mitchell, 2011), which is built on evidence from nurse experts in global health.

In a qualitative study to better understand the key elements of global health nursing, Leffers and Mitchell (2011) interviewed 13 global health nurse experts. The outcomes of analysis of the interviews led to the development of a conceptual model for partnership and sustainability. The nurse experts, whose experiences included roles as researchers, educators, clinicians, and consultants, all emphasized the importance of collaboration and partnership as well as the ongoing sustainability of the program or nursing intervention. Emergent themes include nurse partner factors and roles, host partner factors, resources, collaboration, cultural bridging, capacity building, organizational factors, leadership, partnership, and sustainability. The model shows the partner factors for partnership, the process for partnership, and sustainability of global health nursing interventions (see Figure I.1).

Nurses most often participate in global health endeavors through an organization, whether governmental, nongovernmental, or academic. As a result, the nurse factors that the individual nurse brings to the relationship, such as his or her cultural perspective, personal attributes, personal expectations, and knowledge of the host country, are also affected by the organization sponsoring the nurse role. Specific attributes that the nurse brings to the global health experiences include needs for personal comfort, space, and privacy; a spirit of adventure; flexibility; openness to the perspective of others; willingness to collaborate with others; and fears. Other nurse factors include the nurse's particular skill set and expertise; expectations of the nursing practice role in the host country; and expectations of the people, lifestyle, and environment of the host country—as well as some degree of previous knowledge of the host country. Furthermore, the nurse's ability to identify personal biases that impact cross-cultural collaboration is central to the nurse and host partner relationship. The mission and philosophy of the organization with which the nurse partner works will reinforce the individual nurse factors as noted above. For example, if the global health organization offers extensive orientation for nurse participants, the expectations and personal biases might differ from those of a nurse who receives no orientation (Leffers & Mitchell, 2011).

Equally important to the nursing role and nurse partner are those factors of the host country partners. Host country partner factors include expectations of outsiders, particularly those from the country where the nurse lives, expectations of nurses who come from other countries, the nursing role overall, and the influence of the political, social, economic, and environmental status of the host country on the host partners. Furthermore, in many low-resource countries, there is a history of colonialism that will impact the host partner's relationship with nurses from other countries. The formation and quality of the partnership is affected by the interaction of the nurse partner factors and the host country factors.

Resources are essential to any program or project to improve health in global settings. Frequently nurses who participate in global health nursing experiences are from higher resource countries and are more likely to share material or financial resources with the host country partners. This might include bringing donated supplies, sharing nursing textbooks

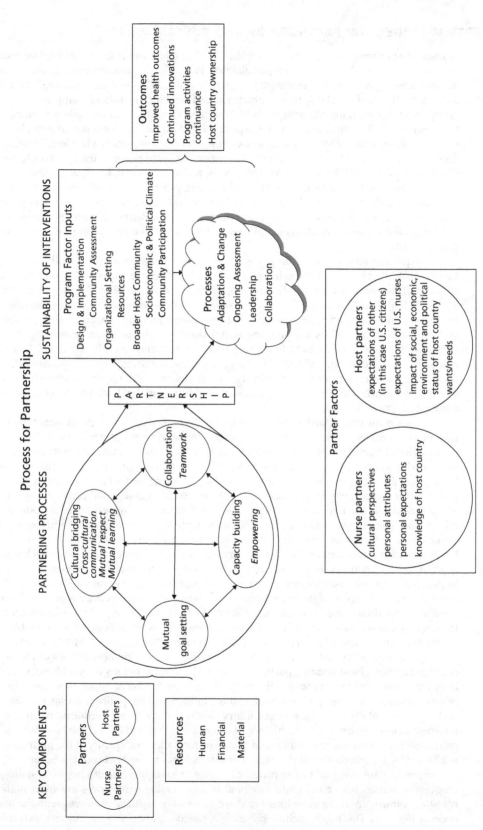

FIGURE I.1 Conceptual Model of Partnership and Sustainability in Global Health (Leffers & Mitchell, 2011). Reprinted with permission.

or materials, or donating their time in service, consultation, or education. For the nurse partners there is often the need to finance the global health experience in part or entirely. Depending on the program, there is a need for necessary equipment and supplies on site in the host country. Material resources can include specific technical or legal support from the sponsoring organization or institution. Human resources include the nurse partner and any other health professionals who serve in the host country setting.

Various themes emerged that addressed processes for building relationships. In the model these are described as cultural bridging, collaboration, capacity building, and mutual goal setting. Together these processes culminate in partnership as an outcome. However, partnership is a process as well, resulting from ongoing interactions between hosts and visitors in global health programs.

Every nurse expert interviewed for the study spoke of culture as essential to any relationship between nurse and host country partners. Terms used by the experts included *respect for cultural differences, cultural competence, cultural sensitivity,* and *language barriers.* The literature also includes terms such as *cultural humility* and *cultural safety* (Foster, 2009; Polaschek, 1998). Leffers and Mitchell (2011) elected to use the term *cultural bridging* that was offered by one of the nurse experts. We use this term as well to address the reciprocity between the nurse partner's cultural perspective and that of the host partners and the host locale. Furthermore, the term addresses the process of promoting cultural humility and cultural safety.

Collaboration is another process for partnership in the model. The term broadly addresses how both the visiting nurse partners and host country partners develop their goals and program outcomes, how they negotiate roles and responsibilities, and how they continue their ongoing work over time to achieve sustainability. In the model mutual goal setting is included separately because most of the participants spoke about setting goals as a distinct concept from collaboration. Often the discussion of mutual goal setting was part of the explanation of community and needs assessment. Collaboration as an essential element of partnership building involves related topics, such as the mandate for mutual respect; assurance that the nurse partners will base the goals on the host partners' needs; and integration of knowledge of culture, host country resources, and limitations. The conceptual model includes collaboration as a process for both building partnerships and creating sustainability.

Capacity building is an essential element for partnership formation and maintenance. Nurses who participate in global health endeavors are likely to enter a partnership developed by the organization or agency that sponsors the program and are likely to become part of an ongoing capacity building project with host partners. This can be an effort to build capacity for nursing or patient education, for nursing research, or for organizational and professional management. In many settings, visiting nurse partners work directly with nurses from the host country—an ideal situation. Thus, the host country nurses are collaborative partners in all aspects of the program. Frequently, nurse partners work with community health workers or nonprofessional host partners. Due to the severe worldwide shortage of human resources for health, nurse partners are likely to be involved with the education and training of nonprofessionals to build the capacity of the host country to meet its own health care needs. Working with nursing organizations or associations is an excellent way to build capacity for health for the host country. In those instances in which nurses join a voluntary nongovernmental organization (NGO) that provides direct care in a low- or middle-income country (LMIC), nurse partners must examine the project to ensure that capacity building is an element of the work.

Relationship building can begin at an individual level between one nurse partner and a host partner who generally serves in a key role in host setting. More likely, the partnership is between a group of visitors, who may not all be nurses, and partners in the host country. For either type of relationship building, the nurse partners should learn or conduct their own community assessment or needs assessment relevant to their program or project. A comprehensive community assessment includes examination of the traditional and existing health care practices and community members' perceived health needs, as well as identification of the host country health care system, community strengths, cultural brokers, and community leaders (Anderson & McFarlane, 2004).

Sustainability has not been well developed in the nursing literature but is more commonly used in global health program planning. To plan for parasite programs in LMICs, the WHO (2002) defined sustainability as "the ability of a project to continue to function effectively, for the foreseeable future, with high treatment coverage, integrated into available health care services, with strong community ownership using resources mobilized by the community and government" (as cited in Amazigo et al., 2007, p. 2071). Shediac-Rizkallah and Bone (1998) add key elements for sustainability that include "(1) maintaining health benefits achieved through the initial program, (2) continuation of the program activities within an organizational structure and (3) building the capacity of the recipient community" (p. 93). The Conceptual Model for Partnership and Sustainability in Global Health (Leffers & Mitchell, 2011) defines the formation and maintenance of partnerships as being essential for sustainability of programs. Outcomes of sustainability include improved health outcomes, continuance of the program or continued innovations, and transfer of ownership from a shared state to host partner control.

ORGANIZATION OF THE BOOK

Using the Conceptual Model for Partnership and Sustainability in Global Health (Leffers & Mitchell, 2011) to guide the focus of this book, we decided to combine chapters and case studies discussing not only *what* the reader can learn about global health nursing but also *how* to use principles of global health, partnership, and nursing to guide collaborative global health nursing practice. Each chapter is followed by one or more case studies from the lived experience of the authors that highlight aspects of the chapter topic. The case studies include examples from nurses whose focuses were on consultation, research, education, academic partnerships, and service. Reflective questions follow each chapter and case study.

Chapter 1, "Selecting and Negotiating Partnerships for Collaboration," discusses the importance of program selection and early partnership experience. In this chapter we discuss types of existing partnerships and how nurses make the selection of an appropriate program to begin a partnership. Specific topics include matching philosophy, mission, and goals. We also discuss how nursing and personal roles are established and maintained during the initiation of a relationship and over time. We speak to how nurses maintain professional roles while building personal relationships with host partners. Using examples of how nurses locate an organization such as Health Volunteers Overseas (HVO) or how an academic or clinical program locates and builds collaborative relationships, we offer guidance for the early partnership experience. We offer comparisons between nurse-to-nurse consultation for education and practice and programs that involve nursing students. The first case study, contributed by Nancy Kelly, executive director of HVO, highlights the mission and goals of an organization, describing how an organization selects programs for nurse participation globally and how the nurse volunteer is integral to the overall partnership in host countries. The additional two case studies provide a student perspective of selecting a graduate program, detailing the experience of being an international student, while the third case study focuses on a locally based U.S. project with global implications.

Chapter 2, "Nurse and Visiting Organization Factors for Global Partnership," addresses how cultural perspectives, personal attributes, expectations, and knowledge of host country influence a volunteer nurse's experience. We address issues of language barriers, interpreters, and the need for language knowledge prior to working in-country. Also, we include information about how the expectations of the organization represented by the nurse impact the partnership. We include a discussion of the organizational vision/mission and the overall return benefit expected by the organization. Michele J. Upvall's first case study illustrates nurse factors related both to the nurse as a volunteer and to the mission of HVO in Bhutan. The second case study, authored by Jeanne M. Leffers and Gale Hull, uses an example of an academic partnership between a college of nursing in the United States and an NGO based in the United States that partners with health professionals in Haiti to meet health needs there. Specific issues related to student, faculty, and nurse mentor expectations, preparation, and in-country experience show the importance of culture, language, knowledge of host country, and personal attributes for building and maintaining successful partnerships.

Chapter 3, "Nursing Practice and Licensure Across Borders," addresses nursing practice issues that extend beyond geography. Nursing roles in host country are addressed, community assessment as essential knowledge is highlighted, and we specifically address ethical issues when nurses practice in host countries, such as the importance of nursing licensure, mutual respect, and partnership. In addition, we address practical issues, such as health promotion while traveling, and travel requirements such as passports and visas. The chapter and case study authored by Diane C. Martins and Alicia J. Curtin describe a long-term collaboration between nurses and nursing students from the United States who partner with local community partners in the Dominican Republic.

Chapter 4, "Host Partner Factors for Partnership and Sustainability," considers factors that the host partners bring to the relationship. Examples include their experience with volunteers or partners from the United States or elsewhere, differences in the scope of practice between nursing partners, and the role of the nurse and nursing profession in host countries. We discuss the impact of social, economic, environmental, and political factors on the host partners, the role of traditional medicine, and social determinants of health. The chapter and case study by Nancy Hoffart, Jenny Vacek, Myrna A. A. Doumit, Judy Liesveld, and Debra Brady highlight host factors in the development of a nursing school in Lebanon.

Chapter 5, "Resources for Global Health Partnerships," emphasizes the importance of resources, whether human, material, or financial, that are essential in developing a partnership. Nurse partners from higher income countries frequently contribute resources to the host partners. We discuss the importance of appropriate selection of resources with consideration of sustainability and fit to the cultural needs in the host setting. Emphasis on the host partners' and resources' needs and constraints guides nurses to prepare effectively for global partnerships. We discuss how to seek funding for projects. The case study contributed by Sarah E. Abrams shows how a partnership between a university in the United States and an NGO in Uganda addresses their partnership in relation to the resources available and the resources required in the host setting. In addition, she highlights factors related to student participation in the project that impact required resources.

Chapter 6, "Capacity Building for Global Health Nursing," provides an overview of capacity building. In particular, we discuss how partners work together to use the human, organizational, and scientific resources of the host setting to strengthen the skills, competencies, and abilities of the host partners. In addition, we discuss how to modify interventions based on area resources. The case study by Marie J. Dreiver, Valentina Sarkisova, Natalia Serebrennikova, Barbara Mandleco, and Janet L. Larson shows how the partnership between nurses from the United States and Russia helped build capacity among nurses to conduct nursing research.

Chapter 7, "Bridging Cultures," addresses the essential requirement that nurse partners seek to bridge cultural differences with respect and cultural humility. We discuss how nurses demonstrate respect for host partners, for example, through communication and dress. We emphasize the importance of mutual learning among all partners. The first case study, by Jessica Larrett-Smith and Luisa Barton, speaks to the topic of culture from the perspective of First Nations in Manitoba, Canada. The second case study, contributed by Jacqueline Maria Dias of the Aga Khan University in Pakistan, addresses how cultural bridges were built between the university and other hospitals and programs throughout the country.

Chapter 8, "Collaboration With International Organizations," addresses specific issues involved with collaboration across international organizations. This includes how nurses work with a ministry of health in another country and the role of nurses who work with

NGOs. We emphasize the importance of empowering and engaging global nursing leaders in other countries. In particular, we discuss the issues involved when an academic institution develops a partnership across international borders and the need to collaborate with a variety of organizations. The first case study by Julia Plotnick describes the importance of working with nurses to facilitate and strengthen nursing organizations globally. In particular, her experience helping local nurses build their nursing associations in Romania during the 1990s and in Rwanda in 1995 demonstrates the importance of nursing organizations. The second case study, by Anne Sliney and Catherine Uwimana, features the collaboration among the Clinton Health Access Initiative, the Rwandan Ministry of Health, and the Rwandan Nurses and Midwives Association for the Rwandan Human Resources for Health program.

Chapter 9, "Making Collaborative Research Work," discusses important aspects of nursing research in international settings. Nursing evidence is essential for the advancement of nursing practice worldwide. Increasingly, nurses are involved with nursing research across international borders. This chapter explores issues of culture, the effect of nurses from high-income countries conducting research in low- and middle-income countries (Harrowing, Mill, Spiers, Kulig, & Kipp, 2010), and ethical considerations for international research (Ketefian, 2000). The case study by Linda Ciofu Baumann features a research partnership to improve diabetes care in Uganda.

Chapter 10, "Maintaining Partnerships Through Leadership," explores the elements of sustainability to address the leadership required to maintain the partnership, how visiting partners must step back and support leadership by host health care providers, and how to continually monitor and assess the project. The first case study, from Marilyn Lotas of Case Western University and Marcia Petrini from Wuhan University in China, describes the development of the relationship of the schools of nursing and the challenges of collaboration. The second case study, written by Leah J. Hart, Peter Johnson, and Geoffrey Menego from Jhpiego (an affiliate of Johns Hopkins University), discusses challenges from the perspective of an NGO working in Kenya.

Chapter 11, "Ongoing Project Support," examines what happens when volunteers return home. The chapter addresses strategies to maintain long-term relationships through the use of technology (including e-health and m-health) to support partnerships when the visiting nurse partners return home. The need for resources for support is also reviewed. The first case study, by Ruth McDermott-Levy and Miguel Angel Estopinan, features a collaborative project in Nicaragua to build the capacity of community health workers using cell phone technology. The second case study, contributed by Jeanne M. Leffers, Speciosa M. Mbabali, Rose Chalo Nabirye, and Scovia Nalugo Mbalinda, highlights how the Internet and communication technology can foster ongoing relationships with host partners in Uganda when the nurse partner returns home.

Chapter 12, "Sustainability of International Nursing Programs," discusses long-term projects that have ended with their outcomes achieved. In particular we speak to the continence of program activities led by the host partners. The case study by Mary E. Riner and Marion E. Broome outlines their collaboration to re-establish nursing education in Liberia.

Chapter 13, "Host Country Ownership," describes the outcome goal for host partners for collaborative projects. The ultimate goal of all projects where visiting partners from higher income countries collaborate with host partners from low- or middle-income countries is host country ownership of the project or programs. This chapter examines this goal in light of program sustainability. The first case study, by Jill B. Derstine and Pamela Hoyt-Hudson, features collaboration between faculty from Temple University in the United States, Hue University in Vietnam, and the Dreyfus Health Foundation. The second case study, written by Manila Prak of Cambodia, shares the challenges to host country ownership in a case study describing a hospital-based in-service program in Cambodia.

In the Conclusion, "Moving Forward for Global Health Nursing," we draw conclusions and make recommendations for the future of global health nursing.

REFERENCES

Amazigo, U., Okeibunor, J., Matovu, V., Zoure, H., Bump, J., & Seketeli, A. (2007). Performance of predictors: Evaluating sustainability in community-directed treatment projects of the African Programme for Onchocerciasis Control. *Social Science & Medicine, 64,* 2070–2082.

American Nurses Association. (2010). *Nursing's social policy statement: The essence of the profession.* Silver Spring, MD: Nursesbooks.org

Anderson, E. T., & McFarlane, J. (2004). *Community as partner: Theory and practice in nursing* (4th ed.). Philadelphia: Lippincott Williams & Wilkins.

Beaglehole, R., & Bonita, R. (2010). What is global health? *Global Health Action, 3,* 1–2. doi:10.3402/gha/v3i0.5142

Bentley, R., & Ellison, K. J. (2005). Impact of service learning projects on nursing students. *Journal of Nursing Education, 4*(10), 433–436.

Brow, T. M., Cueto, M., & Fee, E. (2006). International to global public health. *American Journal of Public Health, 96,* 62–72.

Campbell, R. M., Pleic, M., & Connolly, H. (2012). The importance of a common global health definition: How Canada's definition influences its strategic direction in global health. *Journal of Global Health, 2,* 1–6. doi: 10.7189/jogh.02.010301

Casey, D., & Murphy, K. (2008). Irish nursing students' experiences of service learning. *Nursing and Health Services, 10*(5), 224–231.

Crigger, N. J. (2008). Towards a viable and just global nursing ethics. *Nursing Ethics, 15*(1), 17–27. doi: 10.1177/0969733007082121

Crump, J. A., & Sugarman, J. (2010). Ethics and best practice guidelines for training experiences in global health, *American Journal of Tropical Medicine & Hygiene, 83,* 1178–1182. doi: 10.4269/ajtmh.2010-0527

Davis, A. J., & Tschudin, V. (2008). Introduction and topic of globalisation. In V. Tschudin & A. J. Davis (Eds.), *The Globalisation of nursing* (pp. 3–11). Oxford: Radcliffe Publishing.

Dyar, O. J., & deCosta, A. (2011, Spring). What is global health? *Journal of Global Health.* www.ghjournal.org/jgh-print/spring-2011-issue/what-is-global-health

Dybul, M., Piot, P., & Frenk, J. (2012, June/July). Reshaping global health. *Policy Review* (173), 3–18.

Fee, E., & Brown, T. M. (2002). 100 years of the Pan American Health Organization. *American Journal of Public Health, 92,* 1888–1989.

Foster, J. (2009). Cultural humility and the importance of long-term relationships in international partnerships. *Journal of Obstetrical, Gynecological & Neonatal Nursing, 38,* 100–107.

Frenk, J., Chen, L., Bhutta, Z. A., Crisp, N., Evans, T., Fineberg, H., . . . Zurayk, H. (2010). Health professionals for a new century: Transforming education to strengthen health systems in an interdependent world. *The Lancet, 376,* 1923–1958. doi: 10.1016/S0140-6736(10)61854-5

Fried, L. P., Bentley, M. E., Buekens, P., Burke, D. S., Frenk, J. J., Klag, M. J., & Spencer, H. C. (2010). Global health is public health. *The Lancet, 375,* 535–537. doi: 10.1016/S0140-6736(10)60170-5

Grace, P. J. (2009). Advanced practice nursing: General ethical concerns. In P. Grace, *Nursing ethics and professional responsibility in advanced practice* (pp. 75–106). Sudbury, MA: Jones and Bartlett.

Harrowing, J. N., Mill, J., Spiers, J., Kulig, J., & Kipp, W. (2010). Critical ethnography, cultural safety, and international nursing research. *International Journal of Qualitative Methods, 9,* 240–251.

Hunter, A., Wilson, L., Stanhope, M., Hatcher, B., Hattar, M., Hilfinger Messias, D. K., & Powell, D. (2013). Global health diplomacy: An integrative review of the literature and implications for nursing. *Nursing Outlook, 61,* 85–92. http://dx.doi.org/10.1016/j.outlook.2012.07.013

Institute of Medicine. (2009a). *The U.S. commitment to global health: Recommendations for the new administration.* Washington, DC: The National Academies Press.

Institute of Medicine. (2009b). *The U.S. commitment to global health: Recommendations for the public and private sectors.* Washington, DC: The National Academies Press.

International Council of Nurses. (1999). *Position statement. Nurse retention, transfer and migration.* www.icn.ch/psretention.htm

Ivanov, L. L., & Oden, M. S. (2013). Public health nursing, ethics and human rights. *Public Health Nursing, 30*(3), 231–238. doi: 10.1111/phn.12022

Ketefian, S. (2000). Ethical considerations in international nursing. *Journal of Professional Nursing, 16,* 257.

Khubchandani, J., & Simmons, R. (2012). Going global: Building a foundation for global health promotion research to practice. *Health Promotion Practice, 13,* 293–297. doi:10.1177/1524839912439063

Koplan, J. P. Bond, C. T., Merson, M. H., Reddy, R. S., Rodriguez, M. H., Sewankambo, N. K., & Wasserheit, J. N. (2009). Towards a common definition of global health. *The Lancet, 373,* 1993–1995. doi: 10.1016/S0140-6736(09)60332-9

Kulbok, P., Mitchell, E., Glick, D., & Greiner, D. (2012). International experiences in nursing education: A review of the literature. *International Journal of Nursing Education Scholarship, 9*(1), Article 7. doi: 10.1515/1548-923X.2365.

Leffers, J., & Mitchell, E. (2011). Conceptual model for partnership and sustainability in global health. *Public Health Nursing, 28*(1), 91–102. doi: 10.1111/j.1525-1446.2010.00892.x

Merry, L. (2012). Global health for nursing . . . and nursing for global health. *Canadian Journal of Nursing Research, 44*(4), 20–35.

Merson, M. H., Black, R. E., & Mills, A. J. (2006). Introduction. In M. H. Merson, R. E. Black, & A. J. Mills (Eds.), *International public health: Diseases, programs, systems, and policies* (2nd ed., pp. xiii–xxiv). Sudbury, MA: Jones and Bartlett.

Novotny, T. E., & Adams, V. (2007). Global health diplomacy: A global health sciences working paper. University of California San Francisco Global Health Sciences. http://igcc.ucsd.edu/pdf/GH_Diplomacy.pdf

Nussbaum, M. (1998). The good as discipline, the good as freedom. In P. A. Crock & L. Lindon (Eds.), *Ethics of consumption* (pp. 312–341). Boulder, CO: Rowman & Littlefield.

Pender, N. J., Murdaugh, C. L., & Parsons, M. A. (2006). *Health promotion in nursing practice* (5th ed.). Upper Saddle River, NJ: Pearson/Prentice-Hall.

Polaschek, B. A. (1998). Cultural safety: A new concept in nursing people of different ethnicities. *Journal of Advanced Nursing, 27,* 452–457. doi: 10.1046/j.1365-2648.1998.00547.x

Racine, L., & Perron, A. (2012). Unmasking the predicament of cultural voyeurism: A postcolonial analysis of international nursing placements. *Nursing Inquiry, 19*(3), 190–201. doi:10.1111/j.1440-1800.2011.00555.x

Reising, D. L., Allen, P. N., & Hall, S. G. (2006). Student and community outcomes in service learning: Part 2 community outcomes. *Journal of Nursing Education 45*(12), 516–518.

Rosenkoetter, M. M., & Nardi, D. A. (2007). American Academy of Nursing expert panel on global nursing and health: White paper on global nursing and health. *Journal of Transcultural Nursing, 18,* 305–315. doi:10.1177/1043659607305188

Rowson, M., Willott, C., Hughes, R., Maini, A., Martin, S., Miranda, J., . . . Yudkin, J. S. (2012). Conceptualising global health: Theoretical issues and their relevance for teaching. *Globalization and Health, 8*(36), 1–8. www.globalizationandhealth.com/content/8/1/36

Ruger, J. P. (2005). The changing role of the World Bank in global health in historical perspective. *American Journal of Public Health, 95,* 60–70.

Schumacher, K. L., & Meleis, A. I. (1994). Transitions: A central concept in nursing. *Image: Journal of Nursing Scholarship, 26*(2), 119–127.

Sen, A. (2004). Elements of a theory of human rights. *Philosophy & Public Affairs, 32,* 315–355.

Sharma, M., & Atri, A. (2010). *Essentials of international health.* Boston, MA: Jones and Bartlett.

Shediac-Rizkallah, M. C., & Bone, L. (1998). Planning for the sustainability of community based health programs: Conceptual frameworks and future directions for research, practice and policy. *Health Education Research, Theory and Practice, 13*(1), 87–108.

Sultan, F., & Khan, A. (2013). Infectious disease in Pakistan: A clear and present danger. *The Lancet, 381,* 2138–2140.

Tyer-Viola, L., Nicholas, P. K., Corless, I. B., Barry, D. M., Hoyt, P., Fitzpatrick, J. J., & Davis, S. M. (2009). Social responsibility of nursing: A global perspective. *Policy, Politics, & Nursing Practice, 10*, 110–119. doi:10.1177/1527154409339528

World Health Organization. (1948). *Preamble to the constitution of the World Health Organization.* www.who.int/about/definition/en/print.html

World Health Organization. (2002). Guidelines and instruments for conducting an evaluation of the sustainability of CDTI projects. WHO/APOC/MG/02-1. African Programme for Onchocerciasis Control, Ouagadougou.

World Health Organization. (2007). *World health statistics 2007.* Geneva: World Health Organization. www.who.int/whosis/whostat2007/en

World Health Organization. (2013). *Public health.* www.who.int/trade/glossary/story076/en/

World Health Organization. (n.d.). *Declaration of Alma Ata.* www.who.int/publications/almaata_declaration_en.pdf

Winslow, C. E. A. (1920). The untitled fields of public health. *Science, New Series, 51*(1306), 22–33.

Unite for Sight. (n.d.). *Colonial medicine.* www.uniteforsight.org/global-health-history/module2

United Nations. (n.d.a). *We can end poverty 2015: Millennium Development Goals.* www.un.org/millenniumgoals

United Nations. (n.d.b). *Universal declaration of human rights.* www.un.org/en/documents/udhr

CHAPTER 1

Selecting and Negotiating Partnerships for Collaboration

Elizabeth Downes

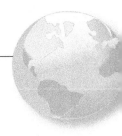

> To create and develop without any feelings of ownership, to work and guide without any expectation and control, is the best quality.
>
> *Lao Tzu*

Nursing has a long heritage of seeking to improve health and prevent illness through collaboration and partnership. Libster (2011) points to nurse-led partnerships with governments, medical and religious communities, hospitals, colleges and universities, and other organizations spanning hundreds of years. As long ago as the 17th century, the Daughters of Charity, one of the earliest established nursing programs, grew from a partnership between a priest named Vincent de Paul and a woman, Madam Louise de Marillac, to care for the sick (Libster, 2011). In the nearly 400 years since the founding of the Daughters of Charity, nursing has extended from caring for the sick in their homes to full engagement in global health partnerships. Nurses have always worked to improve health and achieve equity in health. Global health is defined by Koplan et al. (2009) as:

> an area for study, research, and practice that places a priority on improving health and achieving equity in health for all people worldwide. Global health emphasizes transnational health issues, determinants, and solutions; involves many disciplines within and beyond the health sciences and promotes interdisciplinary collaboration; and is a synthesis of population-based prevention with individual-level care. (p. 1995)

This example demonstrates the longstanding involvement of nursing in successfully partnering toward health promotion, illness prevention, and care of individuals and populations. This chapter discusses the initiation of a partnership and explains how nursing and personal roles are established. It also explores important components of seeking a partnership, approaching potential partners with whom you have never worked, and dealing with unrealistic expectations while in a host country.

The American Association of Colleges of Nursing (2010) compiled a summary of literature on successful partnerships in nursing that is congruent with the Leffers and Mitchell partnership model (2011). Central to these partnerships are:

- Mutual trust and respect
- Communication

- Shared vision
- Commitment

These components are not necessarily separate and distinct steps, but rather mutually supportive and interdependent aspects of successful partnerships. For example, the process of creating a shared vision can strengthen (or weaken) a trusting relationship. Trust can support open communication and vice versa. However, each of these components is worth discussing separately.

MUTUAL TRUST AND RESPECT

Partnerships are voluntary collaborative agreements wherein parties agree to work together, sharing benefits and risks as well as competencies and responsibilities. Wheeler (2012) compares trust to trusting relationships. Trust is defined as "a psychological state in which positive expectations are held regarding the motives and intentions of another actor" (Ruzicka & Wheeler, 2010, p. 70). A trusting relationship involves acting on that trust and has been defined as "one into which actors enter in order to realize benefits which would otherwise not be available to them. They do so in the knowledge that this increases their vulnerability to other actors whose behavior they do not control, with potentially negative consequences for themselves" (as cited in Wheeler, 2012). Although it is important that nurses maintain professional roles, trusting relationships with host partners are key to successful partnerships.

Personal Relationships

Research on successful partnerships points out that it is helpful to have a personal relationship. In fact, personal relationships can be foundational to a partnership (Beal et al., 2011; Breslin et al., 2011). It is interesting to note that Mikhail Gorbachev pointed to the personal relationship he and President Ronald Reagan developed as being essential to ending the Cold War. In his memoirs, Gorbachev called it "the human factor" (as cited in Wheeler, 2012). Many articles on partnerships in nursing, especially articles addressing programs abroad, speak to the importance of face-to-face contact (Breslin et al., 2011; Hope, 2008; Sostman et al., 2005). Furthermore, visiting the location can also help build context for the collaboration. These interactions can go a long way toward developing comfort and trust.

For effective interpersonal relationships, it is important to share information about yourself and, if applicable, the institution you represent. There must be a clear understanding of all partners' roles and responsibilities. The process of establishing these roles is discussed in subsequent chapters. However, it is important to keep in mind that governments and institutions are not capable of entering into *personal* relationships. Embedded trust can develop from personal relationships and extend to the institutions (Notter, 1995). This, in turn, can facilitate expansion in terms of participants and programs. Although embedded trust can be a distinct benefit (as is evident in the relationship between Gorbachev and Reagan), it will not substitute for personal face-to-face interaction. That is not to say that a partnership should be limited to two or three individuals. In fact, a web of relationships can strengthen the partnership and facilitate sustainability—but initially it may start with one or two motivated individuals.

COMMUNICATION

Good communication is essential to successful partnerships. According to Ross (in Kanani, 2012), "Partnership failures can usually be linked to some level of miscommunication. This can range from misperceptions about the objectives, expected results, operating approaches and/or roles and responsibilities" (p. 2). Clearly, communication means more than just language. Diversity in language, cultures, and perspectives is to be expected when working globally. And as diversity increases, so do the communication challenges.

Working with partners from other cultures requires cultural humility and fluency, as explained elsewhere in this book. Culture can have a powerful effect on communication. Anthropologist Edward T. Hall's theory of high- and low-context culture can help anticipate challenges in communication (Hall, 1976). Although we are all individuals, we are acculturated from a very young age. Hall's theory of intercultural communication can help when used as a general approach for communication. For example, high-context cultures (Latin American, African, Asian, Mediterranean, Slav, Native American) are generally cultures of few words. Much is left in between the lines, to be understood through context and nonverbal clues. People from high-context cultures generally are collectivist, intuitive, and relational, valuing interpersonal relationships. Low-context cultures (North America and Western Europe) value communication that is straightforward and direct. People from these cultures are individualistic, logical, and action-oriented (Fussell, Zhang, & Setlock, 2008; Goman, 2011). Views on time can also affect communication. Cultures that have a sequential approach to time speak of it almost as money ("waste time," "spend time," "save time," even "buy time"). Synchronistic cultures do not see time as something to be bargained for, but rather as something to be experienced. The work of Triandis (1995) added the dimension of task versus relationship orientation (whether people focus on accomplishing tasks or on establishing rapport). The additional challenge of computer-mediated communication (CMC) can potentiate these challenges. Fussell, Zhang, and Setlock (2008) show that cultural background affects CMC. This reinforces the need for face-to-face encounters in developing partnerships. Studies on partnerships point to the need for open and free communication (Beal et al., 2012; Bosworth et al., 2006; Breslin et al., 2011; Everett et al., 2012; MacPhee, 2009). This can be more complicated when relying on CMC but is worth the extra effort.

SHARED VISION

Shared Decision Making and Problem Solving

Partnerships are driven by a need or desire to accomplish something that a partner cannot accomplish alone (Long & Arnold, 1995). This begs the question, "What is the goal of the partnership?" This is the first step of the initiation phase. The other two phases (execution and closure/renewal) are all based on the goal. All stakeholders must be involved in the initiation phase. Understanding and sharing each other's mission and values provides a foundation for developing congruent goals for the partnership. Personal expectations of the partners are explored in the next chapter.

In her book *Expanding the Pie* (2012), Susan Rae Ross posits an eight-step "Partnership Decision-Making Process," depicted in Table 1.1. Six of the eight steps are related to the initiation phase, an indication of its importance. Although Ross's work was developed specifically to facilitate work between businesses and nongovernmental organizations (NGOs), the steps outline key considerations when entering into any partnership. Step 1, "conduct an internal assessment," is appropriate for large and small organizations—even individuals. What are your reasons for entering into this partnership? What can you bring to the partnership? If you are part of a larger organization, does the effort dovetail with your broader mission? This self-exploration will help you to move through the identification of partners (Step 2) and with your approach to selected partners (Step 3). What is the basis for the partnership? Can individual goals of each partner be aligned?

Step 4 (due diligence) is essential to both creating a shared vision and developing trust. It also aids identification of any potential risks to the partnership. It is important to recognize that partner incompatibility is a potential pitfall. Why does this partner wish to engage with you? What are the risks? Are there any conflicts of interest? What do you know about the partner organization's structure and decision-making processes (Cohen, 2003; Ross, 2012)?

TABLE 1.1 Steps in the Partnership Decision-Making Framework

Steps	Task
Step 1: Conduct an internal assessment	• Determine rationale for the partnership • Determine type of partnership desired • Assess organizational capacity to support partnership
Step 2: Identify, research, and short-list potential partners	• Develop selection criteria • Research potential partners
Step 3: Approach potential partners and make the business case	• Leverage key contacts • Identify decision makers • Organize the initial meeting • Make the business case
Step 4: Conduct a due-diligence process to select an appropriate partner	• Create a due-diligence process • Use a due-diligence matrix • Select partners
Step 5: Negotiate the partnership	• Determine the element of partnership agreement • Decide on partner structures • Decide on partner systems
Step 6: Initiate the partnership	• Create plan to launch the partnership
Step 7: Execute and implement the partnership	• Execute work plans • Communicate; hold regular meetings • Redesign strategies as needed
Step 8: Evaluate and reassess the partnership	• Assess indicators to measure partnership effect and value created • Assess indicators to measure partnership efficiency

From *Expanding the Pie*, Susan Rae Ross. Copyright © 2012 Susan Rae Ross. Published by Kumarian Press, an imprint of Lynne Rienner Publishers, Inc. Used with permission of the publisher.

The Community-Campus Partnerships for Health (CCPH), based out of the University of Washington (http://depts.washington.edu/ccph), provides a rich resource for partnership development that can be adapted even if neither partner is university based. CCPH speaks of the "glue" that holds partnerships together. This can include policies, procedures, and processes developed in collaboration. But the first principle of partnership is to have a shared mission. Cauley (2000) lists three stages in the development of a partnership—identification, development, and maintenance—and cautions against trying to rush the mission statement. As stated above, the process of articulating a shared mission can provide opportunity to build trust. As with Ross's work, begin with, *What do I bring to this partnership?*

Green-Moton, Palermo, McGranaghan, and Travers (2006) give an example of an exercise that may aid the development of a shared vision. It is designed for both small and large groups:

Participants take 15 minutes to generate a list of key words and phrases that characterize a common vision for their partnership(s), based on the issue(s) they are addressing or hope to address. Small groups report what they have listed and the large group identifies common themes.

COMMITMENT

After the initial work is done and the partnership is developed, the hard work of sustaining commitment to the partnership begins. During this time it will be necessary to "check in" with partners. It is particularly important to be aware of power inequities that can develop

(Green-Moton, Palermo, Flicker, & Travers, 2006; Tierney et al., 2013). As partnerships evolve, it may be necessary to restate the mission and revise policies, procedures, and processes. There may even be an opportunity for expanding or contracting the partnership itself. It is always important to remain inclusive even at the risk of expedience—it is at this point that the trusting relationship gets further reinforced through open communication and sustained commitment.

Over time, partnerships can be expected to evolve. The evaluation process can be used to strategize and plan for sustainability. Process evaluation is normally done to monitor a program (e.g., number of immunizations given, number of patients served, number of students taking part in an exchange program). In addition, process evaluation offers the opportunity to revisit the mission and policies and to monitor the health of the partnership. Resources for developing process evaluation questions can be found through the various websites of the Centers for Disease Control and Prevention (www.cdc.gov/healthyyouth/evaluation/pdf/brief4.pdf) and the CCPH (http://depts.washington.edu/ccph/cbpr/index.php).

Process evaluation can determine whether goals and objectives are well aligned. Anonymous surveys or reflective discussions can help identify areas of strength and for growth. However, threats and weaknesses will also be identified and should not be ignored.

When problems arise in partnership, it is important to address them. Conflict resolution is rarely simple. Add a cultural dimension, and things are further complicated. The process of team development is well known to nurses (forming, storming, norming, and performing). Research on teams indicates that successful teams are comfortable dealing with conflict and are committed to, and learn from, resolution.

Unfortunately, that research was done on mostly North American organizations. For some cultures, the group is more important than the individual. Harmony and group conformity is sought, sometimes at the expense of personal interests. Although everyone may seek to avoid conflict to some degree, persons from individualistic societies may be more direct in dealing with conflict ("meet it head on"; "take the bull by the horns"). In fact, culture may determine whether conflict even exists. An elderly Chinese man in Canada denied having had any conflict at all in the past 40 years. Consistent with his Confucian upbringing, he saw the world with a vision of harmony rather than of conflict (LeBaron & Grundison, 1993).

In her essay "Culture and Conflict," Michelle LeBaron speaks of cultural fluency as "a key for disentangling and managing multilayered, cultural conflicts" (LeBaron, 2003, para. 25). In addition to awareness of distinctions in communication as articulated by Hall, cultures have different ways of "naming, framing, and taming" conflict. It is important to understand the context of a perceived conflict. Cultures have different ways of meaning-making, and not knowing these may make it easier to attribute negative motives to a behavior.

Working to develop partnerships across cultures can be rewarding and challenging. How we approach the partnership and whether the inevitable changes involves "recognizing and acting respectfully from the knowledge that communication, ways of naming, framing, and taming conflict, approaches to meaning-making, and identities and roles vary across cultures" (LeBaron, 2003, para. 25).

As stated above, partnerships are voluntary collaborative agreements wherein parties agree to work together, sharing benefits and risks as well as competencies and responsibilities. This voluntary nature of relationships does not mean, however, that partnerships are self-sustaining. The steps toward negotiating and maintaining a relationship are succinctly elaborated by Ross (2012) in Table 1.2. Through a literature review and interviews with NGOs and business leaders, Ross has identified 10 elements of a partnership agreement that include everything from creating a shared vision and maintaining communication to deciding to end a partnership.

INTERNATIONAL STUDENT EXPERIENCES

All the elements for developing a partnership are necessary for a successful international student experience. However, as these types of experiences become more common, special attention should be given to promoting true partnerships among students and faculty. Kulbok,

TABLE 1.2 Elements of Partnership Agreement

Partnership area	Key questions	Key considerations
Formality of the agreement	How formal/informal should the partnership be?	Memoranda of understanding (MOUs) may or may not be legally binding.
Vision	What is the vision of the partnership?	Does it benefit everyone? Has everyone "bought into" the vision?
	What is the effective time frame of the partnership?	
Partnership objective	What are the objectives of the partnership?	Objectives should be SMART (specific, measurable, achievable, realistic, and time-bound).
	How does each organization contribute to the objectives?	Agreement on key indicators, as well as how they will be measured, is essential. For example, will the partners use third-party auditors or independent evaluators?
Roles and responsibilities of each organization	Clearly identify the assets and resources each partner will provide, including financial human resources, skills, products, office space, intellectual property, and networks.	A specific scope of work statement can be included in the body of the agreement or provided as an attachment.
Exchange of resources	If either partner is going to provide specific resources to the other partner, such as a grant, then the funding amount and activities should be clearly articulated, along with payment agreements, schedules, and reimbursement policies. This can be discussed in the agreement, and a separate legally binding document can be developed and attached.	
Partnership management	How will the partnership be managed? Is a specific structure required? What systems are needed to support the partnership?	This may be as simple as agreeing to a monthly or quarterly meeting in which to approve activities and monitor progress. It should include who should be represented at the meetings, responsibilities for note-taking, and communication among the partners.
	Which department or staff will be the key liaisons for the partnership?	
Partnership decision making	How will decisions be made between partners?	
Partnership communication	How will partners communicate within their organizations?	Use of intranet, newsletters
	How will the partners communicate with each other?	Updates from partner meetings
	How will the partners communicate externally?	What information can be put on each partner's website?

(continued)

TABLE 1.2 Elements of Partnership Agreement (*continued*)

Partnership area	Key questions	Key considerations
	What permissions are needed from each organization to allow their partner organization to use their logos? Co-branding?	What is the approval process for each organization's discussing the partnership with external parties?
	Who owns the data about the partnership? With whom can the data be shared?	
Grievance/Dispute process	What are the levels of grievances?	
	How will each level be settled?	Mediation vs. arbitration
	Who will represent the organization in a dispute process?	
	What makes a fair grievance?	
Termination parameters	Under what conditions can either organization terminate the partnership?	What type of notification is required to terminate the partnership?

From *Expanding the Pie*, Susan Rae Ross. Copyright © 2012 Susan Rae Ross. Published by Kumarian Press, an imprint of Lynne Rienner Publishers, Inc. Used with permission of the publisher.

Mitchell, Glick, and Greiner (2012) reviewed the literature on student international experiences from 2003 to 2010. Their findings highlight the need for published reports that discuss two-way exchanges between students of higher and lower income countries. Too often emphasis is placed on the student from the high-income country going to another country with a high UN development index rating (e.g., European countries, Australia, Japan, Norway) rather than countries considered low-income that are struggling with the issues of poverty and other social determinants of health. Second, published reports of the student experience should include authorship from the country hosting the international student. Including authors from all countries involved in the partnership can increase the capacity for conducting research and developing scholarship. Third, all students, including those from the host country, should receive additional education addressing the cultural differences among all the partners. Finally, experiences that extend beyond the university setting should be considered partnership opportunities for students. Students can benefit from working with NGOs and other agencies active in low-income countries. There is tremendous opportunity for international student partnerships that challenge students to extend themselves beyond providing basic clinical procedures, moving them away from "us and them" to true partnerships.

Three case studies follow that highlight the processes of selecting and maintaining partnerships. The first case study provides the perspective of an NGO, Health Volunteers Overseas (HVO), in developing relationships with partners outside of the borders of the United States. Practical information on the process of volunteering is shared, including the role of volunteers and dealing with the challenge of continuity.

The second case study offers the perceptions of an international student pursuing a doctoral degree in the United States. Having a dream, facing the reality of living and studying in a land completely different from her home country, and wondering how her life will be changed when she returns home are all discussed in a spirit of openness and honesty. Themes from this case study can be compared to the research of the Arab/Muslim international student experience from entry to the United States to reentry in the home country by McDermott-Levy (2011, 2013).

The final case study focuses on a community partnership in existence for over 20 years. Although this partnership has evolved over the years, some of the pioneering individuals are still involved, as are some of the original institutional partners—but the program itself has expanded.

REFERENCES

American Association of Colleges of Nursing. (2010). Summary of literature related to academic-service partnerships. Retrieved June 12, 2013, from http://www.aacn.nche.edu/leading-initiatives/academic-practice-partnerships/SummaryLiteratureAcademic.pdf

Beal, J. A., Alt-White, A., Erickson, J., Everett, L. Q., Fleshner, I., Karshmer, J., . . . Gale, S. (2012). Academic practice partnerships: A national dialogue. *Journal of Professional Nursing, 28*(6), 327–332. doi: 10.1016/j.profnurs.2012.09.001

Beal, J. A., Breslin, E., Austin, T., Brower, L., Bullard, K., Light, K., . . . Ray, N. (2011). Hallmarks of best practice in academic-service partnerships in nursing: Lessons learned from San Antonio. *Journal of Professional Nursing, 27*(6), e90–e95. doi: 10.1016/j.profnurs.2011.07.006

Bosworth, T. L., Haloburdo, E. P., Hetrick, C., Patchett, K., Thompson, M. A., & Welch, M. (2006). International partnerships to promote quality care: Faculty groundwork, student projects, and outcomes. *Journal of Continuing Education in Nursing, 37*(1), 32–38.

Breslin, E., Stefl, M., Yarbrough, S., Frazor, D., Bullard, K., Light, K., . . . Lowe, A. (2011). Creating and sustaining academic-practice partnerships: Lessons learned. *Journal of Professional Nursing, 27*(6), e33–e40. doi: 10.1016/j.profnurs.2011.08.008

Cauley, K. (2000). Principle 1. Partners have agreed-upon mission, values, goals and measurable outcomes for the partnership. In K. Connors & S. Seifer (Eds.), *Partnership perspectives.* http://depts.washington.edu/ccph/pdf_files/summer1-f.pdf

Cohen, A. (2003). *Multiple commitments in the workplace: An integrative approach.* Mahwah, NJ: Lawrence Erlbaum Associates.

Everett, L. Q., Bowers, B., Beal, J. A., Alt-White, A., Erickson, J., Gale, S., . . . Swider, S. (2012). Academic-practice partnerships fuel future success. *Journal of Nursing Administration, 42*(12), 554–556. doi: 10.1097/NNA.0b013e318274b4eb

Fussell, S., Zhang, Q., & Setlock, L. (2008). Global culture and computer mediated communication. In S. Kelsey & K. St. Amant (Eds.), *Handbook of research on computer mediated communication.* Hershey, PA: Information Science Reference.

Goman, C. (2011). Communicating across cultures. https://www.asme.org/engineering-topics/articles/business-communication/communicating-across-cultures

Greene-Moton, E., Palermo, A. G., Flicker, S., & Travers, R. (2006). Unit 4: Trust and communication in a CBPR partnership—Spreading the "glue" and having it stick. *The Examining Community-Institutional Partnerships for Prevention Research Group. Developing and Sustaining Community-Based Participatory Research Partnerships: A Skill-Building Curriculum.* https://depts.washington.edu/ccph/cbpr/u4/documents/section.pdf

Hall, E. T. 1976. *Beyond culture.* Garden City, NY: Anchor Press.

Hope, K. L. (2008). The development of a medical service learning study-away program. *Journal of Emergency Nursing, 34*(5), 474–477. doi: 10.1016/j.jen.2008.06.011

Kanani, R. (Interviewer), & Ross, S. R. (Interviewee). (2012). *How to design the perfect partnership for social change.* www.forbes.com/sites/rahimkanani/2012/06/14/how-to-design-the-perfect-partnership-for-social-change/2

Koplan, J. B., Bond, T. C., Merson, M. H., Reddy, K. S., Rodrigues, M. H., Sewankambo, N. K., & Wasserheit, J. N. (2009). Towards a common definition of global health. *Lancet, 373,* 1993–1995.

Kulbok, P. A., Mitchell, E. M., Glick, D. F., & Greiner, D. (2012). International experiences in nursing education. *International Journal of Nursing Education Scholarship, 9*(1), article 7. doi: 10.1515/1548-923X.2365

LeBaron, M. (2003). Culture and conflict. In Guy Burgess & Heidi Burgess (Eds.), *Beyond intractability*. Boulder, CO: Conflict Research Consortium, University of Colorado. www.beyondintractability.org/bi-essay/culture-conflict

LeBaron, M., & Grundison, B. (1993). *Conflict and culture: Research in five communities in British Columbia, Canada*. Victoria, BC: University of Victoria Institute for Dispute Resolution.

Leffers, J., & Mitchell, E. (2011). Conceptual model for partnership and sustainability in global health. *Public Health Nursing, 28*(1), 91–102. doi: 10.1111/j.1525-1446.2010.00892.x

Libster, M. M. (2011). Lessons learned from a history of perseverance and innovation in academic-practice partnerships. *Journal of Professional Nursing, 27*(6), e76-81. doi: 10.1016/j.profnurs.2011.07.005

Long, F., & Arnold, M. (1995). *The power of environmental partnerships*. Fort Worth, TX: Harcourt Brace College Publishers.

MacPhee, M. (2009). Developing a practice-academic partnership logic model. *Nursing Outlook, 57*(3), 143–147. doi: 10.1016/j.outlook.2008.08.003

McDermott-Levy, R. (2011). Going alone: The lived experience of female Arab-Muslim nursing students living and studying in the United States. *Nursing Outlook, 59*, 266–277. doi: 10.10016/j.outlook.2011.02.006

McDermott-Levy, R. (2013). Female Arab-Muslim nursing students' reentry transitions. *International Journal of Nursing Education Scholarship, 10*(1), 1–8. doi: 10.1515/ijnes-2012-0042

Notter, J. (1995). Trust and conflict transformation. *The Institute for Multi-Track Diplomacy, Occasional Paper Number 5*. http://imtd.server295.com/pdfs/OP5.pdf

Ross, S. R. (2012). *Expanding the pie*. Sterling, VA: Stylus.

Ruzicka, J., & Wheeler, N. (2010). The puzzle of trusting relationships in the Nuclear Non-Proliferation Treaty. *International Affairs, 86*(1), 69–85.

Sostman, H. D., Forese, L. L., Boom, M. L., Schroth, L., Klein, A. A., Mushlin, . . . Gotto, A. M. Jr. (2005). Building a transcontinental affiliation: A new model for academic health centers. *Academic Medicine, 80*(11), 1046–1053.

Tierney, W. M., Nyandiko, W. N., Siika, A. M., Wools-Kaloustian, K., Sidle, J. E., Kiplagat, J., . . . Inui, T. S. (2013). "These are good problems to have . . .": Establishing a collaborative research partnership in east Africa. *Journal of General Internal Medicine, 28*, S625–S638. doi: 10.1007/s11606-013-2459-4

Wheeler, N. (2012). Trust-building in international relations. *Peace Prints: South Asian Journal of Peacebuilding, 4*(2). Retrieved from http://www.wiscomp.org/pp-v4-n2/nick%20wheeler.pdf

Selecting an International Project Site: Health Volunteers Overseas

Nancy Kelly

CONTEXT

It is generally recognized that one of the most serious systemic problems in the delivery of health services in developing countries is the lack of appropriately trained health care providers. The World Health Organization focused on this problem in its 2006 World Health Report, *Working Together for Health*, and Health Volunteers Overseas (HVO), a private nonprofit organization dedicated to improving the availability and quality of health care in developing countries through the training and education of local health care providers, is actively addressing this concern (www.hvousa.org/whoWeAre/mission.shtml). By investing in education and training, HVO is focusing on building local capacity and empowering local health personnel. A key concept underlying the implementation of all of HVO's projects is that of sustainability.

HVO has developed a series of dynamic institutional partnerships with a wide variety of nongovernmental organizations, government ministries, and teaching institutions around the world (for a list of these partnerships, visit www.hvousa.org/whereWeWork/institutions.shtml). These partnerships are the result of years of relationship building and provide HVO with the opportunity to develop and sustain its educational programs. The initiation of a new partnership may come from one of several sources—a HVO volunteer may recommend pursuing an opportunity with a new organization, or HVO may receive a request from an organization that has heard of HVO's work in other settings. It is not uncommon for a facility to seek additional projects in other program areas after a project has been successfully established and the value of the educational input has been demonstrated. For example, HVO recently established a series of new projects (nursing education, physical therapy, and orthopedics) at a hospital in Bolivia. The request came from a contact who had previously worked with HVO at a hospital in Cambodia. Her familiarity with HVO's mission and her understanding of HVO's methods were critical factors in her decision to ask HVO to consider this new partnership.

HVO depends on the commitment and skills of dedicated volunteers to accomplish its goals. These volunteers bring different backgrounds, experiences, and perspectives to their assignments but all share a commonality: HVO volunteers understand that the long-term solution to the health care problems found in developing countries depends on the training and education of the health professionals in those countries. Faced with serious resource constraints, as well as an immense burden of disease, developing countries must deal with enormous needs in the health care sector but have limited ability to educate and support the workforce needed.

HVO operates under the premise that only through the development of local expertise and institutional capacities will countries be able to handle the health care challenges they face. Countries must develop the expertise to identify and address their own health care problems and to create their own appropriate solutions. The training and education of health professionals is the critical component in this process. Projects must be carefully planned from the outset. Resources in developing countries—whether human, financial, or technological—are extremely limited, and demands for basic services go unmet. Planners thus must rationally, practically, and efficiently allocate these scarce resources based upon realistic objectives and sensible priorities.

Good Intentions Simply Are Not Enough

We must look critically at the needs of a country to decide what can reasonably be accomplished at a site within a certain time frame. Then we must ask whether HVO is the organization best suited to undertake the project. These are difficult questions that are sometimes glossed over or ignored entirely in the initial enthusiasm of starting a project. Unfortunately, this can result in a disappointing project with few tangible results, disgruntled volunteers, and little in the way of long-term effects.

THE HVO MODEL

Unlike many organizations involved in international development and relief efforts, HVO relies almost exclusively on short-term volunteers to staff its projects. The short time frame of the assignments (generally 1 month) facilitates the participation of many medical, dental, and health professionals who would otherwise be unable to share their knowledge and skills overseas.

What are the fundamental components of the HVO model?

1. HVO projects are developed, monitored, and staffed by *volunteers, HVO's primary resource.*
2. Projects are designed to *share knowledge and skills* with professionals in developing countries.
3. Volunteers are encouraged to teach skills that are appropriate to a given country's level of development and with an understanding of the serious competition for resources that exist in this setting. The use of *appropriate technology and local materials* will lessen the developing country's dependence on a foreign organization.

Basic Parameters

Over the years, HVO has learned that there are certain conditions that must be present in order to facilitate the development of a new project. Without these conditions in place, an HVO project, no matter how needed or wanted, simply will not work.

First, a certain amount of *political stability* is essential to setting up an effective training project. Consider the realities of starting a project in a country mired in a difficult and draining conflict. Will personnel be able to participate in training activities under these circumstances? The government or local hospital authorities may not be able to spare them from active duty. They may be physically unable to come to the training site as a result of fear and intimidation. They may wonder what the point is of additional training, seeing that they have no supplies, no equipment, no support staff, no money, and, most importantly, no hope for the future.

Second, there must be *local support* at all levels for the initiation of an HVO project. HVO should not be seen as a threat or as an avenue of professional advancement at the expense of others. Too often, expatriate volunteers become pawns in the local politics found in any medical or educational institution. This can be avoided through a careful assessment of the degree and strength of local support. If the dean or any other person in a leadership position at a potential project site is against a project being started, that person's feelings should be taken into serious consideration. This lack of interest or support can translate into serious problems when the project is being implemented.

Third, *the primary language of instruction must be English, or else adequate translators must be available* at the site. Although some HVO volunteers are fluent in other languages, HVO is not in a position to undertake a training project in a country where volunteers need to speak French, Portuguese, or other non-English languages unless funds are available for translation services.

Fourth, *volunteers must want to go* to a site. A project, no matter how well designed, will be a complete failure if no one signs up to go. This lack of interest is often the result of perceptions (and misperceptions) about a country or the result of strong emotions generated by a past event. Repeated wars, floods, famines, and other natural or manmade disasters can create an image of despair and desperation that leads volunteers to think that their efforts will be for nothing.

Finally, *volunteers must believe that their time and efforts are going to make a difference.* This must hold true throughout the volunteer experience—before, during, and after their service. For most HVO volunteers, their assignments are life-changing experiences that broaden their understandings of the world, of their profession, and of their own capabilities. As one HVO volunteer wrote in a post-trip report:

> I think I have become not only a different person but a better
> person because of this opportunity. My eyes were opened to a whole new world
> where a population doesn't have much in regards to resources but has a lot of
> heart and graciousness. (Jantzi, 2008)

Successful Selection of a Site

The process of identifying a possible project site and assessing the viability of a potential partnership is a critical first step in the design of a project. This phase of the project development requires a significant investment of time and requires that the site assessor have strong communication and cross-cultural skills as well as a commitment to key values and concepts such as partnership and mutual respect, mutual goal setting, and collaboration. HVO's mission is grounded in the concept that capacity building and sustainability are the keys to long-term effects. Working from that premise means that all HVO projects are by definition partnerships involving intense collaboration between HVO and the host institution and the personnel at the site. Decisions about the design of the project—what to teach, whom to teach, how to teach—must be the product of dialogue between the partners. This dialogue needs to be open, frank, and ongoing. This can be a challenge in a cross-cultural setting where linguistic differences may contribute to miscommunication or where cultural or social expectations are not in alignment.

A critical part of the assessment is asking a series of open-ended questions and listening carefully to the responses. Asking follow-up questions for clarification is essential. By the end of the assessment, the following questions should have been answered:

- Is there a genuine need?
- Is the project desired by the intended beneficiaries?
- Do the objectives of the project fall within the scope of HVO's mission?
- Is the project likely to achieve its objectives?
- Is the project technically appropriate and economically viable?
- Will the project survive the test of time? Will it be sustainable?
- What are the constraints? Can they be overcome?

It is also important when planning a training project to determine whether the problems being addressed can be resolved through education and training. Many training projects attempt to address problems that really result from a lack of resources, not inadequate skills.

HVO projects are to be established with the full knowledge, support, and consent of the host government and institution. HVO attempts to ensure that each project is consistent with the national strategy for health and human resource development. HVO projects should complement the existing health structure and reinforce national health priorities and goals.

Project Design

After this input has been gathered and assimilated, the next step is to start conceptualizing the project. Again, this should be a collaborative process with input regarding whom should be trained and the type of training/education needed. Any independent training effort should be fully integrated into the country's health and education systems to ensure that those who participate are appropriately recognized and compensated. It does no good to teach someone new skills if he or she is not allowed to use them.

There will need to be discussions about what kind of volunteers are needed to staff the project—type of experience, years of clinical experience, emphasis on clinical or teaching credentials, and so forth.

Finally, there should be agreement on how to define success. What changes (both short- and long-term) are expected in terms of attitudes, behaviors, knowledge, skills, or level of functioning of the beneficiaries? What will be the effects of this project?

Develop Goals and Objectives

After these components have been identified, develop an explicit set of goals and objectives. This requires determining (1) a time frame for the project and (2) a realistic assessment of what can be accomplished in that time frame—the intended results.

These goals and objectives will serve as a yardstick to determine whether the project has been successful over time. Evaluation of a project is impossible without clearly defined and quantifiable goals and objectives. Setting goals and objectives should be done in consultation with the developing country partners. They need to agree with and be supportive of the proposed activities. If there is only lukewarm support for these goals and activities, the project is not likely to succeed.

Goals and objectives should be reviewed annually and, if necessary, revised to ensure that they match site needs and situational changes. Projects in developing countries are often subject to unexpected problems or constraints. Rather than ignoring these developments, a realistic reassessment is critical to be effective.

Objectives should be simple, clear, and easy to understand and quantify. Both HVO and the partners must have a clear understanding of what the project will accomplish over a specific period of time—2, 3, or 4 years—and annual reviews are necessary to determine whether a project's design needs to be modified or totally revamped.

Project Implementation

After HVO and its partners have defined the project, it is time to roll it out. As with the design and development phases, it is essential to communicate frequently with partners in the field to ensure that what was envisioned and discussed is in alignment with the actual implementation of the project. The same cross-cultural sensitivity, active listening, and attention to the collaborative aspect of the partnership is just as necessary during this phase of the project as it is in the design phase.

One of the keys to a successful project is to ensure that volunteers are properly briefed and that they have access to appropriate background materials as part of that process. HVO has addressed this need by creating an online platform, the *HVO KnowNET*, that serves as a central repository of documents, orientation materials, class notes and lectures, assessment reports, and curricula. Prospective volunteers can read past trip reports, access contact information from recent volunteers to a site, and participate in online discussions. Access to the extensive materials on the *HVO KnowNET*, combined with conversations with the project director, staff, and other returned volunteers, serves to frame expectations for the volunteer. Realistic expectations are critical to a volunteer's ability to be effective once at the site.

CONCLUSION

HVO has developed a reputation for designing strong, effective clinical education programs in developing countries that successfully use short-term volunteers. It must be acknowledged, however, that there are some serious limitations to the HVO model, including issues related to continuity of volunteer coverage and coordination between volunteers. There can be problems with volunteers adjusting to the challenges at a site—both on personal and professional levels. Proper vetting and briefing of volunteers is an essential component of this process, and most issues are related to inappropriate expectations or misplaced assumptions.

There are limited resources in developing countries to support the training and education of health care professionals. Educational materials that are taken for granted in the West (textbooks, journals, access to the Internet, models, charts, slides, and the like) are usually not available or are woefully out of date. There are few, if any, opportunities for continuing education for clinicians in the field, nor any real opportunities for faculty development. Health care providers often work in professional isolation, unable to network or communicate with other professionals in nearby countries faced with similar problems and constraints.

Against this backdrop of significant need sometimes comes a tendency to think that input from any organization or well-meaning (and qualified) health care professional is of value. After all, resources are so scarce that surely something is better than nothing. There is ample evidence in the literature and plenty of anecdotal evidence from well-meaning but flawed projects that have been in fact a barrier to progress (Easterly, 2007; Maren, 1997; Moyo, 2009; Riddell, 2008).

A Focus on Resiliency

HVO continues to focus on developing resiliency, seeking partnerships to leverage the synergy that occurs through collaborative efforts. Working together, HVO and its partners are building resiliency in individuals, in professions, and in health care systems. With each new development, HVO is striving to improve the availability and quality of health care for patients in resource-scarce countries. Ultimately, of course, it is the patients—both current and future—who benefit.

As one HVO trainee stated,

After knowing HVO's work, I saw that I could do more. There was hope and there are things that we have managed to change. The training aspect is the most exciting and the most important. (Nakakeeto, 2011, p. 3)

REFLECTIVE QUESTIONS

1. The author outlined several preconditions that must be present at an institution under consideration. Are there any other preconditions you would add to this list? What, and why?

2. What do you foresee as possible difficulties in making a site assessment to determine whether an institution might be a viable project site?
3. How might cultural competence, language barriers, and cultural differences affect your ability to accurately assess the information you collect?
4. Why do you think setting "realistic expectations" is so important to a volunteer's ability to be effective during his or her assignment?

REFERENCES

Easterly, W. (2007). *White man's burden: Why the West's efforts to aid the rest have done so much ill and so little good*. New York, NY: Penguin Press.

Jantzi, M. (2008). *Trip report: India*. Washington, DC: Health Volunteers Overseas.

Maren, M. (1997). *The road to hell: The ravaging effects of foreign aid and international charity*. New York, NY: Free Press.

Moyo, D. (2009). *Dead aid: Why aid is not working and how there is a better way for Africa*. New York, NY: Farrar, Straus and Giroux.

Nakakeeto, M. (2011). *History of health volunteers overseas 1986–2011*. www.hvousa.org/pdfs/hvo-history.pdf

Riddell, R. (2008). *Foreign aid: Does it really work*? New York, NY: Oxford University Press.

World Health Organization. (2006). *Working together for health*. www.who.int/whr/2006/en

Seeking Higher Education: From Egypt to the United States

Nermine Elcokany
Azza Hussein

It takes much courage to decide to live in another country far from home for an extended period of time. It becomes even more complicated when differences in language and culture are so vast. For me, Nermine Elcokany, the nursing profession is what provides cohesion with my nursing colleagues despite these differences. I hope my story of how I decided to come to the United States for further study and my experiences dealing with tremendous cultural change will give courage to others who are thinking about making this same change. To begin, it is important to provide a sense of the different worlds of nursing, academics, and women in Egypt compared to the United States.

CONTEXT: NURSING IN EGYPT

History

Egypt was colonized by the British people from the end of the 18th century to the mid-19th century, and trained nurses from England and France were working in the hospitals at that time. British physicians also replaced Egyptian professors in medical schools across the country, establishing a tradition of English as the language of choice for medical and university education (Ma, Fouly, Li, & D'Antonio, 2012).

Throughout this period, nursing involved two levels of education. The first level of education included students who joined nursing school after completing the 9th grade of education. After graduation, they worked as nursing assistants or aides. The second level of education involved 5 years of graduate training with these nurses, called *Hakima*. After graduation, they were licensed to practice nursing and midwifery or physical therapy (Ma et al., 2012).

Nursing Education in Egypt Today

There are seven types of nurses in Egypt, but three types dominate. The first level is at the secondary level of education. Students can join these schools after completing 9 years of elementary preparatory education. Nursing in these schools is taught by qualified nurses (those who have a bachelor's degree of nursing) and some physicians who teach the medical courses—for example, anatomy and physiology. These high schools are controlled by the Egyptian Ministry of Health and Population and provide markets with nurses equivalent to auxiliary nurses. The students who join these schools are usually from poor families who select a fast and cost-effective way of working and practicing nursing. The curriculum in these schools is not based on strong clinical reasoning or a theoretical base for nursing skills. The subjects taught are basic sciences of physics, chemistry, biology, health education, hospital administration, nutrition, and psychology, in addition to fundamentals of medical, surgical, obstetric, and mental health nursing. The curriculum in these schools is taught in Arabic in addition to an English-language course and requires the students to spend 3 days in hospital practice and 3 days in class each week (Farag, 2008; Ma et al., 2012).

After completing this program, the students should apply for the nursing license and join the Egyptian Nursing Syndicate. Employment is guaranteed to those nurses after at least 2 years of nursing practice in the governmental hospitals in a particular geographic location selected by the Egyptian Ministry of Health and Population (MOHP). Some graduates choose to join the technical nursing institute, considered a higher level of nursing education; others choose to practice as general nurses. Some nurses apply for 6 months of training to be specialized nurses in a specific area—for example, anesthesia, surgery, or normal labor and delivery. The secondary technical nursing education is considered the largest source of nursing graduates, providing approximately 94% of the available nursing workforce (El-Noshokarty, 2004). Moreover, those nurses are very young, ranging from mid-adolescence to young adulthood; the MOHP has identified these nurses as not being adequately prepared.

The second category of nursing education is carried out in the technical health institutes. The study at this level consists of 2 years of education and, after completion, on to general secondary school or nursing secondary school. This type of education was established in Alexandria in 1972 and in Cairo in 1973. The graduate gets an associate degree from one of these institutes. It is controlled by the Egyptian Ministry of Education. The courses taught in this curriculum are more in-depth than those in secondary nursing education.

In 1955, the Higher Institute of Nursing was established in Alexandria as the first higher institute in the Middle East and Africa. It was established by an agreement between the faculty of medicine and the World Health Organization (WHO). The teaching staff consisted of five visiting American nurses and a director assigned by the WHO. It was affiliated with the Faculty of Medicine. In 1992, the Supreme Council of Egyptian Universities granted independence to the Higher Institute of Nursing from the Faculty of Medicine (Ma et al., 2012). The institute, directed by the Egyptian Ministry of Higher Education and Scientific Research, offers a baccalaureate degree of nursing. It consists of a 4-year program in addition to 1 year of internship offered by the nursing faculties in collaboration with university hospitals. The bachelor's degree is not awarded to the nursing students until they have completed the internship year. In the internship year, the student receives a small stipend and each month practices in different units affiliated with a university or teaching hospital. Each student is under the supervision of an assigned preceptor on different shifts and is evaluated each month before moving to the next month of practice or continuing in the same practice for another month.

Some faculties of nursing also offer three postgraduate programs—diploma, master's degree, and doctorate degree—in nine nursing specialties. The diploma program takes 1 year after the bachelor's degree. The master's program takes from 3 to 4 years after the bachelor's degree or the diploma degree. The doctorate program takes 5 years after earning the master's degree.

Implications for Advancement of Egyptian Nursing

Nursing in Egypt is a skilled profession that has seen little change over the past 30 years. The primary challenges in nursing are centered on education, performance, accommodation, an image that is not highly appreciated, and a lack of motivation due to low salaries and incentives. The existing weaknesses in legislation regarding nursing have left nurses with minimal social and human rights benefits (WHO, 2012, www.emro.who.int/images/stories/cah/fact_sheet/Nursing_Profile.pdf).

The challenges facing nursing in Egypt are addressed through the collaboration between the Egyptian MOHP, the WHO, and other partners and universities who provide technical and financial support. Among these challenges are ensuring and supporting the upgrading of nurses' performance in the health services through education and reviewing and updating existing regulations through supporting existing nursing syndicates (WHO, 2012, www.emro.who.int/images/stories/cah/fact_sheet/Nursing_Profile.pdf).

Obstacles to Nursing Advancement in Egypt

Achievement of goals is important, but many obstacles impair the advancement of professional nursing in Egypt, which in turn may inhibit personal goal acquisition. The obstacles that impair the advancement of nursing are similar to those faced in other countries: supply and demand for nurses, education level of nurses, long hours, working conditions, and low wages (Rashdan, 2007).

Supply and Demand for Nurses

One of the obstacles affecting the nursing workforce is the supply of nurses. "Egypt suffers from a severe shortage in the number of nurses in hospitals and public clinics. There are 276 nurses for every 100,000 people" (United Nations Development Program, and the Institute of National Planning, Egypt, 2005, p. 76). The distribution of nurses is not equal throughout Egypt. Unfortunately, there is a severe shortage in the governorates of Upper Egypt (rural area). The WHO (2006) estimates that approximately 2.36 million health care providers will be needed to deliver health care. Without action from countries addressing the supply and demand, the shortage of health care providers will worsen.

Education Level of Nurses

As we mentioned before, the majority of Egyptian nurses are diploma graduates from the nursing secondary schools (El-Noshokarty, 2004). In addition, they are very young. As a result of the multiple levels of entry into practice and various ages associated with admission to programs, there is a lack of role delineation for each graduate, which creates the mentality of "a nurse is a nurse." It may be beneficial to determine the minimum level of entry into practice. To accomplish this task, there is a need to open channels of communication with all nursing education venues to ensure a sufficient number of nursing faculty possessing advanced degrees and willing to educate the professional nurse (Rashdan, 2007).

Long Working Hours

The research clearly documents staff nurse fatigue and its impact on patient safety (Balas et al., 2004; Rogers et al., 2004). Studies link fatigue to slow reaction times, lapses of attention, and errors of omission that compromise problem-solving ability (Tabone, 2004). In Egypt, nurse fatigue exists due to the shortage of nurses to handle the number of patients and the long hours worked because of the lack of enforcement of labor laws (Rashdan, 2007). The schedule of technical nurses sometimes contains 30 days of night shifts, which can be exhausting.

Working Conditions

Due to the financial constraints that face some hospitals and clinics in Egypt, especially those belonging to the governmental sector, some basic supplies can be unavailable, such as gloves and hygienic products for hand washing, which can lead to a high turnover of nurses (Farag, 2008; Rashdan, 2007).

Low Wages

In 1999, wages stood at 116 Egyptian pounds per month at minimum, with an average of 928 Egyptian pounds per month during 2004/2005. Many foreign companies related to Gulf hospitals offer high wages (10 times more than standard Egyptian wages) to attract workers (American Chamber of Commerce in Egypt, 2008). In some governmental hospitals, nurses who double a shift can get only 90 piasters, which is frustrating (El-Noshokarty, 2004).

After the Egyptian revolution of January 25, 2011, all Egyptian nursing categories have called for salary increases to counter high living expenses. The MOHP is currently responding to the call for improved wages.

A Call for Advancement in Egyptian Nursing

In order to meet the dynamic demands of Egypt's booming population growth, there is a need to increase the number of competent professional nurses that are available to deliver health care. More attention should be paid to educating nurses to allow them to broaden the impact of nursing knowledge in a hospital or clinic, similar to how a pebble ripples across a body of water (Rashdan, 2007).

Regulation of Practice

A clear and specific Nursing Practice Act defining the scope of nursing practice that defines professional nursing is important to advancing the nursing profession in Egypt. Development of a Nursing Practice Act will safeguard the public health by shielding the public from unqualified and unsafe nurses. Creating a Nursing Practice Act will define entry into nursing practice, specify the scope of practice, and establish disciplinary procedures (Rashdan, 2007).

From Syndicate to Nursing Board

After graduation from the nursing secondary schools, technical nursing institutes, or the faculties of nursing, the graduates have to register automatically in the nursing syndicate to legally practice nursing in the hospitals. This syndicate is responsible for providing service of all the nurses all over the country. It provides social activities and workshops—continuing education programs that can help nurses improve their practice. Sometimes ceremonies are held to honor exemplary nurses from around the country. Nurses in Egypt are not required to pass a board exam to practice nursing.

Encouraging the Egyptian Nursing Syndicate to adopt an agency mission is very important. However, the nursing board needs to be responsible regarding all nursing practice–related issues in Egypt. This can offer protection to the citizens of Egypt and promote their welfare by ensuring that each person practicing as a nurse in the country is competent to practice safely. Moreover, the Egyptian Nursing Syndicate should adopt and enforce rules that regulate the practice of professional nursing, establish standards of professional conduct for those nurses who practice nursing in Egypt, and determine the health activities constituting the practice of professional nursing. The nursing board should delineate the scope of practice for each level of professional nursing (Rashdan, 2007).

Advancement and Growth of Continuing Education Programs

On successful completion of the nursing exam conducted by the MOHP in Egypt, nurses hold a lifetime license to practice. Consider a paradigm shift in the practice of nursing whereby continuing education is a requirement to maintain and continue practicing as a nurse within Egypt. Continuing education can be required, thereby to assure the public that each nurse has current and updated knowledge of nursing science and the skills necessary for protecting the safety of patients receiving nursing care. Education is the most powerful weapon we have for changing the world (Rashdan, 2007).

Foster Curriculum Changes in Nursing Education Programs

Nurses are trained as generalists with little time spent in specialty areas. Curriculum changes will be required. Education should be learner-focused rather than teacher-centered. Curriculum changes need to incorporate the subspecialty areas—for example, oncology nursing, pediatric nursing, and neonatal intensive care nursing (Rashdan, 2007).

Perform Needs Assessment in Current Nursing Education Programs

It is important to perform an assessment of academic institutions to assess the number of graduates per year and their anticipated capacity of students. A needs assessment should be completed to analyze the fundamental needs of nurses and the locales of learning institutions. Educational programs are not meant to teach everything to students but rather to provide them with the skills to learn how to find information through problem-solving accomplished with simulation laboratories, clinical decision modules, critical thinking scenarios, and integration of evidenced-based practice (Rashdan, 2007).

Improve the Image of Nursing in Egypt

Nurses must continue to improve the image of nursing in Egypt by demonstrating to the public the professionalism of nurses there. Positive media coverage of events could make use of newspapers, magazines, television, or other forms of media. Nurses must seize the opportunity to highlight their contributions by writing letters to the editor to discuss what nurses do and how important nurses are to the delivery of health care for the people of Egypt. Nurses must position themselves at strategic levels of policy decision making to help develop policy and legislation to benefit the image of nursing and impact the delivery of health care (Rashdan, 2007).

Advance Gender Roles in Nursing

Nursing in Egypt is primarily a female occupation, and very few men are admitted to nursing programs in the university sector. In 2007, the Egyptian military sector graduated its first class of male subofficers, with a graduating class of 60 nurses. The employment of male nurses represents a positive advance in gender roles for Egypt (Rashdan, 2007). Male nursing students joined university nursing education in 2004. This has helped nursing become a more gender-balanced profession. Females continue to dominate the profession, and male nursing students display a lack of desire and enthusiasm attributable to the image of nursing in Egypt and a general feeling that nursing is a female job. From our experience with our nursing students, it was difficult for a male to become a nurse, taking on what is considered a female job. In the beginning, male students felt ashamed to tell others that they would be nurses, but after the first group of students graduated and entered the workforce, this image began to change, and male students are now more positive about the profession.

Challenges to Egyptian Health Care Within the Context of Culture

There are many challenges within any health care system, and cultural context always plays a role regardless of country. In Egypt some of the factors influencing health and the nursing profession include:

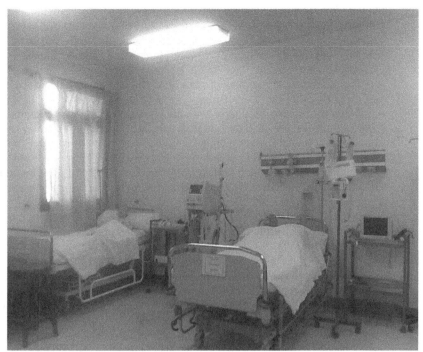

Critical care nursing training lab in the Faculty of Nursing, Alexandria University. *Credit*: N. Elcokany

- Female patients prefer to be examined by a female physician, especially for gynecological or obstetric purposes. Women feel shy and embarrassed talking about private issues like sexual issues with a male physician, so they prefer female doctors.
- Egyptian patients like to hear good news about their health, but if they have a serious illness, it is better to report the seriousness of illness and its consequences to a selected member of the family.
- Most Egyptian people don't seek medical care unless they are in need. They don't like routine checkups, lest they discover a disease—though the educated people have regular checkups.
- Herbal medicine use is a common precursor to seeking medical advice.

THE DREAM: STUDYING NURSING ABROAD

In light of the challenges to nursing in Egypt, as a nursing educator, I was looking for new information that I could apply in my field. I wanted to develop my career, expand my nursing skills, and learn more about conducting nursing research. My story began 5 years ago when I started to think of studying nursing abroad. These years were spent comparing nursing in my country (Egypt) and nursing in Western countries. I had many ideas about nursing abroad from the media as I watched the television series *Grey's Anatomy* and *ER*. They motivated me to practice nursing in my country and I noticed in these series that the nurse has an important role in the medical team. Essentially, the media and Internet were the instigators of my search.

AWARENESS AND SEARCH FOR INTERNATIONAL PROGRAMS OF STUDY

My first problem was to find a university for study. To do this, I contacted many universities to find a professor who matched my area of research. A second problem was to find a way (grant or scholarship) to cover my study and living expenses. The Internet was the only way to look for a professor who matched my specialty in critical care nursing with an emphasis on pulmonary problems. In Egypt, I was a student in the PhD program at the University of Alexandria and had completed the coursework and data collection for my dissertation. The studies I envisioned would add to what I had learned and enable me to take this information back to my country.

I contacted many schools of nursing in the United States, and each school suggested another school for me. I was surprised to find that they read e-mails from people abroad. I felt that the nursing professors were helpful and willing to attract international students and help them succeed. After I found a professor (Dr. Leslie Hoffman) at the University of Pittsburgh, I was in contact with her for more than 18 months before receiving my scholarship. My dream then was not just to come to the United States as a visiting scholar, but to earn a degree in the United States. The value and quality of studying in the United States is well known and includes exposure to advanced technology in research, teaching, and nursing practice.

At our university, located in Alexandria, Egypt, we usually receive many announcements about scholarships, grants, and exchange programs between our university and other universities. The scholarship that I applied for was offered by the mission sector, which was managed by the ministry of higher education and scientific research. Major requirements for receiving support included being an assistant lecturer at the university, being younger than 30 years old, obtaining professor acceptance from a foreign university, having an acceptable TOEFL score, and completing the PhD coursework, along with other requirements. I learned that prior successful applicants were primarily from the medical field and other majors, such as engineering, agriculture, and veterinary medicine. Undeterred, I submitted my application. I was finally accepted during the revolution of January 25, 2011, 10 months after I applied. The scholarship provided me a small stipend to cover my living expenses.

Next came the process of obtaining a visa, and for that, I needed to journey to Cairo from my hometown of Alexandria, a 135-mile trip (3 hours by car or train). I had to leave at 5 a.m. each morning to arrive at the visa office at 8 a.m., but I persisted through all the paperwork and the required interview process.

EXPECTATIONS AND FEELINGS ASSOCIATED WITH STUDYING NURSING IN THE UNITED STATES

When first arriving in the United States, I had mixed feelings that included happiness and worry. I was happy because it was one of my dreams to go abroad, but at the same time I was worried about the language. In Egypt, we study nursing in English, but we do not use English when speaking with each other. Therefore, we learn a more formal way of speaking that does not include slang or common expressions used with each other. I was worried that I would be misunderstood by the people around me, including my advisor, if I didn't catch the correct meanings of words. In addition, I worried about being away from my family and was concerned about the weather in a different climate. Before traveling to Pittsburgh, I had not been in a country with four distinct seasons, and I had never experienced snow.

REFLECTIONS ON IMMERSION IN A NEW CULTURE

Personal Feelings

I thought that living in a culture totally different from my home culture would be difficult. I was also concerned about communicating with different people. I decided from the start that as long as I was in a different country with a different culture, I must respect new rules, beliefs, and cultural differences. This attitude helped me a lot. At first, I was happy and impressed with the change. However, I did not feel that I truly "fit in." My culture shock was not evident to the people around me, though. I knew my name, where I was living, and who I was talking to, but at the same time I felt I had some clouds in front of my eyes. I was a little bit confused, but I was also excited by this new experience and new environment. I felt I had finally seen the other half of the world.

I was fortunate that I attended a class in my PhD courses in Egypt about cultural diversity. I remembered what our professor, Dr. Amany Gamal El-Din, said when she explained the concept of culture shock in detail. She had also earned her PhD from the University of Pittsburgh, so she was able to transfer her knowledge and experiences to me. I spoke with her often before leaving, and she gave me the idea of what life would be like in the United States.

In the beginning, I was excited and happy, feeling I had "made it." I did what I was dreaming of: I came to the United States, my dream, but this enthusiastic moment didn't last forever. After all the excitement, enjoyment, and happiness I initially experienced, I felt loneliness, homesickness, frustration, and anxiety and had trouble concentrating and being organized. I started to blame myself and wonder why I had come.

I missed my family and friends. I blamed myself for not reading more about American culture before arriving. The hardest thing for me was to understand what Americans were saying in the street. English is not my native language, and I found American slang extremely difficult. I was no longer able to express myself the way I wanted—this was the hardest adjustment for me.

Everyday life activities were different for me as well, and required significant adjustment. Transportation in the United States is different from in my home country. I solved this problem by trying to get the bus with friends and learning the maps for going from place to place. I found it funny that the people who were using maps included both international students and American citizens. I didn't use a map in my country but found doing so was normal in the United States. When I went food shopping, I could not find what I liked, especially traditional Egyptian food, and I found myself using different units of measurement. I didn't have a conception of an ounce, a pound, or a degree Fahrenheit—we usually use kilograms for weight, centigrade for temperature, and liters or milliliters for volume. The coins were also difficult for me to distinguish. Which coin was higher in value? I couldn't find numbers on coins, so I assumed that the larger in size, the higher the value. Unfortunately, I learned, there is the dime! Over time, though, I learned the differences between coins and at the same time was encouraged by the new things I was learning—I liked the challenge and the new experiences I was having.

Socializing in the United States

There are big differences in social situations in Egypt and the United States. For example, in the United States I found that hand shaking is common when anyone is introduced. In my country, male friends can hug each other. In the United States a man can hug a woman, which is something not allowed in my country. I found that Americans have a very high degree of transparency. For example, on the bus, I can listen to an entire story told by someone speaking with a loud voice. In my country, we keep things private and say little in public.

I also observed that Americans like to have frequent parties in their houses. In addition, they go many places on weekends with others to the nearby park or stores, enjoying their day off. They use their weekend time to the maximum. I also found parks well equipped for many activities, which I found strange at first but now think amazing.

Because Egyptian culture is very different from American culture in many ways, in the time I have been in the United States I have also changed internally. I found that in the United States, people do not have time to look at each other or to judge each other, so they can do as they like in the street without any comment or judgment from nearby people. In Egypt, public behavior is judged by others. For example, clothing is different, for many reasons—such as religion, gender, and weather—influencing dress in Egypt. Most of the women in Egypt cover their body completely. If a woman has uncovered any of her body parts, she will be seen as attractive to people in the street, whether male or female. For some this is in accordance with Islamic doctrine, but Christians also usually cover their bodies. Wearing shorts can be seen as disrespectful even in hot weather, except in some places such as beaches. Finally, another notable difference in social life is dealing with becoming an adult. Egyptian girls and boys are cherished and looked after by their parents until they get married, regardless of age. In the United States, however, it is possible to find many young persons living independently away from their families while unmarried.

Academic Life in the United States

I was shocked when I found that some students refer to their professors by name without using a title such as "doctor"—something not accepted in my country. In Egypt, I use my colleagues' titles when saying their names. This is viewed as respectful to one's senior colleagues. Also, in Egypt as a sign of respect, one does not speak to an older man or woman without adding "uncle" or "aunt" to the name.

Freedom in the classroom is also worlds away from my experience. For example, in Egypt we can't sit in front of the teacher with crossed legs. To do so is considered disrespectful to the teacher—students who do so are considered impolite or thought to have grown up in a poor environment. In the United States, students are free to just sit or to do another activity while attending class. Students may eat in class or engage in other activities while attending the lecture. For example, I attended a class with PhD students and found one of the students knitting while attending the class—and the professor didn't comment, leading me to consider this commonplace. But such students also engage in lecture discussions while doing these things—meaning that they are fully concentrating.

I was eager to gain experience from the United States and to know more about the actual practice of nursing. I asked my mentor to find an undergraduate course I could help teach as a volunteer in the lab or in the hospital. This was a great opportunity for me to learn more about clinical teaching, and my mentor facilitated this as well as other experiences, always offering to help me even without my having asked.

I gained experience in clinical teaching in the hospital by dealing with patients, seeing the hospitals and their many different machines, working with different categories of nurses, and seeing how nurses deal with the patients—and also dealing with different students. One memorable event was hearing the nurses sing to the patients before discharge. My initial impression was that the hospitals are like hotels, they are so advanced and so comfortable. Nurses here are required to do everything for the patients and it seems they have time to provide psychological support as well as physical care. They are talking, singing, smiling, and listening with the patients. I am now assured in my belief that the psychological aspect of care is more important than the physical part and can help in recovery.

Unfortunately, in Egypt nurses have multiple duties and responsibilities. First, we don't have respiratory therapists, so our nurses perform all the pulmonary activities patients need. Second, we have few or, at times, no nursing assistants. Egyptian nurses are also required to care for the mechanical ventilator and the other machines. All these responsibilities add stress to the nurses and can lead to burnout.

Observing and Adjusting to Life in the United States

As part of becoming adjusted to life in the United States, I started to observe everything around me, trying to collect ideas about Americans and American culture. One significant observation that continually amazed me was that I found Americans to always seem happy and positive. Their reaction to different situations is totally different from what I am used to in my country. I'm not sure whether this is a result of the natural environment—with all the green land in Pittsburgh—or whether all Americans behave so.

I also started to find people from other Arab countries, including Egyptians, to help me in my adjustment. Many are immigrants here and gave me hints about the culture and American people. I could see that they were happy, and they were a support to me, helping me realize that I'm not alone here in such a different culture.

After 5 months, I started to adjust. I used my sense of humor to adjust and I found help from others. My American academic advisor gave me a lot of support, guidance, and direction. I felt understood by my advisor. For example, she was driving us somewhere and a male Indian student started to sit beside me in the car, but she asked him to sit in the front seat instead. I can't express the great feeling of happiness that I felt in that situation. I was so happy that my advisor recognized that sitting next to a male student was not considered appropriate in my culture and handled the situation so smoothly.

I also found many of my fellow students here to be totally independent, and so I started to be more independent. I lived for a long time with students from different cultures, including China and Russia, and being with them helped me deal with people in general. We were exchanging cultural differences together. I do find that people in Pittsburgh are friendly and welcoming toward international students.

CONCLUSION

In nursing education, students learn about differences between cultures and religions, so the teachers, students, and classmates probably knew a little bit about my traditions. I remember when I attended a clinical session with the undergraduate students in the simulation center and the teacher gave them many scenarios about different cultures and religions and how to deal with these differences. These activities help nurses deal with humanity with extra care and inspire others to serve without discrimination. I will always remember when I was in my undergraduate class on nursing ethics. The first rule I learned in the code of ethics was to accept the patient as he or she is, regardless of race, religion, and culture.

I like Americans, and yet I know that during my stay I was touched by only a few sides of America—in particular, academic and professional life. My perspectives are subjective, and I know I cannot uncover everything about the United States during my brief stay of 18 months.

I have seen a number of things I would like to take back with me as goals for change in Egypt:

- An effective board of nursing to control the practice of the nursing profession
- Passage of an exam such as NCLEX as requisite to beginning a nursing career
- Standards of practice for each category of nurses
- Increased funding in support of research
- Websites providing ideas and dialogue about nursing practice

Finally, I'm thinking seriously about how I can be helpful in my country when I return, and about how I will adjust when I go back. Can I be effective in changing something in the curricula? Can I be a factor of change in the nursing profession in general? If so, how? I have a lot of plans and ideas, but I will need strong support from the administrative level and the decision makers in my home institution. I don't know if the people around me will motivate or frustrate me (probably both at times), but I'm hoping I can be a force for change.

REFLECTIVE QUESTIONS

1. What factors do you think would be important to you if you were selecting a nursing program in another country?

2. Think about study abroad for a prolonged period in another country. What challenges do you think you would face? How would you cope?
3. Compare the profession of nursing in Egypt with your country. How is nursing similar? How is it different?

REFERENCES

American Chamber of Commerce in Egypt. (2008). Doing business in Egypt. Retrieved from http://www.amcham.org.eg/dbe/General_Info.asp

Balas, M. C., Scott, L. D., & Rogers, A. E. (2004). The prevalence and nature of errors and near errors reported by hospital staff nurses. *Applied Nursing Research, 17*(4), 224–230.

El-Noshokarty, A. (2004). The job of mercy. *Al-Ahram Weekly.* http://weekly.ahra.org/eg/print/2004/690/fe2.htm

Farag, M. (2008). *Economic analysis of the nurse shortage in Egypt.* Working Paper Series. Dubai School of Government (08-06), 1–24.

Ma, C., Fouly H., Li J., D'Antonio P. (2012). The education of nurses in China and Egypt. *Nursing Outlook, 60*(3): 127–133. doi: 10.1016/j.outlook.2011.08.002

Rashdan, T. (2007). *Implications for advancement of Egyptian nursing: Input equals output.* Paper for Fulbright Academy Workshop in Doha, March 23–25.

Rogers, A. E., Hwang, W. T., Scott, L. D., Aiken, L. H., & Dinges, D. F. (2004). The working hours of hospital staff nurses and patient safety. *Health Affairs, 23*(4), 202–212.

Tabone, S. (2004). Data suggest nurse fatigue threatens patient safety. *Texas Nursing, 78*(2), 4–7.

United Nations Development Program and the Institute of National Planning, Egypt. (2005). p. 76.

World Health Organization. (2006). The global shortage of health workers and its impact (Fact Sheet No. 302). Retrieved March 9, 2008, from http://www.who.int/mediacentre/factsheets/fs302/en/index.html

World Health Organization. (2012). Egypt nursing profile. WHO country office in Egypt. Retrieved from http://www.emro.who.int/images/stories/cah/fact_sheet/Nursing_Profile.pdf

Developing and Sustaining Partnerships Through Global Health in Local Communities

Elizabeth Downes
Judith Lupo Wold

CONTEXT: FARMWORKER FAMILY HEALTH PROGRAM, UNITED STATES

Global health practice does not always require a passport. The United States is a remarkably diverse nation, where over 300 languages are spoken. In fact, over 55 million people speak a language other than English at home (Shin & Komanski, 2010). It is essential that health care workers be prepared to work with diverse cultures. This case study describes a "domestic as global" academic–community partnership that has been in existence for longer than 20 years. Clients of this partnership are largely migrant workers and their family members from Mexico, who are not necessarily working in the United States with appropriate documentation. They primarily speak Spanish, but some speak indigenous dialects. These workers harvest fruits and vegetables by hand, grueling work. We ask no questions of clients regarding documentation status during our 2-week summer rotation. However, for the sites where care is provided, migrant status is virtually 100% assured. Federally funded migrant health clinics can only treat clients who meet their definition for migrant status. Because of the fluidity of this population, there is little collaboration between these clinics.

The initial Farmworker Family Health Program (FWFHP) partnership, which began with one small group of undergraduate public health nursing students and one faculty member from a single school who engaged with a single south Georgia farmworker clinic, has evolved to encompass over 100 students and faculty members from five different universities along with community partners. The number of community partners has expanded to include not only the initiating federally funded migrant farm clinic, but also a summer school program, day care centers, two area health education centers (AHECs), businesses, faith communities, and, of course, the farmers and growers. Dental hygiene, nursing, pharmacy, psychology, and physical therapy students, volunteers, and faculty travel to a rural area of a southeastern state as part of a 2-week service learning cultural immersion experience, each adding to the overall scope of services.

PROGRAM OVERVIEW

The FWFHP is a collaboration of the federally funded Ellenton Health Clinic (hereinafter referred to as the Ellenton Clinic), located in Ellenton, Georgia, and five Georgia universities: Emory University (lead university), Georgia State University, Clayton College and State University, Darton College, and the University of Georgia. Other partners include the Colquitt County Health Department, the Colquitt County Board of Education, the Southern Pine Migrant Education Agency, and the owners of farms and packing houses in the Colquitt County area. Additional budget-relieving in-kind support comes from churches and community organizations in the area. The FWFHP, coordinated by the Lillian Carter Center for Global Health and Social Responsibility in the Nell Hodgson Woodruff School of Nursing at Emory University, has served over 13,000 individuals in its 20-year history. Using students and faculty in the health professions, preventive and episodic health care is delivered over a 2-week period each summer in an intensive outreach setting that also serves as part of the clinical training programs of the universities. Each participating university pays the salaries of its faculty and makes some arrangement with its students regarding housing costs. Although the program is intermittently funded by small grants, no single current funding source covers all program expenses.

The team provides care for farmworker families to live, work, and go to school. In the mornings the team sees children enrolled in a migrant summer program at a local elementary school and day care. In the evenings the team caravans to various locations, including packing sheds, farmworker camps, and local neighborhoods. While the Ellenton Clinic is responsible for communication with and arranging for the various locations for our nightly schedule, the faculty is responsible for making sure students arrive at the farms or service sites together and on time. Participants meet in the parking lot of the hotel where we are housed at a designated time and all leave together for our destination. The leader of the caravan knows the directions to each farm, and a "caboose" faculty car also follows with the directions. Country roads are extremely dark, and the farms and their entrances are spread over four very rural counties. Earlier years without cell phone service posed a challenge, but improvements in technology have helped significantly.

Services provided at the migrant summer school program in the morning are structured around comprehensive physical examinations of children and adolescents. Parental permission is required for a child to be seen. Outreach workers from the Southern Pine Migrant Education Agency work alongside the Colquitt County Board of Education to sign children up for the summer school, and the Ellenton Clinic provides existing charts from their files and makes new charts for children without records. All records are property of the Ellenton Clinic, and all HIPAA regulations are observed. Undergraduate nursing students (BSNs) complete screenings of height, weight (body mass index [BMI]), blood pressure, hemoglobin, vision, and hearing. Nurse practitioner (NP) students do full physical examinations. Developmental assessments are carried out by physical therapy (PT) students. Dental services, including application of sealants and fluoride, are provided by dental hygiene (DH) students. Pharmacy (PharmD) students provide health education in the classrooms. Meanwhile, a small team of students and faculty work at the partnering farmworker clinic seeing patients and preparing the pharmacy. If health-related problems are detected, children who do not have a Medicaid provider listed on their permission form are referred to the Ellenton Clinic for follow-up. Health status letters in both Spanish and English are sent home to the parents of each child seen, whether a referral is necessary or not. Ellenton Clinic outreach workers handle emergent problems on an as-needed basis.

In the evenings BSN students complete height, weight, blood pressure, BMI, hemoglobin, and blood glucose screenings. A foot care station is staffed primarily by BSNs but also with other team members' participation. DH, NP, and PT students have separate stations for their respective practices. The evening focus of care is acute complaints rather than comprehensive examinations. NPs can prescribe with collaborative practice protocols, and PharmD students operate a pharmacy dispensary on site out of the clinic's mobile unit. Patients with chronic conditions are referred to the clinic for follow-up, with on-site clinic outreach workers arranging appointments and transportation. The clinic staff has provided interpretation services subsidized by one of the AHECs at the evening clinics. The need for more interpreters has led to inclusion of an additional team partner, the Emory Volunteer Medical Interpretation Services. This is a student-run organization made up of bilingual students formally trained as medical interpreters. The team starts seeing patients in the evening clinics before sunset, often staying out past midnight. All members wait until the last patient and provider are done. Then we caravan home together, and in the morning we get up and do it again.

PROGRAM HISTORY OF DEVELOPING TRUST AND A SHARED MISSION

The executive director of the clinic and the lead faculty came to trust each other through a shared vision of improving access to health care for migrant farmworkers and their families. The FWFHP extends the work of the clinic and adds to the numbers of new annual visits they need to continue their federal funding. As the need for additional expertise became obvious, they jointly decided to invite other disciplines to join the nursing students, thus expanding the program's services. The grueling work and conditions of farm labor result in multiple musculoskeletal complaints, and the benefit of having PT students on site became apparent. The nursing faculty reached out to the physical therapy department. A similar situation occurred with psychology, where an identified need carved out a role for an additional discipline.

A good exemplar of dovetailing interests is the example of dental hygiene. Dental disease is among the top five health problems in this population (Lombardi, 2001). Both the clinic executive director and nurses saw a great need for dental services for both the children and the migrant workers. About the same time, many of the dental hygiene programs in the state were transitioning to bachelor-level programs, needing sites for community rotations. These needs allowed for great synergy. Even more importantly, the application of dental sealants and fluoride has probably been the most positive measurable outcome of the program.

Mutual trust and respect has grown over the years. The program's collaboration with the churches each summer has done much to raise community awareness regarding the plight of the farmworker. Because farmworkers are basically an "invisible" population working and living in these outlying rural areas, citizens of the four focal counties rarely see the labor or living conditions of these workers up close.

Two of the individuals who were founding partners have either retired or moved on, but leadership has not been lacking. The strong foundation built by years of work has fostered embedded trust between the involved institutions and has in fact led to a web of new personal relationships that have spun off to additional partnerships in different locations. For example, a member of the FWFHP nursing faculty runs a clinic caring for the uninsured and underinsured population of Atlanta. A member of the PT faculty now brings students to this clinic.

After 20 years of working together, even the site visits have evolved. Initially program faculty drove to the rural area for a day meeting a few months before the annual event. Then all participants (including all students) had a full-day orientation in Atlanta. Communication in preparation for the event now includes e-mails and conference calls and occasional "off-season" site visits. Medical records (the point of which is, after all, good communication) are developed by the Ellenton Clinic to meet their reporting requirements, with interstation transit front sheets developed in collaboration by all partners.

The 20 years together have not been without conflict. Working with partners requires compromise and negotiation. For example, the school system at the partner site determines the dates of the program. These may not always coincide with the best times for academic faculty and students, but as their guests and partners, it is imperative that we work with them based on their needs. In fact, one year the funding for the program was cut, and at the end of the first week we were told the last day would be the following Monday. We took this as an opportunity to look for new partners, which is when we began working with child care centers. This conflict thus turned into a benefit as NP students were able to complete physical examinations on children age 6 months to 3 years at a migrant Headstart program.

An ongoing conflict exists in the broader context of the program. We ask ourselves whether a program that provides care for migrant farmworkers perpetuates the inequities and conditions that put them at risk. Health care is rarely neutral or innocent. Placing

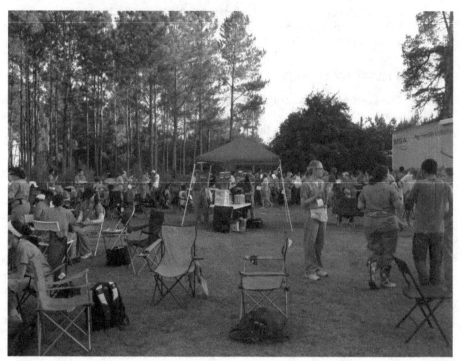

Evening activities from the Farmworker Family Health Program. *Credit:* J. Wold

care in its full context is an important consideration for all health care providers. The act of delivering health care, like providing assistance in complex humanitarian emergencies, isn't that complicated. It's the operational context in which the assistance is provided that is the complicated part. In caring for farmworkers with health problems exacerbated by the working conditions, are we doing all we can to solve the problem? This question is put to students and faculty and provide for self-reflection and ethical discussion. The FWFHP objective is to care for as many people as possible. As we work through this conflict, it may lead to a review of our vision.

The program is evaluated by each student and faculty member every summer. Undergraduate student nurses use this course as the clinical component of their public health nursing course and are evaluated on both didactic and clinical standards used by the Emory School of Nursing. Reflection journals are kept by undergraduate student nurses, and interprofessional reflection groups meet each morning prior to beginning the day covering various questions reflecting on the previous day's experiences. Other students' clinical expertise is evaluated by their respective faculty and credit allocated accordingly. Annual student and faculty evaluations through a questionnaire combining Likert scale and open-ended responses are tallied at Emory School of Nursing. The results are distributed to the other participating schools and considered as a whole by the program faculty. The operations of the program are enriched by suggestions from both seasoned faculty and staff and fresh student participants. We seek continued improvement in the efficacy and efficiency of this important work. Other evaluation comes in the form of thesis or dissertation projects of students from varying disciplines that request use of our anonymous clinical data collected each year on all clients.

Unforeseen collateral benefits include the interprofessional education. Continuity of faculty from year to year fosters faculty role modeling of interprofessional teamwork and partnership. Through the FWFHP, students from the various disciplines collaborate and consult with each other on all sorts of patient conditions. This interprofessional program predates the calls from the World Health Organization (2010) and the Institute of Medicine (Greiner, 2003) for increased interprofessional education.

CONCLUSION

The FWFHP is a unique interprofessional service-learning program that promotes student learning, improves knowledge and skills, and impacts students' attitudes. By partnering with a local clinic to support and expand its capacity at peak harvest season, health care professional students provide care for a vulnerable population. Students learn with, from, and about each other and the community they serve. The FWFHP is an example of a successful academic–community partnership.

REFLECTIVE QUESTIONS

1. Considering that farmworkers are often exploited by their crew bosses, is offering free health care to the workers helping or hindering those workers' cause for just employment and access to health care?
2. Should health care professionals providing health care to migrant workers attempt to lobby for them in the political arena? How do you think this would affect the ongoing development of the partnership?

REFERENCES

Greiner, A. (Ed.). (2003). *Institute of Medicine report: Health professions education: A bridge to quality.* Washington, DC: National Academies Press.

Lombardi, G. (2001). *Dental/oral services.* www.ncfh.org/docs/01%20-%20dental.pdf

Shin, H., & Komanski, R. (2010). Language use in the United States: 2007. *American Community Survey reports, ACS-12.* Washington, DC: U.S. Census.

World Health Organization. (2010). *Framework for action on interprofessional education and collaborative practice.* Geneva, Switzerland: World Health Organization.

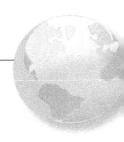

CHAPTER 2

Nurse and Visiting Organization Factors for Global Partnership

Michele J. Upvall

Relationships embody the essence of successful global partnerships, with *all* nurses bringing their beliefs, attitudes, values, and life experiences to the partnership. Establishing and maintaining relationships is often challenging in circumstances and surroundings familiar to nurses, but challenges can be easily magnified in global health when nurses find themselves in potentially extreme circumstances of dissonance. Alone and surrounded by the unfamiliar, the nurse may lose confidence in professional skills, misinterpreting behaviors and comments from partners, unsure of whom to ask for clarification. However, positive relationships are fundamental to successful partnerships. A sense of trust and respect, along with a commitment to the relationship through ongoing evaluation, is crucial from the perspective of both nurse and host partner (Hodgkinson & Holland, 2002; Kulbok, Mitchell, Glick, & Greiner, 2012; Sochan, 2008). Nurses are well positioned to develop such partnerships, as relationship building is fundamental to nursing practice with individual clients or within the community.

In the global health partnership process identified by Leffers and Mitchell (2011), nurse partner factors include cultural perspectives, personal attributes and expectations, and knowledge of the host country. This chapter explores these nurse factors from the perspective of the nurse as an individual and the nurse situated within an organization. Knowledge of self, organizational mission, host, and the environment of the host are precursors to developing strong relationships. This introspective, although broad-based, may help mitigate the challenges inherent to global partnerships.

BRINGING SELF TO THE GLOBAL HEALTH EXPERIENCE

Nurses seeking opportunities for global health experiences demonstrate particular personal attributes that include curiosity, a willingness to serve and extend compassion to others, flexibility, and perhaps even the simple love of adventure. As professionals, these nurses enjoy being challenged in their work and appreciate variety. These personal and professional attributes are shared by other health care professionals as well. In a study of allied health professionals in British Columbia, Canada, researchers found the following factors to be primary motivators in the decision to work in rural or remote communities:

- Past positive experiences
- Preference for professional variety
- Opportunity for challenges, including development of new skills
- Need for adventure

Research participants perceived themselves as adventurous, sociable, confident, resourceful, independent, and flexible. However, there was also recognition of changing values over time. Family needs were reported to take precedence over career goals. Age and stage of life also affect decision making for both coming to the remote area and determining how long the individual stays (Manahan, Hardy, & MacLeod, 2009). Attributes for success in global nursing partnerships are not dissimilar from other health professionals. Leffers and Mitchell (2011, p. 95) identify the following as factors for success:

- Willingness to live in less than comfortable conditions
- Openness to the perspective of others
- Flexibility
- Willingness to share or give leadership to host partners
- Energy to take personal risks to advocate for social justice and achieve morally sound outcomes

Some nurses enter the profession with the intention of being a global health provider, while others experience critical incidents as students or have an *aha* moment at a time in their career when they can make a commitment to global health. Confidence or cultural self-efficacy can be developed through various educational and clinical practice experiences (Jeffreys, 2010), but intrinsic factors or the internal motivation of the nurse provides the foundation for ongoing successful partnerships. These partnerships may extend to become true friendships, more than just professional relationships. Baumann (2012) identifies this approach as one of honoring the nurse in a low-resource country where the voice of the nurse is heard and a feeling of respect and hope for the future emerges. However, the beginning of the relationship is internal to the nurse. Identifying the desire or will to develop the relationship and having the self-awareness to understand relationships with others begins within the self.

The Will to Serve

More than 2 decades ago Ram Dass and Paul Gorman asked the question "How can I help?" (Dass & Gorman, 1985). The desire to help is often a reflex. For example, a car accident occurs and the nurse in the car behind leaps into helpful action; or a nurse, remembering what it was like to be a patient, is especially sensitive to the patient experiencing pain and offers comfort measures. Caring emanates from the action and is a response to the call for help, recognition that everyone experiences suffering as well as joy. The belief that "we are all in this together" and unifying notions of a common humanity inspire nurses' will to serve others. Specific theoretical constructs such as compassion, curiosity, courage, and cultural humility strengthen the will of the nurse to be of service and to extend the self in relationship to all global health partners, including colleagues from the same organization as the nurse.

Compassion, curiosity, and courage have been identified as principles of program development in global service-learning programs (McKinnon & Fealy, 2011). However, these constructs may also reside within the individual nurse pursuing the path of global health partnerships.

Compassion implies empathy with another's suffering. A compassionate nurse brings a fully present self to the encounter with an open mind and heart, willing to be engaged in alleviating suffering. Pity, also known as "idiot compassion" (Cash, 2007), is the antithesis of compassion and implies a relationship of "us" versus "them." We feel sorry for others but do very little to alleviate the suffering. True compassion is action-oriented.

Curiosity is an attitude that fosters exploration and ongoing learning. The curious nurse is comfortable asking questions and observing behaviors in pursuit of knowledge. However, curiosity is meaningless without internalizing the new knowledge for use in future situations.

Courage denotes an inner strength to face difficulties. In the context of global health, the nurse with courage confronts unknown people and places with confidence. Feelings of fear may surface, but the nurse with courage acknowledges the fear and vicissitudes with an attitude of acting "as if": as if the fear will be resolved or as if the change in situation will result in a positive outcome.

Cultural humility, defined as "a lifelong commitment to self-evaluation and critique" (Tervalon & Murray-Garcia, 1998, p. 123), extends models of cultural understanding and skill by acknowledging power structures within health care provider relationships. An attitude of cultural humility is a true partnership wherein all partners benefit from the relationship without a sense of paternalism. Humility as a virtue leads to self-reflection and change (Crigger & Godfrey, 2010).

Realizing these constructs in the personal and professional self is an ongoing process requiring commitment to action. Connecting to others in a global health partnership requires more than superficial compassion. The nurse brings a developing self, with all its imperfections, into the partnership along with expectations. Examining the self and expectations is the beginning of true partnership.

Self-Awareness

Understanding the self is a crucial prelude to effectively reaching out to others. How we see ourselves affects our response to others. If we feel that we do not have enough to give or that we do not have the ability to give what is required, then no action is taken and the question "How can I help?" is not ever asked. In the context of cultural and global health, self-awareness is defined as:

> a deliberate and conscious cognitive and emotional process of getting to
> know yourself: your personality, your values, your beliefs, your professional
> knowledge standards, your ethics, and the impact of these factors on the various
> roles you play when interacting with individuals different from yourself.
> (Purnell & Salmond, 2013, p. 45)

Uncovering motivational factors for choosing global health service is a life-long journey of introspection, action, and reflection. Self-assessment tools are available to measure potential for pursuing global experiences. A broad-based approach developed by Leffers and Plotnick (2011) includes deep reflection of motivation to serve, commitment to others and time available, physical ability, emotional stamina, social issues, clinical expertise, and professional skills.

Boyle and Andrews (2011) promote the concept of cultural self-assessment, asking the individual to determine his or her level of comfort in approaching specific cultural groups. A faculty self-assessment is available from Jeffreys (2010, p. 120) incorporating questions about students as well as the faculty member. Examples of questions include:

- What are my own cultural beliefs?
- What do I know about students' cultural values and beliefs?
- How do I feel when a student's cultural beliefs are different from mine?
- What is my motivation for engaging in the process of becoming culturally competent?
- What is my level of commitment in developing cultural competence in myself, peers, administrators, and students?

SITUATING SELF IN THE CONTEXT OF ORGANIZATIONS

Congruency among personal attributes explored through self-assessment, identifying personal expectations, and understanding sender and host organizational values solidify the global health partnership. The organization's mission and goals are strong indicators of the level of support that the nurse may be able to rely on when seeking global health experiences. In academic organizations, the institution's mission can influence coursework and types of affiliations with host organizations (Powell, Gilliss, Hewitt, & Flint, 2010; Riner, 2011).

There is a trend toward hospitals' and universities' collaborative agreements developing with global partners, and corporate volunteer opportunities continue to increase annually (Ketefian & Redman, 2013; www.gooverseas.com/6-companies-will-pay-volunteer-abroad).

Nurses employed by hospitals or other health care organizations may seek financial support from the employer, or even just time away from the job, but may be unsure of the administration's receptivity to the concept of a global health experience. In such a case, the nurse can assess the degree of cultural competency within the organization by using selected Health Resources and Services Administration indicators (HRSA, 2002):

- Organizational values: What are the perspectives and attitudes regarding the significance of culture and commitment to providing culturally competent care?
- Communication: Does the exchange of information between the organization/staff and organization/client population promote cultural competence?
- Staff development: Is there a commitment to training staff in delivering culturally competent services?
- Services/interventions: Are services provided in a culturally competent manner?

Another assessment tool of organizational diversity offers an even simpler approach to thinking about the significance of culture within the organization (Murry, 2010):

1. Does your leadership team represent the diversity of the population served?
2. Does your agency provide awareness training to sensitize staff on diversity?
3. Does your agency recruit staff by accessing cultural resources?
4. Does your agency consider diversity when planning clinic services?
5. Does your agency host multicultural celebrations or activities?

Responses to these yes/no questions can provide some measure of possibility for the acceptance of global health experiences and can also be a guide for nurses in leadership positions to strategize cultural competence development.

Nurses seeking to volunteer in agencies outside of their employment setting should carefully evaluate the organization and its expectations. Organizational factors to assess include (Leffers & Plotnick, 2011):

- Philosophy and mission
- Organizational history
- Nursing's role within the organization
- Focus of nursing interventions
- Location
- Expenses
- Meeting personal needs such as providing transportation, housing, and safe water

The volunteer organization's philosophy is perhaps the most important element to consider. An organization clearly stating a commitment to partnership would be ideal for the nurse seeking to create and sustain global health partnerships. However, the nurse should conduct a deeper analysis by seeking current examples of partnership within the organization and determining how these partnerships are maintained. Asking to speak to or e-mail current volunteers would provide even further information about the work of the organization and how its philosophy is realized in the field.

Guidelines for ethics and best practice in global health training provide direction for academic organizations and host organizations (Crump & Sugarman, 2010). A well-structured program does the following:

- Ensures that both sender and host institution derive mutual and equal benefit
- Considers local needs and priorities

- Provides an opportunity for long-term relationships to enable nesting of short-term experiences
- Promotes transparency regarding the motivation for developing the program
- Contains clear goals, expectations, and responsibilities using explicit agreements that are periodically reviewed
- Develops current training materials for the trainees and mentors within the sending and host institutions
- Encourages nonthreatening communication to resolve ethical conflicts in the field as they occur
- Selects trainees who are adaptable and motivated, sensitive to local needs, and willing to listen and learn
- Promotes the safety of trainees in the field
- Monitors costs and benefits to the sender and host institutions
- Establishes effective supervision and mentoring of trainees while in the field
- Establishes a feedback method for trainees while in the field and on their return home to evaluate the impact of the experience

These best practices do not weaken the responsibility that trainees have toward the global health experience and expectations of sponsors. Organizations focused on developing and sustaining strong global partnerships will be clear in how they achieve high-quality outcomes in their programs and on the role of the nurse as part of the process.

BUILDING A KNOWLEDGE BASE

Attributes and expectations intrinsic to the nurse are essential to developing a successful global partnership. Clarifying the nurse's role within the organization provides the boundaries of the partnership, and knowing what to possibly expect on arrival and throughout the partnership facilitates ongoing understanding of the partners within the context.

Cultural assessment is the process of discovering the health beliefs and patterns of individuals within a family, community, or organization. Examples of comprehensive assessment tools are prominent in nursing literature and include tools developed by Boyle and Andrews (2011), Giger (2013), Leininger (1991), and Purnell (2013). These assessments are useful for determining individual variations within cultural belief systems and provide direction for culturally competent nursing interventions. Dayer-Berenson (2011) discusses each of the cultural models used for deriving the specific cultural assessment tools allowing for comparison. The Purnell Model (Marrone, 2013) was developed for assessing organizational cultural competence from a broad perspective and includes 12 domains. These domains serve as a framework for designing cultural competency programs, assessments, organizational planning strategies, and interventions at the individual, family, and community levels.

Communication

All assessment tools derived from the cultural models address the importance of communication. However, Giger (2013) includes communication as a distinct component in her model. The model details the following communication elements:

- Verbal communication: vocabulary, voice quality, intonation, rhythm, speed, pronunciation, and silence
- Nonverbal communication: touch, facial expression, eye movement, and body posture
- Patterns combining verbal and nonverbal communication: warmth and humor

Nurses fluent in the language of the host partners should remain cognizant of the nonverbal cues of the partners as well as appropriate use of humor and conveying warmth.

Translation and interpretation are distinct concepts with translation related to written documents while interpretation takes place between individuals. Using family members and friends as interpreters is not recommended because of the potential sensitivity of the communication and the undue burden it places on the family member to remain as objective as possible. The following video provides tips for working with interpreters: www .youtube.com/watch?v=Q4voquDnkbM.

Often, host partners may speak English as a second or even third or fourth language if at all. Or, they may understand English, but are unable to speak fluently. Regardless, communication can be a major frustration for all global health partners as well as among partners from the nurse's own cultural background (Bednarz, Schim, & Doorenbos, 2010). Assessing level of communication is a priority when initiating the partnership as well as assessing for understanding on a regular basis. Culturally-appropriate communication strategies should be developed with all partners and communication materials should be tested for readability when possible. (National Institute of Environmental Health Sciences, U.S. Department of Health and Human Services, 2012)

Public health nursing is another source for building a knowledge base for enriching global health partnerships. The Public Health Nursing Assessment Tool (PHNAT) promotes assessment of the individual, community, population, and system and is available in an online format allowing tables to be formed and assessment data to be compared with national and international databases (Truglio-Londrigan & Lewenson, 2011). PHNAT consists of five parts:

1. Assessment of determinants of health: biology (population, age, race, and gender distribution), behavior (health behaviors, employment, industries, income, education levels), physical environment, social environment, policy and interventions (organizational structure of community, political issues), access to care
2. Analysis of health status: vital statistics, communicable and noncommunicable diseases, leading causes of death
3. Prioritize public health issues
4. Plan, implement, and evaluate using Minnesota intervention strategies: population-based health intervention strategies and levels of practice
5. Reflection

Completing a cultural assessment and determining strategies for communication promote knowledge specific to the health and facilitate understanding of the health care focus of the partnership. However, health care does not exist in isolation from the cultural context. The well-informed nurse partner has knowledge of the country and popular culture. Historical literature can also provide context for understanding present-day political conflicts. For example, the book *Freedom at Midnight* (Lapierre & Collins, 1997) provides compelling background for analyzing the often tense relations between India and Pakistan. Reading novels and literature related to the country and its surroundings promotes a deeper understanding for strong partnerships.

FACILITATING ONGOING DEVELOPMENT

Developing skills to manage challenging situations in any partnership requires continual effort and learning. Neither of the partners in the relationship can achieve complete knowledge or understanding of the other, and to expect such a degree of knowledge is unrealistic. For example, the nurse may be fluent in the language, but not growing up within the culture will prevent complete understanding of the cultural nuances behind the words. Florczak (2013) recommends approaching each person with an open mind. This approach was substantiated by Callister and Cox (2006) in their phenomenological study of the long-term meaning of international nursing experiences for students. The theme of "opening our minds and hearts" was expressed by students as they discussed the deep impact from having a clinical experience overseas that culminated in life-changing events.

Listening

> But he learned more from the river than Vasudeva could teach him. He learned from it continually. Above all he learned from it how to listen with a still heart, with a waiting, open soul, without passion, without desire, without judgment, without opinions. (Siddhartha as quoted in Dass & Gormman, 1985, p. 112)

The ability to be actively present and listen with an open mind and heart requires patience and practice. Listening and reflecting understanding of the message are reassuring to the one trying to be heard. There are many ways in which the nurse can listen in relation to the partner. Mindfulness and reflexivity are two practices that promote deep listening with presence. The practice of mindfulness is "both a way of being aware, and the intentional practice of cultivating such awareness. . . . The practice of mindful awareness in the present can support reflective listening by allowing one to be less swayed by one's own thoughts and need to reply" (McCaffrey, Raffin-Bouchal, & Moules, 2012, p. 95). Reflexivity is key to demonstrating cultural humility and is characterized by actively engaging in self-reflection to promote understanding and self-awareness. Reflexivity facilitates recognition of different worldviews and belief systems and promotes respect and negotiation within the partnership (Clark, Calvillo, Dela Cruz, Fongwa, Kools, Lowe, & Mastel-Smith, 2011).

A Metaphor for Entering Into Partnership

The use of metaphors is not common in nursing literature, but it is a way to illustrate complex ideas in a meaningful way to the reader. The metaphor of "nurse as guest" provides a unique way of describing nurse in relation to community (Milton, 2012) and, by extension, nurse in relation to global health partnership. Milton (2012) explicates the meaning of nurse as guest through expressing common characteristics of a guest within the community:

- The guest should be invited into and not force his or her way into the community.
- No demand should be made to the community to adhere to predefined biomedical standards.
- Self-serving attitudes should be replaced with an attitude of other-serving when participating in projects.
- Coparticipation of nurse and community members is required when identifying changing patterns of health.

Nurse as guest may not always understand the choices community members make, and there may be only transitory moments of understanding, but nurse as guest signifies movement away from the nurse as expert model of care. Nurse as guest appreciates the opportunity to be invited into the community and is honored to coparticipate in community decisions regardless of the consequences of community decision making.

MOVING TOWARD CRITICAL CONSCIOUSNESS IN GLOBAL PARTNERSHIPS

Power and nursing's demonstration of power in relation to partners often remain unrecognized but can covertly influence the partnership. Nursing's modern-day story has been characterized as one of powerlessness, and yet examples of professional imposition and imperialism are noted by Racine and Perron (2011) in their discussion of cultural voyeurism embedded in the global health experiences of student nurses. Cultural voyeurism creates distance in partnerships where partners are seen as exotic "others." While this view was promulgated by early anthropologists in their quest for recognition as a science, it can also be seen in the attitudes and stories of nurses participating in global health experiences. These stories usually begin with the words "Those people . . .".

The "us versus them" attitude is mitigated when global health programs are structured from a postcolonial feminist framework. This approach mirrors the metaphor of nurse as guest as the subjective experience of the partner is valued. Faculty operating within a postcolonial feminist framework discuss issues of inequality, race, gender, and class with students, and they examine power structures within global relationships.

Cultural safety extends the discussion of the postcolonial feminist framework to health. Developed in the 1980s by the Maori people of New Zealand, cultural safety focuses on engaging with people from a genuine desire to respond to health needs without being condescending or patronizing (Mkandawire-Valhmu & Doering, 2012).

Promoting cultural safety and dialogue from a postcolonial feminist perspective facilitates development of critical consciousness. Kumagai and Lypson (2009) trace the historical roots of critical consciousness to the Frankfurt School and Friere (1993). Critical consciousness is the beginning of the call to social action as we view the self in relation to the world. It requires reflective awareness and exploration of power and privilege, the foundation of social justice.

The standards of practice for culturally competent nursing care (Douglas et al., 2011) relevant to global health partnerships include:

- Standard 1: Social justice
- Standard 2: Critical reflection
- Standard 3: Knowledge of cultures
- Standard 9: Cross-cultural communication

This chapter has addressed these standards within the context of the nurse in relation to global health partners. The nurse who has a clear understanding of underlying motivational factors for entering into partnership and operationalizes the philosophy and mission of the sponsoring organization has greater potential for developing and sustaining long-term partnerships in global health.

The following case study provides the perspective of the individual nurse consultant entering into a partnership. However, nurses may also be part of a team providing direct health care services or bringing students into a partnership through educational exchange programs or service-learning initiatives.

SUGGESTED WEBSITES

http://nccc.georgetown.edu/foundations/assessment.html provides assessment tools for individuals and organizations and publications related to cultural competence

http://sis.nlm.nih.gov/outreach/multicultural.html#a0 contains multiple sources for developing cultural competency skills

https://www.aacn.nche.edu/diversity-in-nursing makes available cultural competencies and toolkits for BSN and MSN programs

https://www.thinkculturalhealth.hhs.gov provides free continuing education opportunities for nurses

www.cahealthadvocates.org/news/disparities/2007/are-you.html provides an explanation of cultural humility within the context of cultural competence as well as exercises in self-reflection and additional resources

www.edchange.org/multicultural/activityarch.html is a practical resource for teaching cultural awareness and promoting dialogue between cultural groups

www.hret.org/quality/projects/cultural-competency.shtml works in partnership with the American Hospital Association to help health care organizations become culturally competent

www.hrsa.gov/culturalcompetence/index.html contains literacy and cross-cultural communication resources

www.icn.ch/publications/free-publications/ offers free publications from the International Council of Nurses

www.intercultural.org/about.php offers resources for teaching and measuring culture and diversity

www.uniteforsight.org offers volunteer opportunities as well as free online courses to develop cultural competencies and low-cost certificates from its Global Health University

REFERENCES

Baumann, S. L. (2012). Dilemmas of international collaborative nursing partnerships. *Nursing Science Quarterly, 25*(2), 182–183. doi: 10.1177/0894318412437954

Bednarz, H., Schim, S., & Doorenbos, A. (2010). Cultural diversity in nursing education: Perils, pitfalls, and pearls. *Journal of Nursing Education, 49*(5), 253–260.

Boyle, J., & Andrews, M. (2011). *Transcultural concepts in nursing* (5th ed.). Philadelphia, PA: Lippincott.

Callister, L. C., & Cox, A. H. (2006). Opening our hearts and minds: The meaning of international clinical nursing electives in the personal and professional lives of nurses. *Nursing and Health Sciences, 8*, 95–102.

Cash, K. (2007). Compassionate strangers. *Nursing Philosophy, 8*, 71–72.

Clark, L., Calvillo, E., Dela Cruz, F., Fongwa, M., Kools, S., Lowe, J., & Mastel-Smith, B. (2011). Cultural competencies for graduate nursing education. *Journal of Professional Nursing, 27*(3), 133–139.

Crigger, N., & Godfrey, N. (2010). The importance of being humble. *Advances in nursing Science, 33*(4), 310–319.

Crump, J., & Sugarman, J. (2010). Ethics and best practice guidelines for training experiences in global health. *American Journal of Tropical Medicine and Hygiene, 83*, 1178–1182.

Dass, R., & Gorman, P. (1985). *How can I help?* New York, NY: Alfred A. Knopf, Inc.

Dayer-Berenson, L. (2011). *Cultural competencies for nurses: Impact on health and illness.* Sudbury, MA: Jones & Bartlett Publishers.

Douglas, M., Pierce, J. U., Rosenkoetter, M., Pacquiao, D., Callister, L. C., Hattar-Pollara, M., . . . Purnell, L. (2011). Standards of practice for culturally competent nursing care: 2011 update. *Journal of Transcultural Nursing, 22*, 317–333. doi: 10.1177/1043659611412965

Florczak, K. L. (2013). Culture: Fluid and complex. *Nursing Science Quarterly, 26*(1), 12–13. doi: 10.1177/089412466741

Friere, P. (1993). *Pedagogy of the oppressed* (20th anniversary ed.). New York, NY: Continuum.

Giger, J. N. (2013). *Transcultural nursing: Assessment and intervention* (6th ed.). St. Louis, MO: Elsevier.

Jeffreys, M. R. (2010). *Teaching cultural competence in nursing and health care* (2nd ed.). New York, NY: Springer Publishing Company.

Health Resources and Services Administration. (2002). *Indicators of cultural competence in health care delivery organizations: An organizational cultural competence assessment profile.* www.hrsa.gov/culturalcompetence/healthdlvr.pdf

Hodgkinson, M., & Holland, J. (2002). Collaborating on the development of technology enabled distance learning: A case study. *Innovations in Education and Teaching International, 39*(2), 89–94. www.gooverseas.com/6-companies-will-pay-volunteer-abroad

Ketefian, S., & Redman, R. W. (2013). Nursing science in the global community. In W. K. Cody (Ed.), *Philosophical and theoretical perspective for advanced nursing practice* (5th ed.) (pp. 279–289). Burlington, MA: Jones & Bartlett Learning.

Kulbok, P. A., Mitchell, E. M., Glick, D. F., & Greiner, D. (2012). International experiences in nursing education: A review of the literature. *International Journal of Nursing Education Scholarship, 9*(1), 1–21. doi: 10.1515/1548-923X.2365

Kumagai, A. K., & Lypson, M. L. (2009). Beyond cultural competence: Critical consciousness, social justice, and multicultural education. *Academic Medicine, 84*(6), 782–787.

Lapierre, D., & Collins, L. (1997). *Freedom at midnight.* New Delhi, India: Vikas Publishing.

Leffers, J., & Mitchell, E. (2011). Conceptual model for partnership and sustainability in global health. *Public Health Nursing, 28*(1), 91–102. doi: 10.1111/j.1525-1446.2010.00892.x

Leffers, J., & Plotnick, J. (2011). *Volunteering at home and abroad: The essential guide for nurses.* Indianapolis, IN: Sigma Theta Tau International.

Leininger, M. (1991). *Culture care diversity and universality: A theory of nursing.* New York, NY: National League for Nursing Press.

Manahan, C. M., Hardy, C. L., & MacLeod, M. L. P. (2009). Personal characteristics and experiences of long-term allied health professionals in rural and northern British Columbia. *Rural and Remote Health, 9,* 1238 (online). www.rrh.org.au

Marrone, S. R. (2013). Organizational cultural competence. In L. D. Purnell (Ed.), *Transcultural health care: A culturally competent approach* (4th ed.) (pp. 60–73). Philadelphia, PA: F.A. Davis Company.

McCaffrey, G., Raffin-Bouchal, S., & Moules, N. J. (2012). Buddhist thought and nursing: A hermeneutic exploration. *Nursing Philosophy, 13,* 87–97.

McKinnon, T. H., & Fealy, G. M. (2011). Core principles for developing global service-learning programs in nursing. *Nursing Education Perspectives, 32,* 95–100. doi: 10.5480/1536-5026-32.2.95

Milton, C. L. (2012). Teaching-learning in community: The metaphor of nurse as guest. *Nursing Science Quarterly, 25*(2), 137–139. doi: 10.1177/0894318412437959

Mkandawire-Valhmu, L., & Doering, J. (2012). Study abroad as a tool for promoting cultural safety in nursing education. *Journal of Transcultural Nursing, 23,* 82–89. doi: 10.1177/1043659611423831

Murry, J. (2010). *Expanding your cultural vision on the organizational level.* Presented January 27, 2010, at the National Care Grantee Conference, Norfolk, VA. www.hhs.gov/opa/familylife/annualconfabstracts/cultural_competency_murray.pdf

National Institute of Environmental Health Sciences, U.S. Department of Health and Human Services. (2012). *Partnerships for environmental public health evaluation metrics manual.* NIH Publication No. 12-7825. www.niehs.nih.gov/pephmetrics

Powell, D. L., Gilliss, C. L., Hewitt, H. H., & Flint, E. P. (2010). Application of a partnership model for transformative and sustainable international development. *Public Health Nursing, 27,* 54–70.

Purnell, L. (2013). *Transcultural health care: A culturally competent approach* (4th ed.). Philadelphia, PA: F.A. Davis Company.

Purnell, L. D., & Salmond, S. (2013). Individual cultural competence and evidence-based practice. In L. D. Purnell (Ed.), *Transcultural health care: A culturally competent approach* (4th ed.) (pp. 45–59). Philadelphia, PA: F.A. Davis Company.

Racine, L., & Perron, A. (2011). Unmasking the predicament of cultural voyeurism: A postcolonial analysis of international nursing placements. *Nursing Inquiry, 19*(3), 190–201. doi: 10.1.111/j.1440-1800.2011.00555x

Riner, M. E. (2011). Globally engaged nursing education: An academic program framework. *Nursing Outlook, 59,* 308–317. doi: 10.1016/j.outlook.2011.04.005

Sochan, A. (2008). Relationship building through the development of international nursing curricula: A literature review. *International Nursing Review, 55,* 192–204.

Tervalon, M., & Murray-Garcia, J. (1998). Cultural humility versus cultural competence: A critical distinction in defining physician training outcomes in multicultural education. *Journal of Health Care for the Poor and Underserved, 9*(2), 117–125.

Truglio-Londrigan, M., & Lewenson, S. B. (2011). *Public health nursing: Practicing population-based care.* Sudbury, MA: Jones & Bartlett Publishers.

Nurse Educator as Guest in Bhutan

Michele J. Upvall

CONTEXT: BHUTAN

Bhutan, a country slightly larger than the U.S. state of West Virginia and a few square kilometers smaller than Switzerland, evokes a sense of mystery to outsiders with its nickname: Land of the Thunder Dragon.

Situated between Chinese Tibet and India, Bhutan appears as a fragile link between two powerful nations. However, Bhutan is a nation that has never been "conquered" or colonialized. Its cultural heritage, rooted in the practice of Mahayana Buddhism, provides strength and resilience and permeates all aspects of daily life.

Like the rest of the world, Bhutan is undergoing rapid change. Television and the Internet were introduced to the country in 1999 and there has been a significant population shift (estimated at from 700,000 to slightly over 1 million) from rural and remote farming areas to urban centers (Nestroy, 2004). The movement in population has increased the demand for cars, and there are now over 50,000 cars in the country—but no traffic lights.

Bhutan is unique in its approach to managing change. The government philosophy of Gross National Happiness (GNH) guides change with its principles, or four pillars:

- Sustainable and equitable economic development, including health, education, energy, and employment
- Conservation of the environment
- Preservation and promotion of culture
- Good governance

GNH is holistic in nature and concerned with the well-being of society, not the individual. It is not happiness as construed by Western standards. Rather, GNH supports nonmaterial wealth that is not at the mercy of any one individual or the "winner-take-all" concept. It is a framework for ensuring that resources are not depleted, health and education are prioritized, and the Bhutanese culture is not sacrificed to development (Centre for Bhutan Studies, 2007).

In ancient times, Bhutan was known as the "Land of Medicinal Herbs" and today, traditional medicine is still highly valued. The Institute of Traditional Medicine Services, located in the capital city of Thimphu, trains both traditional doctors and traditional compounders (Tobgay, Dorji, Pelzom, & Gibbons, 2011).

Western-style health care in Bhutan has experienced significant growth and change with the development of more primary care centers, regional hospitals, and referral hospitals. The Ministry of Health (2012) also reports progress (see Box 2.1) in achieving the Millennium Development Goals (MDGs).

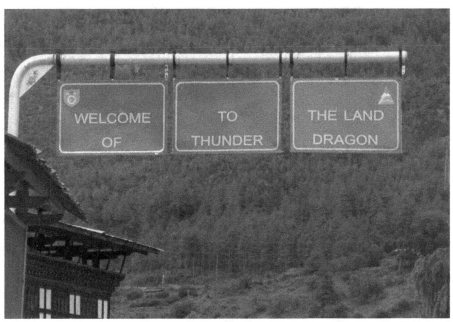

Road sign welcoming visitors to Bhutan as they leave the airport.   *Credit*: M. Upvall

---

BOX 2.1 Progress In Meeting Millennium Development Goals

- Eradicate extreme hunger and poverty

  Underweight children younger than age 5 decreased to 9%

- Reduce child mortality

  Younger than age 5 mortality decreased to 69 in 1,000 live births

  Infant mortality decreased to 47/1,000 live births

  Over 95% of children were immunized against measles at age 1

- Improve maternal health

  Mortality decreased to 146/100,000 live births

  Increase of births by skilled attendant by 69%

- Combat HIV/AIDS, malaria, and other diseases

  Increased incidence of HIV from 38 in 2000 to 176 in 2011

  Relatively low number of cases of TB at 176 in 100,000

  Malaria decreased to 5 in 10,000

- Ensure environmental sustainability

  96% of population has access to safe drinking water

  95% of population has access to sanitation

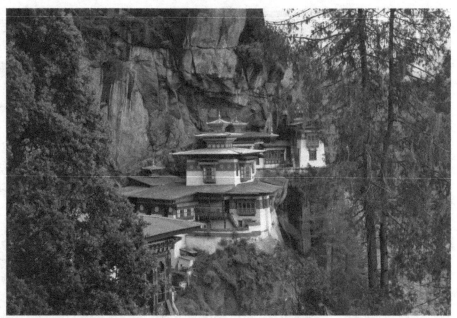

Taktsang Monastery (Tiger's Nest), Paro, Bhutan. *Credit*: M. Upvall

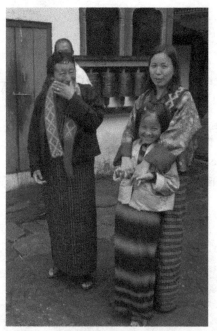

Three generations of Bhutanese women.
Credit: fritz16/Shutterstock.com

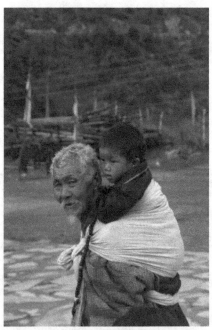

Bhutanese man carrying a young boy.
Credit: fritz16/Shutterstock.com

Nursing in Bhutan has not remained static in its development since its conception in 1961. During the 1960s and 1970s young girls were trained on the job at hospitals or sent to India, the UK, and New Zealand for diploma nursing courses (Wangmo, 2005). Significant events in nursing development include:

- Establishment of the Royal Institute of Health Sciences (RIHS) in 1974; www.rihs.edu.bt
- Introduction of the diploma program for the general nurse midwife (GNM) in 1982
- Diploma to bachelor of science in nursing and midwifery (BSNM) conversion program initiated in 2001 under the direction of LaTrobe University, Australia
- BSNM conversion formally under the direction of the RIHS in February 2012.
- Preservice (generic) BSNM program established July 2012 with diploma program maintained concurrently

Graduate education is also in nursing education's future (personal conversation, Wangmo). However, the preservice BSNM remains a top priority, and no program planning for the MSN is expected until the first class of the BSNM program completes its study.

PERSONAL ATTRIBUTES AND EXPECTATIONS

My assignment in Bhutan was to assess the RIHS as a site for nurse educators from Health Volunteers Overseas (HVO). I attempted to complete this assignment twice: for 2 weeks in June 2011 and for 5 weeks in April 2012. My association with HVO began like so many pivotal moments in my life, serendipitously. I was attending nursing meeting where HVO sponsored a table and, with my previous background in global health, decided to speak with them. After the first meeting, I found myself in Cambodia on a HVO assignment but also discovered that a nurse from a neighboring university was working with HVO. If I categorized my social interactions, I would consider myself an introvert, unlike the list of volunteer characteristics previously discussed. However, my commitment to social justice and ongoing learning as well as my love of adventure and all things spiritual provided a foundation for the experience. In addition, I consider myself to be flexible and enjoy changing circumstances. Challenges intrigue me, and given enough time to reflect and process the circumstances, I can usually adapt to dynamic situations.

My neighboring colleague provided copious amounts of information about Bhutan and nursing at the major referral hospital in Thimphu. Specific information, from names of people to contact at the hospital to names of cafés providing the best Internet service, was useful in helping to adjust my expectations once in country. My expectations were also shaped by previous HVO volunteers and their reports. E-mailing and speaking (via Skype) with nurses and physicians recently in Bhutan or still on site generated further intrinsic motivation—there were specific medical supplies needed; could I please bring them with me? Life experience from other global health assignments also influenced my expectations. I relied on the resilience I learned having spent 5 years in Pakistan and program planning skills acquired after having spent 4 years among the Navajo implementing an on-site bachelor of science in nursing (BSN) program.

VOLUNTEER ORGANIZATION AND EXPECTATIONS

HVO is a nonprofit organization based in the United States for the past 25 years. The mission of HVO is to improve availability and quality of health care through educating, training, and providing professional support to health care providers in low-resource countries. HVO has developed partnerships in 25 countries all over the world, as well as more than 80 programs. Over 4,000 individuals have served with HVO, among them physicians (50%), physical therapists (15%), nurses, including nurse anesthetists (12%), and dentists/oral surgeons (11%). HVO has had a presence in Bhutan since 1990 and currently offers volunteer assignments of varying lengths in internal medicine, emergency medicine, pediatrics, mental health, orthopedics, and nurse anesthesia. HVO's website (www.hvousa.org/index.shtml) provides rich detail for the aspiring volunteer. Specific country program information, including details of obtaining visas, previous volunteer reports, and a volunteer toolkit, support the work of the volunteer before leaving and while in country. HVO staff members remain a valuable resource, willing to e-mail or telephone whenever needed.

My assignment derived from the work of my nurse anesthesia colleague was also supported by the HVO Nursing Education Steering Committee. No nursing educators were present in Bhutan, and committee members felt that this assignment would be timely and at least serve to explore the possibility of supporting nursing education in Bhutan.

KNOWLEDGE OF HOST COUNTRY

As soon as I realized that I would be going to a place where few volunteers or even tourists (tourism is highly controlled and expensive) had gone, I quickly started my quest for information. Aside from the Lonely Planet guide for practical information, I discovered introspective literary works from others who had spent more than a few months volunteering and living with the people. Carpenter and Carpenter (2002) describe Bhutan as "improbable . . . the place will seem exotic, and a long way from home. Later, your sense of place will change. Bhutan will emerge as an extraordinary laboratory in which to examine questions of culture and values" (p. 1). In their book of essays, *The Blessings of Bhutan*, historical and contemporary Bhutan is portrayed through important symbols and deities, offering a glimpse into the heart of the nation.

Jamie Zeppa (1999) is a familiar name to many Bhutanese and opens the door to conversation. Her experience as a novice teacher in remote eastern Bhutan in 1989 provides clues to understanding teaching and learning in present-day Bhutan. Why is memorization and rote learning so important in the learning styles of students? Why is having only one answer so important? Zeppa offers her experience with her junior high school students and helps inform the nurse educator working with young nursing students.

Buttertea at Sunrise (Das, 2007) documents the story of a physiotherapy volunteer, again in eastern Bhutan. Das's story of learning, improvising, teaching, making friends, and falling in love begins with the overwhelming sense of being a guest and ends with change as a

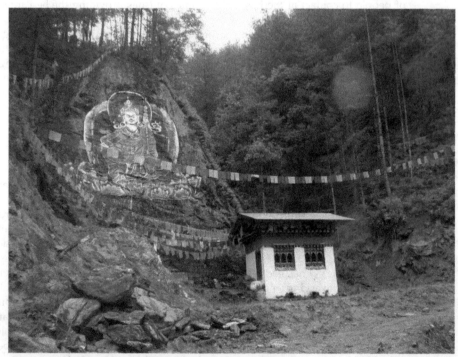

Rock painting of Guru Rimpoche on the trail to Tango Monastery, Bhutan.　　　*Credit*: M. Upvall

new beginning. Das described her first encounter meeting a young girl who spoke English and invited her to dinner "there"—where the mountain meets the clouds. Das accepted the invitation, thinking she would learn more of the local language, but there were some surprises waiting. She wondered about the proper role of a guest when she was left alone for an extended period of time while her host made buttertea. More tea and rice appeared as Das finished each portion. Her host continued to come and go from the room and Das remained alone. Finally, Das was requested to sing. Her thoughts of learning the local language diminished further when her host sang a song in Hindi. Her host requested another song before leaving the room again. Das wrote, "What can I do but agree to her wish? I am the guest after all, and this seems to be the expected behavior. . . . Unwilling to leave before I have at least thanked my young host, I set out to search for her. I find her beside the barn . . . apparently, she is not interested in my gratitude speech. 'I am so sorry. We have nothing to offer,' she says instead, and then slips two clean brown eggs into my hands. 'Please come back next week, okay?'" (p. 43). Rules of etiquette differ, but expressions of giving are humbling for both host and guest.

LIVING THE NURSE EDUCATOR-AS-GUEST EXPERIENCE

Bhutan emerged as a place like none I had ever been to before; far different from my years in southern Africa, among the Navajo, or in Pakistan. Colorful, wind-torn prayer flags decorate the mountainsides while the golden Buddha sits peacefully on a high peak overlooking the city of Thimphu, a constant reminder that I can never reach complete understanding of Bhutan and its people, a symbol of failure and peace.

For my first stay in Bhutan, I was armed with all the questions I needed to ask in assessing the potential for future nurse educator volunteer opportunities. On the surface, my assignment appeared straightforward. However, having the opportunity to ask the questions of individuals who had the answers was problematic. Unknown to me before arriving, faculty and administration were away at a conference and planning the new BSNM program. I was able to manage only one brief meeting before returning to the United States. However, I shared an apartment with a NICU physician experienced in global health. She introduced me to the health care system and I found myself observing in the operating room on the second day of my arrival, a place unknown to me since my days as a diploma student nearly 30 years before. I was just as uncomfortable in the operating room in Bhutan as I was as a student. However, it was an opportunity to see the operating room team in action and observe patient and family behaviors.

I left Bhutan the first time, making new friends with HVO volunteers and knowing that I would need to return to finish the assessment, at my own expense. My second stay was longer and I was able to be immersed in the everyday life of the RIHS. This was the direct outcome of a previous visit by the HVO director and chair of the HVO board. They provided me with names and e-mail addresses, so I felt more prepared than on my first visit. When I arrived, I immediately noted changes in the area—new buildings, new cafés, even a second airport in the center of the country.

On my first day, I was able to meet with the director only to discover that he was leaving for an extended stay in the United States to explore academic partnerships. I then worked with the interim nursing administration and discovered the "conference culture." Educated nursing faculty are in demand by nongovernmental organizations who require their skills in developing educational materials for the country. I was able to fill the void when faculty were called away, teaching a week-long course in administration and management and proctoring for exams. I was also invited to speak with the BSNM conversion students (diploma- to bachelor-level students) and evaluate their presentations in another class. On my last day at the RIHS I was able to meet once again with the director, who had recently returned from the United States and another conference in eastern Bhutan. We shared observations and I began to appreciate the challenge he faces in meeting multiple responsibilities.

As a guest nurse educator, I saw the need to set aside my own agenda much like Das before me. It was not possible to complete a formal assessment, but when asked how I could be of help, I found multiple opportunities. I was unprepared for the "conference culture" and how disruptive it can be for faculty trying to teach and plan future programs. Flexibility was required of all of us within RIHS. Journaling was an important tool to track daily events and for me to reflect on these events. Staying in the country for a more extended period of time than my first visit was also helpful.

REFLECTIVE QUESTIONS

1. How would you react to meetings that are canceled? How would you handle future interactions?
2. Think about your spiritual/religious beliefs. How would they impact the development of a global health partnership in a country that may have very different beliefs than your own?
3. How would personal and professional factors affect your ability to volunteer? How would the factors impact your length of stay?
4. What is your comfort level in returning home without accomplishing all the stated objectives for the visit? What factors would influence your return?

REFERENCES

Carpenter, R., & Carpenter, B. (2002). *The blessings of Bhutan.* Honolulu, HI: University of Hawaii Press.

Centre for Bhutan Studies. (2007). *Rethinking development: Proceedings of the second international conference on gross national happiness.* Thimphu, Bhutan: Author.

Das, B. (2007). *Buttertea at sunrise.* Toronto, ON: The Dundurn Group.

Ministry of Health. (2012). *Annual report 2012.* Thimphu, Bhutan: Royal Government of Bhutan.

Nestroy, H. (2004). Bhutan: The Himalayan Buddhist kingdom. *Asian Affairs, 35*(3), 338–352.

Tobgay, T., Dorji, T., Pelzom, D., & Gibbons, R. V. (2011). Progress and delivery of health care in Bhutan, the land of the thunder dragon and gross national happiness. *Tropical Medicine and International Health, 16*(6), 731–736.

Wangmo, N. (2005). *An analysis of public policy on the development of nursing profession in Bhutan.* Master of Public Health thesis, La Trobe University, Australia, March 2005.

Zeppa, J. (1999). *Beyond the earth and the sky: A journey into Bhutan.* New York, NY: Riverhead Books.

Building and Sustaining an Academic Partnership in Haiti

Jeanne M. Leffers
Gale Hull

The service learning partnership between the University of Massachusetts–Dartmouth (UMD) College of Nursing in Massachusetts and Partners in Development, Inc. (PID), in Haiti offers an example of why a particular program and country are selected, how collaboration begins, and what elements of partnership are essential to building relationships. The collaboration grew from host country factors as well as partner factors in the college of nursing and the university.

CONTEXT: HAITI

The Republic of Haiti shares the island of Hispaniola with the Dominican Republic and is located in the Greater Antillean Archipelago of the Caribbean. It is the third largest country in the Caribbean, totaling 11,000 square miles and a population of almost 10 million people. Locally called *Ayiti*, which means *land of high mountains*, it is mountainous land in a tropical climate. Once lush, the mountains have been deforested to supply fuel to the people, leaving the country vulnerable to erosion and landslides (Farmer, 2011). In the most economically disadvantaged country in the Western Hemisphere, more than 80% of Haiti's population live in poverty (on less than US$2 per day) and more than 50% live in extreme poverty (less than US$1.25 per day) (World Bank, 2013).

Hispaniola was originally inhabited by Taíno/Arawak Indians prior to the arrival of Christopher Columbus in 1492 (Poole, 2011). Once the Spanish invaded the island, most of the native Indians died from diseases brought by the Spanish. The eastern two-thirds of the island came under Spanish colonization and is the current Dominican Republic. In 1697 Spain ceded the western third of the island to France and the French colony became Saint-Domingue, now known as Haiti. The French landowners brought thousands of slaves from Africa to work in the sugar and coffee plantations that produced much of the world's supply during the early colonial period. Today relations between the two countries continue to be both cooperative and strained. Differences in language and culture have divided the nations since colonial days. At the governmental level, there is cooperation in terms of health and travel, but the startling differences in infrastructure, economy, and environment sharply divide the experiences of the people living on each side of the border (Farmer, 2011). In response to the earthquake, the government and the people of the Dominican Republic offered help to Haiti. However, the divergence in economic prosperity has led many Dominicans to claim superiority over the Haitians, who often come to the Dominican Republic to find work in sugar plantations, called *bateys* (Dubois, 2012).

As the first country to free itself from slavery with the slave-led rebellion against French colonization in 1804, Haiti's history has been fraught with political violence that has led to political instability. Payment of reparations to France, occupation by British, German, and U.S. forces, and the almost 30-year dictatorship by the Duvaliers left Haiti economically and politically unstable. The years following the overthrow of the Duvaliers in 1986 have been filled with efforts to democratically elect government leaders, often accompanied by rebellion and violence (DuBois, 2012). Fortunately, since the election of Michel Martelly in March 2011, the country has not experienced the turmoil of years past.

Adding to the political upheavals of the recent decades, Haiti suffered destruction and devastation from hurricanes Jeanne, Gustav, Hanna, and Ike from 2004 to 2008 as well as from an earthquake that affected Port au Prince and surrounding regions in January 2010. The loss of lives, property, and infrastructure continues to affect Haitians today. Furthermore, when humanitarian forces from around the world and from the UN arrived in Haiti in the months following the 2010 earthquake, thousands of Haitians were exposed to cholera that arrived with the international military personnel (Farmer, 2011).

The cholera epidemic has claimed almost 8,000 lives since the outbreak began in 2010 owing to rapid spread caused by water contamination. Less than 25% of Haitians have access to clean water. Lack of clean water and waste disposal facilities, inadequate housing, and crowded and unsanitary living conditions contribute to the high risk for infectious disease in Haiti. The burden of cholera added to the already serious effects of other waterborne diseases, malaria, tuberculosis, and HIV/AIDs (Farmer, 2011).

Haiti's high rate of infectious disease contributes to the high maternal death rate (35 maternal deaths per 1,000 births) and infant mortality rate (70 infant deaths per 1,000 live births), but the lack of access to health services also contributes to Haitians' morbidity and mortality (UNICEF, 2013; see www.unicef.org/infobycountry/haiti_statistics.html). It is estimated that less than half of Haitians have access to health care (WHO, 2013; see www.who.int/countries/hti/en).

HOST PARTNER: PARTNERS IN DEVELOPMENT, INC.

Gale Hull's Perspective

PID, with offices in Ipswich, Massachusetts, was founded by my husband, James, and me in 1990. PID's mission is to serve those living in extreme poverty in Haiti and Guatemala, and PID provides educational, financial, and material resources that "enable the poor to construct and implement their own programs for development" (PID, 2013). Using a broad empowerment approach, the organization offers a child sponsorship program to advance education; a housing program to enable Haitians to move from inadequate housing in Cite Soleil or post-earthquake tent housing into their own homes with access to clean water and sanitation; a small business program to help families develop their own economies, establishing good credit through payback to be eligible for mortgages; and the health program to provide preventive care, health education, and basic medical treatment. Each of these programs is led by a Haitian coordinator and supported by visiting volunteers in a direct partnership model.

Health Care Services at PID in Haiti

The health program of PID in Haiti, for example, includes Haitian medical staff (one physician, two nurses, two medical assistants who are enrolled in nursing programs in Haiti, laboratory staff, pharmacy staff, and interpreters), a clinic licensed by the Haitian Ministry of Public Health and Population that operates 5 full days each week to provide basic health care services, support social services provided by a full-time social service staff, and health educational services conducted in a newly completed education building.

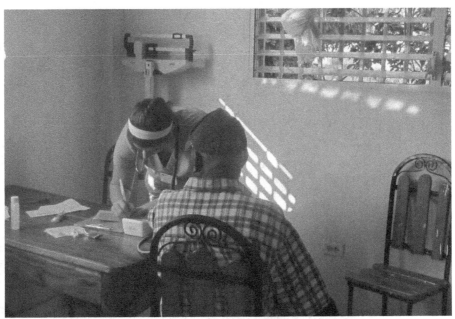

UMD College of Nursing student assisting with health assessment at the PID clinic.   *Credit*: J. Leffers

In collaboration with the Haitian staff and an advisory board of health professionals in the United States, PID has developed a medical formulary that is sustainable, appropriate to the needs in Haiti, and manageable to maintain and administer, as well as a health care protocol that emphasizes prevention and nonpharmaceutical therapies when appropriate. PID coordinates any donations of medications and medical supplies to fit the needs for clinic operation, ensuring the most cost-effective, appropriate, and manageable use of resources. When visiting volunteer service teams arrive to assist PID in accomplishing our mission, the full-time on-site field director as well as the nurse clinic coordinator on rotation for that time frame orient the visitors to their role in supporting the Haitian staff and clinic operation. These practices ensure continuity of care, collaboration with the Haitian staff, and the appropriate use of short-term volunteers to support a sustainable model of care. As our name indicates, the philosophy of PID is to empower the Haitian people to build and sustain their own programs using supportive human, material, and financial resources from PID volunteers, donors, sponsors of children, and U.S. staff.

Through connections between local Massachusetts volunteers, UMD students have participated in service experiences with PID over the past 6 years. Since Massachusetts is the third most popular U.S. residence for Haitian immigrants, with a population exceeding 40,000 (Menino, 2007), the UMD has a sizable student population of Haitian American students in the undergraduate and graduate programs, making Haiti a logical location for service learning programs.

NURSE FACTORS: EXPECTATIONS, KNOWLEDGE, AND PREPARATION

Jeanne Leffers's Perspective: University of Massachusetts Nursing and PID Partnership

As a UMD College of Nursing faculty member who had been involved with nursing student international nursing experiential learning for more than a decade, I was familiar with the importance of partnership, service learning criteria, and global health concerns for any

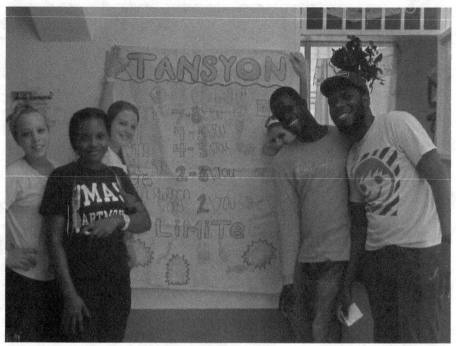

UMD College of Nursing students with PID staff members.   *Credit*: J. Leffers

academic programming. During those years I had taught more than 50 nursing students in global experiential learning. In addition, I had been to Hispaniola 10 times with an organization called Intercultural Nursing, Inc., and lived in Las Matas de Farfan, the Dominican Republic, a community located about 10 miles from the Haitian border. Because of the location where I worked and the number of Haitians living in the western region of the Dominican Republic, I learned about Haitian culture, history, and politics over the course of my visits to this region of the Dominican Republic. I was even there on January 12, 2010, to experience the earthquake's effects at our location, approximately 50 miles from the epicenter in Port au Prince, Haiti. Subsequent to the earthquake, many Haitians made it to our area for health care services. As a result, I learned more about Haiti's people and culture.

Additionally, as a nurse with many years of global health experience both with students and on my own in other countries such as Honduras, Guatemala, and Uganda, I have developed an approach whereby I study the country's history, politics, and culture but keep my expectations at a minimum. I have learned that approaching a new experience, whether at home in my public health work or in global settings, requires the ability to listen well and learn from others, as well as flexibility, cultural humility, and the commitment to build partnerships.

For a variety of reasons I was open to making a change for our college service learning opportunity to develop a stronger partnership with an organization doing collaborative, sustainable work. As a faculty member, it is imperative that I ensure that programs achieve a balance between the students' learning needs and our ability to provide needed services for our host partners. Often, it can be challenging to keep that balance while avoiding negative outcomes for both partners. My years of experience working in local communities allowed me to create a program that could meet divergent but essential needs for all parties. When approached by a Haitian American nursing student in our college who had worked with PID in creating a partnership with PID to assist with their post-earthquake long-term needs, I began the assessment process. PID's established clinic in the Blanchard neighborhood of Port au Prince was originally designed to provide approximately 6,000 visits per year for the Haitians they served in Blanchard and Cite Soliel. However, as one of the unharmed and functioning health facilities immediately after the earthquake, the clinic served more than 50,000 patient visits during the following year (PID, 2013). Although our Haitian American and other university students were eager to help in Haiti, I was aware that as visitors we must be of sufficient help and not detract from the needs of the Haitian population for acute post-trauma care, food, water, and adequate shelter. In conversation with Gale Hull, president of PID, we determined that a team from UMD comprised of nursing students, nurse and nurse practitioner mentors, and students from across campus sponsored by the Haitian American Student Association (HASA) would be helpful for construction, clinic assistance, and language interpretation needs. Indeed, we would advance the services to Haitians and not interfere with disaster response efforts. That first trip was made 5 months after the January 2010 earthquake.

Selecting a Team

Nurse partner factors were essential to building a partnership. To build the visiting team, I solicited four other nurses to assist in student mentorship and to serve in the clinic in Haiti to support the Haitian physician, two Haitian nurses, and the laboratory and pharmacy staff. This first team of five U.S. nurses included another full-time faculty member who is a nurse practitioner, has an MS in community health nursing who served with another organization in Haiti for many years, and two undergraduate alumnae, one of whom made her original service-learning trip to the Dominican Republic 5 years previously and who had continued her global service-making volunteer trips each year, and one of whom was a current MS student, and me. Careful selection of nurse team members was critical to the evolving partnership. The team of nurses were all known to our university as faculty or students, exhibited nonjudgmental attitudes, worked well with other people, demonstrated requisite flexibility, and were passionate about helping those most in need. Currently, each of the original team members has returned with the students at least three times, and two of the nurses have become part of PID's team of nurses rotating service to Haiti's clinic several times a year to provide continuity to new medical and nurse volunteers. This is evidence that this pilot team was ideal for the partnership.

In addition, nursing students made application to participate in a nonacademic service experience. The application included a letter of intent and faculty references that addressed their abilities to think critically, make sound clinical judgments, demonstrate flexibility, be self-directive, and communicate effectively and assessed their nonjudgmental attitudes. Seven rising senior students participated during the first summer trip. In addition, another seven students from the HASA on campus joined our group, totaling 19 volunteers from the university. Meetings were held for the two groups (although there was some overlap of the one nursing student who served as president of HASA) to learn about Haiti, the anticipated work, and how to best prepare for the experience. Each participant was required to read about Haiti's history and culture and to learn essential Kreyòl words. In addition, our meetings focused on the students' expectations, concerns, and fears. We prepared for the possibility of living in tents and learned how to best manage our own health and safety needs.

As leader of the UMD team, I ensured that all members had completed all health, university, and PID requirements as well as undergone careful preparation for their first immersion into a country in which the majority of people live in poverty. The use of personal reflective journals to process the experience was highly encouraged. In addition, since I had not made a preliminary trip to Haiti as I had done prior to leading student groups to the Dominican Republic, my first visit would also be one of assessment for future planning. Therefore, prior to the first trip, I talked to as many people as I could who worked with or had volunteered with PID. Assessment was a critical factor for planning the first service experience in Haiti.

BUILDING RELATIONSHIPS

Our first visit served as the first step in building a partnership. As nurses and nursing students from the College of Nursing (in addition to a diverse team of students from the Colleges of Arts and Sciences, Engineering, Business, and Visual and Performing Arts), we learned from Haitian partners, other PID staff and volunteers in Blanchard during our visit. Our team members worked in the construction program to build homes for Haitian families, many of whom had been living in substandard homes, even tent cities, following the earthquake. Our nursing team worked in the clinic and in mobile sites to do outreach work to those who could not travel to the clinic. As extra support to the Haitian staff we joined their team to serve more than 1,000 people in need who arrived at the clinic early each day, frequently from a great distance, to seek continuing care for earthquake trauma, for emergent conditions, and for common health problems that could not be handled elsewhere due to the destruction of the majority of health facilities in Port au Prince. We completed patient assessments with the help of the PID interpreters, consulted with the nurse practitioner or Haitian physician for therapeutic care, consulted with the PID social service team as needed, and ensured that patient teaching and follow-up were complete. Nursing students worked alongside licensed health personnel to ensure that each team member practiced within the boundaries of his or her license in the United States. After clinic hours we helped with supplies and pharmacy organization.

Each evening at our meeting we shared significant experiences of the day and met with local community members or PID staff members to learn about the community, Haitian history, Kreyól, and PID program services. These meetings were essential for the visiting team to process their experiences as well as to learn from our partners. For me, it was an opportunity to learn more about the region, the local population, their health care needs, and the PID staff and services. Although the continuing post-earthquake crisis changed PID's work from that of a community clinic, meeting the needs of the families in PID's child sponsorship, small business, and housing programs, to that of a busy urgent care clinic, I was able to observe how the organization advanced its mission of partnership and empowerment.

What We Do

Since that first trip in June 2010, UMD has strengthened our work with PID. The current field director in Haiti, Lizzy Barnes, is a 2009 graduate of the UMD College of Visual and Performing Arts. She participated in service learning trips in 2009 and 2010 as part of our team and returned several times before assuming her current role in 2011. In addition, we began to attract a larger number of nursing students and nurse mentors for the program. During the following years and changes in leadership of the HASA, the UMD program grew to include more nurses, nurse practitioners, and nursing students when the HASA students pursued other priorities for their work.

We were able to transition the experience into our undergraduate community health nursing practicum, NUR 331 Experiential Learning: Community Health Nursing, creating a special clinical option for a global experience. Using the course objectives, we developed activities for students prior to the experience in Haiti as well as after they returned to help them prepare for and disseminate their experience. Please see Table 2.1 for a description of the course and course objectives.

Embedding the experience into a required course in our curriculum strengthens the preparation phase of the experience, allowing 5 or 6 weeks for intensive preparation prior to the in-country experience and another 5 or 6 weeks post-experience for follow-up and dissemination. During the preparation students are required to complete a community assessment based on data collection available through the World Health Organization, UNICEF, and the World Bank, among other sources of international demographic and health data. Each student interviews a Haitian American key informant living in Massachusetts. In addition, they read two books about Haiti, usually *Mountains Beyond Mountains* (Kidder, 2003) and *Haiti After the Earthquake* (Farmer, 2011), and they complete the book *Volunteering*

TABLE 2.1 Nursing Course Description and Objectives for Haiti Clinical Option

University of Massachusetts–Dartmouth

College of Nursing

COURSE: NUR 331—Experiential Learning: Community Health Nursing

CREDITS: 3 credits clinical (9 hours per week)

This experiential learning course prepares nursing students to promote health and provide care for individuals, families, groups, and populations in the community, with a special emphasis on vulnerable populations. Principles of epidemiology, demography, environmental sciences, community organization, and health care and political, economic, and legal influences are integrated with nursing concepts and principles to provide the basis for community nursing practice. Community and aggregate strengths and risks are identified through community health nursing process. Students will implement strategies designed to promote the health of populations, guide populations to reduce identified health risks, and shape health policy consistent with ANA Scope and Standards of Public Health Nursing Practice (2007) and AACN (2008), *The Essentials of Baccalaureate Education for Professional Nursing Practice*.

COURSE OBJECTIVES:

1. Demonstrate integrity, honesty, accountability, and collegiality for professional nursing practice in the care of individuals, families, groups, and populations in the community.
2. Demonstrate understanding of the influences of culture, race, age, sexual orientation, and gender in planning nursing care for individuals, families, groups, and populations in the community.
3. Establish a caring partnership to promote health with persons, groups, and /or the community through respect for cultural diversity and patterns, spiritual needs, values, and health beliefs.
4. Implement health promotion and education strategies, including the use of information technology, when planning care for individuals, families, groups, and populations in the community.
5. Use evidence to plan, implement, and evaluate nursing interventions for individuals, families, groups, and populations in the community.
   - International student learning will be specific to the community in Haiti served by PID.
6. Apply sociopolitical, public health, and nursing science concepts to promote health and guide care for individuals, families, groups, and populations in the community.
7. Employ effective communication strategies with culturally diverse individuals, families, groups, and populations in the community to promote health.
8. Use epidemiological principles to assess, plan, implement, and evaluate nursing interventions in the community.
   - International student learning will include data from the PID database to identify priority health concerns in the population they serve.
9. Promote health policy development to shape an accessible and equitable health care system.
   - International student learning will identify health policy issues for global health.
10. Advocate for access and equity among vulnerable persons within the health care delivery system.
    - International student learning will compare issues of access and equity between the U.S. and Haitian health care systems.
11. Develop collaborative relationships with professionals, nonprofessionals, and groups in the community to promote the health of individuals, families, and groups in the community.
12. Evaluate the outcomes of nursing interventions in the community setting in relation to professional standards including the Healthy People 2020 objectives.
    - International student learning will include targets for Millennium Development Goals.

CLINICAL FACILITIES:

Communities and community health agencies in southeastern Massachusetts have been selected by faculty for clinical learning experiences. Communities most often used include but are not limited to Dartmouth, Fall River, New Bedford, and Taunton.

- International student learning will include clinical activities designed to prepare the learner for service in Haiti in collaboration with PID and community members in Port au Prince, Haiti. Preparation for experiential learning in Haiti, an 8-day clinical experience in Haiti, and follow-up activities on return serve as the clinical setting.

(continued)

TABLE 2.1 Nursing Course Description and Objectives for Haiti Clinical Option (*continued*)

CLINICAL ACTIVITIES:

- Compile an overview of a selected community through completion of community assessment.
- Collect and analyze data regarding a selected population group.
- Identify implications of specific demographic and bio-statistical data for the health of the selected population group.
- Formulate and prioritize nursing diagnosis for a selected population group.
- Collaborate with community representatives in planning an appropriate nursing intervention at the community level.
- Using principles of teaching/learning, screening, and community organization, carry out the selected nursing intervention(s).
- Evaluate the outcomes of the nursing intervention in the meeting the health needs of the population group.

Clinical activities for students in the international option for Haiti include:

1. Collaboration with Haitian Americans in the local community prior to trip.
2. Complete key informant interview.
3. Collaborative work with PID to determine health priorities using their clinic database.
4. Learn Haitian Creole words for basic communication.
5. Prepare educational materials to use for teaching in Haiti.
6. Read and learn about Haitian history, culture, and health issues.
7. While in Haiti, clinical experiences will include but are not limited to:
   - Complete a community assessment of the Blanchard neighborhood.
   - Complete second key informant interview.
   - Participate in various clinic activities.
   - Assist with well child assessments.
   - Participate in daily teaching activities.
   - Assist with construction program.
   - Make a home visit in local community (this may be to a tent city resident).
   - Plan a diet plan and price foods to meet the plan for individuals with diabetes.
   - On return follow-up activities will be completed.
   - Students will present to their classmates in the Global Health class.

University of Massachusetts–Dartmouth College of Nursing (2013), adapted for use.

at Home and Abroad: Essential Guide for Nurses (Leffers & Plotnick, 2011). This latter book contains general information helping nurses prepare for global health experiences, including broad topics such as cultural, ethical, and responsible practice and details about health, safety, packing, and travel.

During the preparation phase, students visit members of the Haitian American community in Brockton, Massachusetts, to learn more about Haiti and Haitian culture. During these visits, UMD students have met with women in a church group as well as teens in a youth group. During the meeting with the youth group members, the Haitian American students were able to interact with college students to learn about the college experience and also completed a community service activity by helping the nursing students complete their health education posters.

Service Learning Considerations

As we built our partnership, the importance of meeting goals of service learning for our students and defined needs for our PID partners took precedence. Revisiting the core principles of service learning, we worked to ensure that we indeed worked in partnership with the PID community in Haiti and that our service focused on the expressed needs of the partner (see Table 2.2).

Service learning as a pedagogy demands that learning experiences occur in partnership with community members, be embedded in an academic course in order to foster

TABLE 2.2 Service Learning Criteria

Service learning criteria	How UMD/PID partnership facilitates criteria	Measurement of criteria
Reciprocal relationship between academic institution and community partners	Partnership between faculty, nurse mentors, and nursing students at the UMD College of Nursing	Ongoing communication and assessment between PID and UMD partners
Clear connection to an academic course	Clinical experience is an option of Nursing 331: Experiential Learning in Community Health Nursing course at UMD	One section of NUR 331 is the clinical option in Haiti
Experiential learning		Students fully participate in clinic and construction activities, community assessment in neighborhood, short trips from Blanchard to areas of Port au Prince and coastal Haiti.
Learning activities to meet a community need	PID makes requests for educational materials and assistance with specific projects	Outcome evaluation of educational materials, teaching on site, and other deliverables
Community partner control of service provision	UMD partners participate in activities as required by PID needs at the time we visit	Verbal feedback from PID partners
Structured reflection to promote active learning and civic responsibility	Course requirement that students write a reflective journal	See reflective journal tool

Created by J. Leffers.

desired student outcomes, and provide opportunities for reflection enabling personal and professional insights. Bringle and Hatcher (2009) define service learning as:

> Course-based, credit bearing educational experience in which students (a) participate in an organized service activity that meets identified community needs and (b) reflect on the service activity in such a way as to gain further understanding of course content, a broader appreciation of the discipline, and an enhanced sense of personal values and civic responsibility. (p. 18)

During recent years, there has been increased attention to service learning in nursing in order to integrate social justice, cultural awareness, and critical thinking into the curriculum (Groh, Stallwood, & Daniels, 2011). The publication of *Global Service-Learning in Nursing* (McKinnon & Fitzpatrick, 2011) confirms that academic partnerships for service learning in global settings has increased and become an integral part of professional nursing (see Table 2.3).

In response to requests from our PID partners, over the following years our partnered projects have included assistance in the preliminary analysis of the patient visit database, development of health education materials, and assessment of locally available foods for nutrition planning. To ensure the sustainability of the posters we created, we purchased sturdy canvas material to create visual educational materials. Haitian American students helped us to address health literacy and cultural appropriateness. During the past 4 years we have developed educational materials on topics such as breastfeeding, basic hygiene

TABLE 2.3 Service Learning Reflective Journal Tool

Service Learning Reflective Journal for Haiti Clinical Experience

Suggestions for reflection

The format below is designed to help you *critically reflect on the experience, assisting you in incorporating what you have learned into your personal and professional life to provide information that you can return to at later points in your nursing career.*

You are free to record a narrative of the day's events if you choose, but we ask that *you select (at least) one significant event or observation from the day to report in your journal.*

Suggested format (not required if you prefer to incorporate these elements into a narrative reflection):

Observation	Service learning reflection	Application to personal life
WHAT	**SO WHAT**	**NOW WHAT**
What happened? Provide as much detail as possible in describing an observation (who, what, when, where, why, and how). This can be one event or a series of events during one day.	How did this incident/observation affect you? How is your experience different from what you expected? How does this apply to the course content? What social, cultural, political, and economic forces impacted the incident?	How does this affect you personally? Which of your values, beliefs, principles, and opinions were challenged or strengthened by the experience? How did this observation affect you professionally? How did these forces intersect with the provision of nursing care in the setting?

HERE ARE SOME QUESTIONS THAT MIGHT HELP YOU AS YOU WRITE YOUR REFLECTIONS

What are the most important social issues here? Discuss how you feel. Do these issues affect your thoughts about power, poverty, inequality, and privilege?

How has this experience affected your opinions about social, cultural, political, and economic issues?

What are your thoughts about PID as an organization? How did this change over the time you were working with them? What can you learn about partnership?

Give an example of a situation at the PID experience in which you felt you were in a reciprocal relationship. How does that help you understand partnership?

What is active citizenship?

What has this service learning experience taught you about citizenship, community engagement, and being a socially responsible citizen?

What was the most personally meaningful moment during this service learning activity?

How has this service learning activity affected your life?

Created by J. Leffers.

and sanitation, prevention of diarrheas, appropriate use of medications, filariasis, breast self-examination, feminine hygiene, hypertension, diabetes, gastrointestinal problems, and sexually transmitted diseases. When we return on subsequent trips, it is rewarding for new participants to see our teaching materials in use. In addition, small group or one-to-one teaching occurs between our team members and the Haitian nurses, assistants, and interpreters serving in supportive health roles such as referral liaison, nutrition program administrator, triage coordinator, and social service assistant.

During the most recent trip, the clinic was undergoing evaluation by the Ministry of Public Health and Populations for clinic licensure. The evaluators interviewed members of the team and made positive comments about the educational materials. In addition, the Haitian staff in Blanchard were thrilled to have posters created not only by the UMD nursing students but by Haitian American youth. Linking U.S. partners of Haitian and non-Haitian background with the Haitian staff in Haiti has strengthened our relationships over the past 4 years.

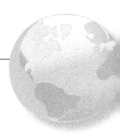

CHAPTER 3

Nursing Practice and Licensure Across Borders

Diane C. Martins
Alicia J. Curtin

The global movement of people, pathologies, technologies, economies, and knowledge is the basis of the international transfer of health risks and opportunities across national borders (Frenk et al., 2010). This globalization of health care gives urgency to addressing the need for nursing care practice and licensure across borders to ensure the safety of individual patients, communities, and at-risk populations. With the nursing shortages in the United States and subsequent recruitment of foreign-born and foreign-trained nurses to the United States, there has been a greater emphasis on the qualification, practice standards, and licensure of nurses recruited for work in developed countries than nurses working in low- and middle-income countries (LMICs) (Fernandez & Hebert, 2004; Rosenkoetter & Nardi, 2007). In addition, with advances in global technologies, economics, and financing have come increasing efforts in higher education to emphasize global citizenship and cultural competency through service learning and humanitarian efforts (Bringle & Hatcher, 1996; Dooley, 2011; Frenk et al., 2010). To meet this need in nursing, there has been a re-emergence of study-abroad programs, including international study tours, voluntary mission trips, and service learning experiences for nursing students in developing countries. Although in the nursing literature researchers have discussed the development, implementation, and impact of these programs, little attention has been paid to nursing practice and licensure of nursing faculty and students across borders (Leffers & Mitchell, 2010; Sloand, Bower, & Groves, 2008).

This chapter first discusses the need for universal standards for education and practice across countries for health professionals including nursing. Second, it presents the discussion on the practice and licensure of foreign-born nurses migrating to LMICs. Finally, it discusses the ethics of nursing practice with short-term international programs in LMICs including international study tours, clinical placements, voluntary missions, and service-learning programs.

GLOBALIZATION OF HEALTH CARE

The need to re-examine and redesign nursing curriculum for opportunities for mutual learning and joint solutions for global issues is very timely. In 2010, a global independent commission (Education of Health Professionals for the 21st Century: A Global Independent Commission) consisting of 20 professional and academic leaders from diverse countries came together to develop a "shared vision" for education in medicine, nursing, and public health reaching beyond national borders and the confines of any one discipline. The commission developed a comprehensive framework considering the connections among education, health systems, and practice. The commission's vision is that

> all health professionals in all countries should be educated to mobilize knowledge and to engage in critical reasoning and ethical conduct so that they are competent to participate in patient-centered and population-centered health systems as members of locally responsive and globally connected teams. (Frenk et al., 2010, p. 1951)

Interdependence in health is growing, and opportunities for mutual learning and shared progress have greatly expanded. This is most evident when examining the global perspective on a number of disease conditions such as HIV/AIDs, pneumonia, tuberculosis, diarrhea, and malaria (WHO, 1999). Nursing professionals are well suited to address these needs globally through collaboration in health prevention and promotion with individuals, communities, and populations. A global perspective improves understanding of the causes and solutions to local problems. In addition, an increasing number of students and graduates from developed and LMICs are moving in both directions creating new networks of knowledge and practice (Frenk et al., 2010).

Global principles of health care professional practice would bring consistency and uniformity across national boundaries. Many international organizations (e.g., World Health Organization, United Nations Education, World Trade Organization, International Council of Nursing, World Federation of Public Health Associations) are setting standards for professional education to deal with transnational threats such as pandemics. One major recommendation of the commission is that all countries should progressively move to align accreditation, licensing, and certification with health goals through the engagement of government, professional bodies, and the academic community. For example, national accreditation systems should develop criteria for assessment and shape the competencies of graduates to meet societal health needs. National standards in licensing and certification of nurses are necessary to protect patients and populations in the face of a globally mobile health workforce (Frenk et al., 2010).

The Institute of Medicine (IOM; 2011) and the World Health Organization (WHO) address international models for nursing. The WHO Task Force on Global Standards in Nursing and Midwifery Education created a report, *Human Resource for Health: Global Standards for the Initial Education of Professional Nurses and Midwives*, which developed global standards. These standards establish educational criteria that (1) are based on evidence and competency, (2) promote the progressive nature of education and lifelong learning, and (3) ensure the employment of practitioners who are competent by providing quality care, and promote positive health outcomes in the populations they serve (WHO, 2009). The IOM (2011) also recommends the creation of an international body to coordinate and recommend national and international nursing workforce policies. They strongly recommend that global health be integrated in the undergraduate and graduate nursing curricula of schools and colleges of nursing.

INTERNATIONAL NURSE MIGRATION

Although uniformity in accreditation, licensure, and certification is necessary globally, there may be unintended consequences, such as ease of professional migration across national boundaries. Migration can be also considered a freedom of choice and an expected result of globalization. Migration is the result of a number of factors, including the search for higher standards of living, personal safety, and improved professional opportunities. However, the migration of nurses from LMICs has resulted in a deepening health care crisis in countries that lack such resources to begin with and leads to further deterioration of inadequate health care systems (Aiken, Buchan, Sochalski, Nichols, & Powell, 2004; Kline, 2004).

Both the short-term and long-term effects of international recruitment require serious consideration (Rosenkoetter & Nardi, 2007). The International Council of Nurses (ICN) condemned the practice of recruiting nurses to countries where human resource planning and problems related to retention and recruitment of nurses have not been addressed. A 2003 study, International Nurse Mobility: Trends and Policy Implications, concluded that inadequate working conditions on one hand and aggressive recruiting efforts on the other contribute to push–pull forces that stimulate what may be unhealthy international nurse migration patterns (ICN, WHO, & Royal College of Nursing, 2003). The extent to which the recruitment of foreign nurses is used to solve the shortage problem raises many questions about nursing and health care globally (Kingma, 2001; Kline, 2004). The ICN recognizes this shortage globally as a critical workplace imbalance of supply and demand, particularly in LMICs (ICN, 2004).

The 2006 World Health Report (WHO, 2006) identified shortages of human resources as a critical obstacle to the achievement of the Millennium Development Goals (MDGs) for improving the health of global populations. It identifies the importance of nursing as an integral element of health systems' infrastructure. Studies have shown a link between nurse staffing levels, service delivery, and health outcomes. According to WHO, a factor that has received considerable attention is the mobility and migration of nurses and their impact on the global delivery of health services.

The legal and professional practice concerns of nurse migration continue to be an issue. The World Health Assembly recently approved a code of conduct for international migration of professions with the goal of establishing and promoting voluntary principles and practices for the ethical international recruitment of health personnel. In many wealthy countries, the import of foreign nurses to meet health care shortages is likely to persist and could even increase (WHO, 2010). International nurses practicing in the United States are held to the same standards of education, training, and testing as U.S. nurses to ensure safe patient care and to meet professional practice standards. International nurses need to successfully complete a screening program prior to receiving an occupational visa. This complex process requires verification of equivalency education; English-language proficiency, a valid nursing license; and successful completion of the National Council of State Boards of Nursing licensure examination or the Commission on Graduates of Foreign Nursing Schools qualifying examination, which predicts a candidate's success on the NCLEX-RN® (Rosenkoetter & Nardi, 2007). Regulation is important in the globalized workplace, but do these same standards and regulatory processes hold true for U.S. nurses practicing in LMICs?

One of the reasons ICN was founded in 1899 was to ensure high-level nursing education and practice worldwide. ICN has a Model Nursing Act Toolkit available to its member countries to aid the development of regulations for licensure and practice. Many countries are at different stages of developing regulations for nursing professionals. In many LMICs, the challenge is differentiating the nurse's scope of practice from that of other health care providers and community health workers (Barry, 2010). The profession of nursing needs to examine the obligations, roles, and responsibilities of nurses in all settings. Nurses also understand that by obtaining and maintaining a license to practice and using the title of nurse, they convey to the public that they are competent to provide care and accountable to uphold ethical codes and practice standards. Accountability is a concept aligned with public trust and confidence with health care professionals and is often described in the international and national professional codes of nursing and in standards of nursing practice (Milton, 2008).

This milieu challenges the nursing profession to carefully examine the emerging licensing and practice issues nationally. The profession's practices and licensing activities must be addressed nationally to assure public safety and increase public trust. Fernandez and Herbert (2004) recommend that there should be clearly stated expectations that professional regulatory agencies continue to contribute to the public policy debate on health promotion, treatment, and prevention, with specific emphasis on maintain competence, measurable outcomes, quality improvement to protect the public interest, and safety.

NURSING PRACTICE IN LOW- AND MIDDLE-INCOME COUNTRIES

In the past decade, interest in providing international education experiences for nursing students has re-emerged with a heightened sense of urgency (Edmonds, 2010; Kulbok, Glick, Mitchell, & Greiner, 2012). Traditional study abroad programs have been difficult for nursing students to access in light of the highly structured, time-consuming nature of nursing programs and the financial resources needed for a sustained period of time abroad (McKinnon & Fealy, 2011). Short-term service learning immersion experiences in another country are seen as one way of addressing this dilemma (Curtin, Martins, Schwartz-Barcott, DiMaria, & Soler-Ogando, 2013; Johansen, 2006; Larson, Ott, & Miles, 2010; Smith-Miller, Leak, Harlan, Dieckmann, & Sherwood, 2010). Identifying the potential impact of these programs is important, especially in light of the longstanding belief that one needs considerable time in another country in order to have any real meaningful, life-changing impact (Curtin, Martins, Schwartz-Barcott, DiMaria, & Soler-Ogando, 2013; Evanson & Zust, 2004; Zorn, 1996). One area that has not been addressed in the development and implementation of international programs is the regulation and licensure of nurses and nursing students practicing in another country and the potential for inadvertent exploitation of the patients. This has often been seen in research endeavors where vulnerable populations have been exploited at the hands of over-zealous researchers (Mkandawire-Valhmu & Doering, 2012).

Most often these ethical issues are raised when conducting research in LMICs. Powell et al. (2010) discuss research relationships that can drift toward a neocolonial model. Research efforts in LMICs should not be hidden in a nursing practice cloak. The host country partner may perceive the academic/nurse developed country partner as providing collaborative research, but in reality very little is gained by the host partners professionally. This was seen in a village in the Dominican Republic where a group of graduate nurse practitioner faculty and students were conducting nutrition studies on the children in a rural village who had been "invited to come to the center" for a free health exam. The nurse practitioner faculty described this as her nutrition research.

Crigger and Holcomb (2007) raise concerns regarding nurses working in another country, particularly LMICs. They raise specific concerns about how nurses interface with the established cultural norms and how nurses handle novel ethical dilemmas that arise from practicing in a different culture.

Milner (2003) also cautioned faculty in the development of experiences for students abroad. In many low-resource countries, students might be tempted to practice outside their scope of practice because the resources are so limited and the needs for health care so great. This may result in students causing unintended harm related to an inadequate understanding of the language or complex cultural issues. It is especially important to work closely with collaborators in the host country when the study abroad course involves clinical experiences. This is demonstrated so clearly in an example used by Foster (2009) in her collaborative nursing partnership in the Dominican Republic, "Stillbirth in the DR." It is clear from this story that professional ethical nursing practice is understood from different perspectives in the Dominican Republic than in the United States. Foster described nursing students working with Dominican nurses in the labor and delivery unit as an example of cultural humility in the Project ADAMES that links maternity nurses in the Dominican Republic with midwifery students from the United States. Through this partnership other students, including undergraduate nursing students, participate at the maternity hospital in the Dominican Republic. She describes a group of U.S. nursing students in the Dominican Republic working with a 19-year-old mother of three who delivered a stillborn girl. The students found the mother sobbing and asked their U.S. instructor whether they could do a psychosocial intervention so the mother could spend time with her deceased newborn (common practice in the United States). The mother agreed. The Dominican nursing staff agreed to let the students proceed. The mother held her baby and cried. The nurses were concerned that the U.S. students were making the mother unhappy. The mother wanted to know whether the baby could be buried in the blanket, but the Dominican nurses said no, "We put all the dead babies together naked in the incinerator." One student left, crying, and the Dominican nurse replied, "You have seen nothing." In the end, both the U.S. and Dominican nurses reflected on each other's practice. The Dominican nursing supervisor said, "You helped the mom psychosocially" (Foster, 2009, p. 102).

This experience shared by Foster demonstrates the sensitive issues culturally and psychologically of stillbirth in maternal and child health care globally. The reactions by the U.S. and Dominican nurses are quite different based on their cultural values and beliefs and nursing experience. It is an excellent example of the self-reflection process in cultural humility and an opportunity of how "cultural bridging" may occur to share perspectives and personal and professional values and be culturally safe in practice.

This scenario also highlights the need to explore the values that influence practice when health care practitioners are practicing cross-culturally. The failure to recognize and understand one's own values and the effect they have on practice can lead to negative outcomes or, as Parfitt notes, "disabling a community rather than enabling it" (1999). "Nurses who persist in practicing in an ethnocentric way with little self-reflection will only reinforce the systems which they believe they are trying to change" (p. 377).

Parfitt explored the influences that cultural values have on the practice of nurses working in LMICs in primary health care. She interviewed 12 nurses who worked for a minimum of 2 years overseas, using an ethnographic approach. The key factors that emerged from her study were related to gender, race, and knowledge. Western values and beliefs had a major influence on the nurses' practice overseas. Parfitt describes the effective expatriate nurse as having a wide range of skills with ability to reflect on practice, not bound by tradition but informed by experience, research, and innovation. Professional knowledge and local knowledge are both important for effective practice. Requirements for effective health care delivery abroad included learning the local language, understanding and appreciating local customs, and, where appropriate, working within the parameters of the host community. Without community involvement, a dependency relationship will occur at all levels. The nurses in this study valued community more than the concept of individuality and saw the community as the focal point for change and development.

Crigger and Holcomb (2007) provide guiding principles for nurses practicing in LMICs. These principles include (1) the common good, (2) beneficence and nonmalevolence, (3) respect for persons, and (4) universality. They describe the common good as the role of a just society to work toward the common good as the good for the individual. Individuals and society are so inextricably joined that actions that may help the individual may be detrimental to the society, and vice versa. Beneficence and nonmalevolence, or to do no harm, are often applied in nursing practice in LMICs—nurses need to critically assess whether giving a client a medication or treatment might do more harm than good.

The third principle that Crigger and Holcomb (2007) describe is respect for persons and autonomy. This is a fundamental principle that undergirds all nursing practice. The American Nurses Association Code of Ethics states:

> The nurse, in all professional relationships, practices with compassion and respect for the inherent dignity, worth, and uniqueness of every individual, unrestricted by considerations of social or economic status, personal attributes, or the nature of health problems . . . the nurse promotes, advocates for, and strives to protect the health, safety, and rights of the patient . . . the nurse participates in establishing, maintaining, and improving health care environments . . . the nurse collaborates with other health professionals and the public in promoting community, national, and international efforts to meet health needs. (Foster, 2009, p. 102)

The final principle described is universality. This is the logical belief that a person should make laws or rules that apply to anyone in a given situation. Nurses often use universality principle to decide on the ethical acceptability of choices and ultimately the care of patients. These principles undergird the professional practice across borders with the ultimate goal of promoting and protecting the health of communities with socially oriented strategies as well as treating individual clients (Crigger & Holcomb, 2007).

The ethical issues raised in providing nursing care in LMICs need to be addressed before nurses and students venture into practicing abroad. In many global settings, visiting partners have been observed to sometimes practice above their level of licensure. This has included a number of professionals, including RNs, NPs, and student nurses who practice in many ways as NPs, MDs, and RNs, respectively. Examples of this include RNs who prescribe medications without consultation with licensed practitioners, NPs who perform minor surgical procedures without oversight or without concern for asepsis, and student nurses who are given the freedom to assess and prescribe common medications without direct supervision by licensed personnel. Levi (2009) describes this practicing above level of preparation with a medical student practicing as an MD as ethically unacceptable. Another concern is practicing without attention to long-term consequences. There are long-term consequences of providing short-term care without attention to things such as antibiotics left by visiting health teams, the possibility that multivitamins may be mistaken for candy, and distribution of ibuprofen with inadequate education, examples given by Levi (2009). In many global settings, some nursing service groups have provided short-term solutions such as the distribution of bags of children's acetaminophen and child vitamins. In some cases, the parents not understanding the instructions as given by the volunteer nurses were later found to give the acetaminophen and vitamins to the children to hold outside while they played. It was clear that the instructions were not culturally sensitive or safe.

Levi also discusses the example of a medical student who used an otoscope and stethoscope that the community had never seen before. The student diagnosed a baby with dehydration and fever and suggested that the family give her fluids and acetaminophen. The unsupervised medical student presented as a physician and did not ask how the baby was fed or about its dietary habits or whether the family had potable water. The baby died within a few days of his visit. The families of the village felt his instruments and medicines caused an "evil eye" and were concerned about the photographs the medical student had taken, worried they may be used for evil means. Lack of understanding of local beliefs, use of unfamiliar technology, and photography without permission of patients may result in unintended harm and border on exploitation (Levi, 2009).

Quality service learning and study-abroad programs for nursing students need to be strategically designed and implemented. There are core elements in the planning, design, and implementation of experiential learning across borders for nurses and students, including strong leadership, strong partnerships with agencies or individuals in the host country, and well-designed curriculum. The success of any international service program is in strong leadership. The leader needs to demonstrate ongoing commitment to the program, value the community partners' perspective, and mentor other faculty, student, and nurse leaders in a continuing commitment to sustain the partnerships and goals of the program (Curtin, Martins, Schwartz-Barcott, DiMaria, & Soler-Ogando, 2013; Leffers & Mitchell, 2010; Levi, 2009; Lotas, 2011).

The success of any international service learning or clinical practice program is in developing strong relationships with host partners. There is also a need for thorough community assessment by the students before visiting any global setting. This assessment is based on secondary data sources for demographic information, health indicators, health services, and social, political, and cultural factors. Some programs have established partnerships with immigrant groups from the host country now living in the country where the academic program is located. Additionally, various academic programs ask faculty and former students to share their previous global health experiences and to serve as key informants. The development of transparent partnerships based on trust, shared learning, and participatory decision making between the nurses and host partners is the foundation for creating an environment of transformational learning for both the nurse partners and host partners (Leffers & Mitchell, 2010; Levi, 2009; Lotas, 2011).

Partnerships transform the traditional perspectives, assumptions, and stereotypes that persist from the colonial era, thus reducing the likelihood of Western health care beliefs and practices being translated into other cultures. Instead a blending occurs that transforms and is transformed by the culture and people in the partnership (De Leo Siantz & Meleis, 2007). Through partnerships, the nurse partners begin to understand the host partners' concerns and professional responsibilities. For instance, in the Dominican Republic, the nurses wondered why we came to the hospital in scrubs instead of the traditional white uniform and cap. They also wondered why we wore our scrubs out of the hospital to return to our homes. Our practice appeared unprofessional to them. We were not bringing a change of clothes, something customary for the local nurses in the Dominican Republic. Such collaboration will only promote the dual goals of providing a transformative educational experience for students while promoting the values of engagement and equality with host communities (Mkandawire-Valhmu & Doering, 2012).

In the development of partnerships, a visit to the host country by the faculty members prior to the scheduled international service learning program can assist in engaging, collaborating, strengthening relationships, and setting mutual goals. This level of preparation can be beneficial to understanding the needs of the community and how the group can support existing resources and to committing to a sustainable program of services (Leffers & Mitchell, 2010; Levi, 2009).

Careful review of the purposes of the service learning experiences/study abroad is essential in selecting clinical sites and determining the level of student engagement. It is necessary to understand the host institution's policies regarding nursing student activities, including policies related to direct patient care. It is equally important to emphasize that the home institution's students/nurses may not exceed the standards and scope of student/nurse practice in the home institution, regardless of the policies existing in the host institution (Lotas, 2011). An example of this is referred to as "drop-in care" whereby practitioners dispense a 30-day supply of antihypertensive medications to persons living in a resource-poor community with limited access to water, food, and health care or dispense antibiotics (Powell et al., 2010). These well-intended interventions could lead to irreversible health problems, including fatal anaphylaxis (Levi, 2009; Miller, 2009). How valuable is intermittent care or "drop-in care" when there is no continuity, limited access to health care, or limited availability of supportive care when the group returns home?

In preparation for international service learning or clinical practice abroad, nurses and students need to be prepared with an understanding of the clinical skills required and expectations as visitors in another country. Visiting nurse partners must resist the temptation to practice beyond their clinical expertise as well as their nursing license or certification. This preparation includes acquisition of language skills and knowledge of the health care problems and solutions abroad, as well as assessment of one's own ability to meet those needs. Nurses and nursing students need to be able to interact with persons who have different beliefs, values, and health care practices (Crigger, Brannigan, & Bard, 2006; Leffers & Mitchell, 2010; Levi, 2009; Lotas, 2011; Miller, 2009). Levi and others (Crigger & Godfrey, 2010; Juarez et al., 2006; Miller, 2009; Tervalon & Murray-Garcia, 1998) address the concept of cultural humility. This requires that nurse education and practice move beyond the concepts of cultural awareness, sensitivity, and competency toward an approach of cultural humility. Cultural humility is defined as:

> [a] process that requires humility as individuals continually engage in self-reflection and self-critique as lifelong learners and reflective practitioners, it requires humility in how [practitioners] bring into check the power imbalances that exist in the dynamics of [provider]–patient communication by using patient-focused interviewing and care, and it is a process that requires humility to develop and maintain mutually respectful and dynamic partnerships with communities. . . . (Tervalon & Murray-Garcia, 1998, p. 18)

Cultural humility is a process that encourages respect for prevailing beliefs and cultural norms and continuous reflection on one's own biases, as well as learning about the culture with which one will interact. This approach is needed to ensure ethical practice across borders but also highlights the continuous need for self-reflection even when one has become bilingual or immersed in a culture/country long term. Leffers and Mitchell (2010) refer to this process as cultural bridging featuring mutual sharing and awareness of the power difference in this cultural exchange. The preparation for any type of international experience or practicing abroad needs to include an opportunity for nurses and students to reflect on their own values and beliefs about cultural differences (Levi, 2009; Lotas, 2011).

In addition to reflection, nurse consultants, practitioners, researchers, and students need to learn about the communities in which they will be providing care. Understanding the political, social, and economic structures impacting the health, education, and resources available to the population is imperative to cross-cultural practice. It is often difficulty to find unbiased interpretations of the countries since authors often write from a Western perspective. Basic safety concerns and any infectious diseases prevalent in the host country should be reviewed and discussed at length. The importance of following all laws and rules of the host country needs to be emphasized. Often students erroneously believe that they are exempted from any local laws because they are U.S. citizens and the U.S. government will intervene if they are accused of any violation or crime (Levi, 2009; Lotas, 2011). Nurses need to successfully interact with culturally diverse individuals and respond appropriately to culture-based cues and situations to meet the needs of our global citizens.

Although reflection is an important component for cultural humility, it is also essential for evaluating the international service experience. The quality of the experience can be understood through reflection. The goal is that transformational learning will occur. It is important for faculty leaders to respond to the reflection for clarification, reinforcement, and reframing. The success is related to extensive planning, reflection, and ongoing monitoring. Maintaining and sustaining the international learning partnership requires clear, open, regular communication among nurses and host partners (Leffers & Mitchell, 2010; Lotas, 2011).

CONCLUSION

Learning about the culture of a population in a country where nursing services will occur requires various levels of assessment, planning, and evaluation. Globalization of health care has magnified the need for communication and collaboration across nations to meet the public health needs of populations. To respond to these needs, the health provider needs critical reasoning that incorporates not only knowledge of the country's needs and resources but also a globally responsible cultural ethic.

The mobility of nurses and other health providers from one country to another clearly supports a need for international licensure and practice standards that will better address societal needs. Migration of nurses from LMICs to higher income countries may weaken poorer countries' health care resources and needs serious critique. Accountability related to nursing practice needs to be in both directions.

Nursing practice issues in LMICs is a pressing issue. Many nongovernmental organizations (NGOs) and nursing programs offer international service opportunities for nurses and nursing students. Scope of practice needs to be consistent across borders. Cultural humility is a requirement of the visiting provider that recognizes the host partner's cultural practices and preferences and allows collaborating in practice that is professional and safe. The effective visiting provider is informed by professional knowledge and local knowledge of the host partner—thus, cultural bridging.

An effective professional nursing practice in a host country also requires ethically based community involvement and collaboration. High-quality service learning will value the host partner's long-term needs and work toward sustainable solutions. This partnership incorporates participatory decision making and engagement that can lead to transformative international service learning for the nurses and students.

REFERENCES

Aiken, L., Buchan, J., Sochalski, J., Nichols, B., & Powell, M. (2004). Trends in international nurse migration. *Health Affairs, 23*(3), 69–77.

Barry, J. (2010). Supporting safe and competent nursing practice: A conversation with Jean Barry. *International Nursing Review,* 409–411.

Bringle, R. G., & Hatcher, J. A. (1996). Implementing service learning in higher education. *Journal of Higher Education, 67,* 221–239.

Crigger, N. J., Brannigan, M., & Bard, M. (2006). Compassionate nursing professionals as good citizens of the world. *Advances in Nursing Science, 29*(1), 15–26.

Crigger, N. J., & Godfrey, N. (2010). The importance of being humble. *Advances in Nursing Science, 33*(4), 310–319.

Crigger, N. J., & Holcomb, L. (2007). Practical strategies for providing culturally sensitive, ethical care in developing nations. *Journal of Transcultural Nursing 18*(1), 70–76.

Curtin, A., Martins, D., Schwartz-Barcott, D., DiMaria, L., & Soler-Ogando, B. (2013). Development and evaluation of an international service learning program for nursing students. *Public Health Nurse,* first published online April 29, 2013. doi: 10.1111/phn.12040

De Leo Siantz, M. L., & Meleis, A. (2007). Integrating cultural competence into nursing education and practice: 21st century action steps. *Journal of Transcultural Nursing, 18*(1), 86S–90S.

Dooley, D. (2011). Transformational goals for the 21st century. The president's 21st century fund for excellence. Retrieved from www.uri.edu/president/Transformational%20 Goals.pdf

Edmonds, M. L. (2010). The lived experience of nursing students who study abroad: A qualitative inquiry. *Journals of Studies in International Education, 14*(5), 545–568.

Evanson, T. A., & Zust, B. L. (2004). The meaning of participation in an international service experience among baccalaureate nursing students. *International Journal of Nursing Education Scholarship, 1*(1), 1–14.

Fernandez, R., & Hebert, G. (2004). Global licensure. New modalities of treatment and care require the development of new structures and systems to access care. *Nursing Administration Quarterly, 28*(2), 129–132.

Foster, J. (2009). Cultural humility and the importance of long-term relations in international partnerships. *Journal of Obstetrics, Gynecology and Neonatal Nursing, 38*(1), 100–107.

Frenk, J., Chen, L., Bhutta, A., Cohen, J., Crisp, N., Evans, T., . . . Zurayk, H. (2010). Health professionals for a new century: Transforming education to strengthen health systems in an interdependent world. *The Lancet, 376,* 1923–1958.

ICN. (2004). The global shortage of registered nurses: An overview of issues and actions. www.icn.ch/glbal/shortage.pdf

ICN, WHO, & Royal College of Nursing. (2003). International nurse mobility, trends and policy implications. http://www.who.int/workforcealliance/knowledge/resources/nursesmobility/en/index.html

Institute of Medicine. (2011). *The future of nursing: Leading change, advancing health* (Appendix J). http://www.iom.edu/~/media/Files/Activity%20Files/Workforce/Nursing/International%20Models%20of%20Nursing.pdf

Johanson, L. (2006). The implementation of a study abroad course for nursing. *Nurse Educator, 31*(3), 129–131.

Juarez, J., Marvel, K., Brezinski, K.L., Glazner, C., Towbin, M., & Lawton, S. (2006). Bridging the gap: A curriculum to teach residents cultural humility. *Family Medicine, 38*(2), 97–102.

Kingma, M. (2001). Nursing migration: Global treasure hunt or disaster-in-the-making? *Nursing Inquiry, 8*(4), 205–212.

Kline, D. S. (2004). Push and pull factors in international nurse migration. *Journal of Nursing Scholarship, 35,* 2, 107–111.

Kulbok, P., Mitchell, E., Glick, D., & Greiner, D. (2012). International experiences in nursing education: A review of the literature. *International Journal of Nursing Education Scholarship, 9*(1), 1–21. doi:10.1515/1548-923X.2365

Larson, K., Ott, M., & Miles, J. (2010). International cultural immersion: En vivo reflections in cultural competence. *Journal of Cultural Diversity, 17*(2), 44–50.

Leffers, J., & Mitchell, E. (2010). Conceptual model for partnership and sustainability in global health. *Public Health Nursing, 28*(1), 91–102.

Levi, A. (2009). The ethics of nursing student international clinical experiences. *Journal of Obstetrics, Gynecologic, and Neonatal Nursing, 38*, 94–99.

Lotas, M. B. (2011). Home institution responsibilities and best practices. In T. McKinnon & J. Fitzpatrick (Eds.), *Global service-learning in nursing* (pp. 53–67). New York: National League of Nursing.

McKinnon, T. H., & Fealy, G. (2001). Core concepts for developing global service-learning programs in nursing. In T. McKinnon & J. Fitzpatrick (Eds.), *Global service-learning in nursing*. New York, NY: National League for Nursing.

Miller, S. (2009). Cultural humility is the first step to becoming global care providers. *Journal of Obstetrics, Gynecologic, and Neonatal Nursing, 38*, 92–93.

Milner, C. (2003). *Global health clinical experiences: Implications for culture, ethics, policy, and standards of practice*. Dissertation proposal, University of Victoria, Interdisciplinary Doctoral Studies.

Milton, C. (2008). Accountability in nursing: Reflecting on ethical codes and professional standards of nursing practice from a global perspective. *Nursing Science Quarterly, 21*(4), 300–303.

Mkandawire-Valhmu, L., & Doering, J. (2012). Study abroad as a tool for promoting cultural safety in nursing education. *Journal of Transcultural Nursing, 23*(1), 82–89.

Parfitt, B. (1999). Working across cultures: A model for practice in developing countries. *International Journal of Nursing Studies, 36*, 371–378.

Powell, D., Gillis, C., Hewitt, H., & Flint, E. (2010). Application of a partnership model for transformative and sustainable international development. *Public Health Nursing, 27*(1), 54–70.

Rosenkoetter, M., & Nardi, D. (2007). American Academy of nursing expert panel on global nursing and health: White paper on global nursing and health. *Journal of Transcultural Nursing, 18*(4), 305–315.

Sloand, E., Bower, K., & Groves, S. (2008). Challenges and benefits of international clinical placements in public health nursing. *Nurse Educator, 33*(1), 35–38.

Smith-Miller, C., Leak, A., Harlan, C., Diekmann, J., & Sherwood, G. (2010). "Leaving the comfort of the familiar": Fostering workplace cultural awareness through short-term global experiences. *Nursing Forum, 45*(1), 18–28.

Tervalon, J., & Murray-Garcia, J. (1998). Cultural humility versus cultural competence: A critical distinction in defining physician training outcomes in multicultural education. *Journal of Health Care for the Poor and Underserved, 9*(2), 17–25.

World Health Organization. (1999). World Health Organization report on infectious diseases. Removing obstacles to healthy development. www.who.int/infectious-disease-report/pages/textonly.html

World Health Organization. (2006). The World Health Report: Working together for health. http://www.who.int/whr/2006/en/

World Health Organization. (2009). Country cooperation strategy at a glance. www.who .int/countryfocus/cooperation_strategy/ccsbrief_dom_09_en.pdf

World Health Organization. (2010). WHO global code of practice on the international recruitment of health personnel. Geneva, Switzerland: World Health Organization. www.who.int/hrh/migration/code/practice/en/index.html

Zorn, C. (1996). The long-term impact on nursing students of participating in international education. *Journal of Professional Nursing, 12*(2), 106–110.

Academic Learning Program in the Dominican Republic: Partnership and Ethical Perspectives

Diane C. Martins
Alicia J. Curtin

CONTEXT: THE DOMINICAN REPUBLIC

The Dominican Republic (DR) occupies the eastern two-thirds of the Caribbean island of Hispaniola and is the second-largest country in the region. Its only border is with Haiti. For political and administrative reasons, the country has three regions and seven subregions, which together total 29 provinces and the National District. The Dominican Republic is home to approximately 10 million people. The country has survived natural disasters, colonization, foreign invasions, and a brutal dictatorship. The original inhabitants, the Taínos, occupied the island until 1492, when Christopher Columbus conquered them and colonized their island for Spain, the first European settlement in the Americas. The Colonial Zone in Santo Domingo celebrates this history. The DR became a French and Haitian country for a while, then an independent country by 1821. The United States occupied the DR from 1916 to 1924. After dictatorships and authoritarian regimes up through 1978, the country developed a representative democracy. The current president is Danilo Medina; the vice president, Margarita Cedeno de Fernandez, is the former president's wife.

The DR is the second largest economy in the Caribbean and Central American region. Its economy is supported by sugar production, resort/travel services, and remittances from the United States (about 1/10 of the GDP) (CIA, 2013). Although there has been major growth in the economy, more than a third of the country's total population live in poverty, and almost 20% live in extreme poverty. The DR is among the countries with the highest disparities in income distribution. In 2002, the wealthiest 20% of the population received 53% of the country's gross income, while the most vulnerable (40%) of the population received only 14% (WHO, 2009).

The highest incidences of poverty and extreme poverty occur in the rural areas along the Dominican–Haitian border regions (Chapin Metz, 2001; PAHO, 2001). The persistence of poverty in these areas is the result of several factors, including the government's focus on developing tourism, industry, and services sectors over the past decade, natural disasters, low agricultural production, and the long history of tenuous relationships between Haitians and Dominicans. The government's investment in social and productive development in the rural areas is limited and the political representation of these areas in government is minimal compared to some of the larger provinces in the DR. Another factor contributing

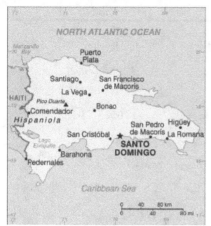

Dominican Republic.   *Credit:* Dominican
Republic Travel Information, www.antor.org

to the poverty in the rural areas is the low agricultural productivity. Although technology is available, it is not always readily accessible to farmers in the rural areas, and the lack of financial resources limits their ability to adopt new technology to improve their productivity and income.

Furthermore the population in this area is affect by the lack of access to health care, adequate housing, sanitation and education. The economy is also strongly affected by the troubled relationship with Haiti over the years. On the one hand, Haitian workers are needed for the harvesting of the coffee and sugar and unskilled construction work, but often the government does not recognize Haitians as working/born in the Dominican Republic. However, over the past decade, both the Haitian and Dominican governments have recognized the need to develop the Dominican–Haitian borderlands as a key factor in freeing this area from the cycle of poverty (PADF, 2010).

Although the social, economic, and political history contribute to the development of the country's identity, the people of the DR are most resilient. The influences of Taino, Spanish, African, French, and English traditions woven together create an intricate complex cultural fabric that flourishes despite the factors that have impeded the economic growth and development of the country.

NURSING PRACTICE, PARTNERSHIPS, AND COMMUNITY ENGAGEMENT IN THE DOMINICAN REPUBLIC

The Early Years of Relationship Building Between Nurse Volunteers and Community Members

This case study describes the movement from participating in a volunteer mission program for health professionals serving a population in the rural areas along the Dominican–Haitian border to the development of a short-term, international service learning program for nursing students in the DR. The key factors in the development of the program are faculty who are committed leaders in the development of partnerships and sustainability in the areas of need; host partners who are invested in the collaboration cross-culturally; knowledge of and respect for the culture, customs, political, economic, and social influences on health outcomes; language acquisition; and institutional support from the university or college of nursing.

The partnership between the nursing faculty and the health care professionals in a small town along the Dominican–Haitian border began more than 20 years ago. The first trip was with a nonprofit organization providing health care professionals the opportunities to serve a rural community along the Dominican–Haitian border. The leaders of the group traveled to the DR and investigated the health care needs in the area. They established a partnership with Catholic Relief Services at the local church and begin to develop 2-week volunteer mission trips to this region, Jose de Ocoa, Bani, San Pedro de Marcoris, and Haiti. The recruitment of health care professionals was often by word of mouth and through a network of dedicated volunteer participants who provided continuity as well as support for other new participants learning about the country and health care needs. In preparation for the trip, the organization would lead a 1-day orientation about the country, including safety tips, political history, and cultural norms. The 2-week trips usually occurred three times a year, in October, January, and June. Participants arranged their own travel and met at the airport to begin their journey. The group stayed together in the local center. The work involved outreach to various rural areas throughout the western border of the DR and also areas of Haiti. As part of the organization's initial mission, partnerships between the local

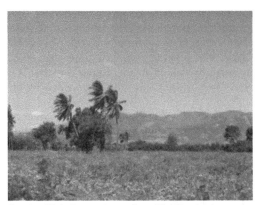

Countryside in the western region of the Dominican Republic.   *Credit*: A. Curtin and D. Martins

church and community health workers (promotores de salud) were established and fostered as an integral component of the commitment in serving the area among the local agencies and the U.S. organization. Often the participants visited the local hospital and nutrition center to help care for children suffering from malnutrition and diarrheal illnesses.

In developing relationships with the local nurses at the hospital, one faculty member became interested in understanding the nursing care and practices at the public hospital. The interest was highlighted through participating in the volunteer mission program and attempting to understand the cultural differences in the presentation of health and illness among the people in the area and the practice of nurses within a U.S./Western framework. This led to obtaining funding for a cultural immersion experience in the DR, which included working with the Dominican nurses at the public hospital and living with a host family in country. During the day, she rotated through hospital units and clinics, including labor and delivery, postpartum, sick care units (where family members cooked for and cared for their relatives), prenatal clinic, TB clinic, breastfeeding clinic, and immunization clinic. During this time the infant mortality rate was high due to the marginal nutritional status of the children and the adopted Western practice of bottle-feeding children. It would take many years for the country's public health initiatives to help mothers return to breastfeeding. Through these initiatives the Dominican nurses were successful in changing the culture and practice through health education and teaching new mothers. Continued economic and social progress has also addressed the lack of clean water sources, sanitation, and other public health initiatives for the people in this region.

The Dominican nurses and public hospital struggle with similar challenges as do U.S. health care systems and professionals. Many health care professionals tend to work in the private urban sectors, where the conditions and the salary are more desirable. This leaves many rural areas without practitioners. The migration of health care personnel poses a dilemma for the health care system as a whole as the competition for positions increases in the larger cities and service to the rural areas declines. This migration also leads to the lack of "licenciadas," professional nurses, in the rural areas. There are three levels of nurses in the public hospital sector: licenciadas, tecnico, and auxiliary. The professional nursing schools require 12 years of general education, 3 years of specialized nursing education, 1 year to obtain the title of "licenciada," and 1 additional year for an advanced license. The second level of nursing, the "tecnico" nurse, requires 9 years of general education and 3 years of vocational training at the secondary school. These technical nurses will receive a "bachillerato" and are supervised by the professional nurse in the in-patient setting. The third level of nursing is the auxiliary nurse, who is required to have 8 years of general education and 4 to 6 months of nursing training. In theory, this educational system appears well organized. The reality is that much of the patient care is delivered by auxiliary nurses who have minimal formal training. Due to the shortage of professional nurses, often the licenciadas assume administrative responsibilities in supervising staff, consulting with physicians, and managing hospital units. Recognizing the important role of nurses within the public health care system, there are a number of initiatives supporting the academic achievement of nurses in the DR. Recently, academic programs have been developed to help auxiliary and technical nurses obtain their licenciado. These programs are very similar to our registered nurse to baccalaureate nursing programs.

Through this experience, relationships were developed and a greater understanding of nursing practice, patient needs, and cultural norms was gained. The nurses were very willing to share their experiences and their perspective on nursing practice. When asked about practice, one nurse replied: "It is a service to the people. When people are sick they have many needs. As nurses we need to meet the emotional, physical and spiritual needs of these patients." Another nurse provided an example of a young boy seeking care for an eye infection. He believed that the infection was a result of not helping a pregnant woman. In reassuring him, the Dominican nurse explained to the young boy that this was not true and instructed him in the correct use of the medication prescribed by the pediatrician.

The relationships developed during this period with the Dominican nurses were an asset to the nonprofit group in their health care services in the rural areas. The Dominican nurses would join us to travel to remote communities and provide health education (charlas) on preventing intestinal parasites, proper nutrition, and preventing dehydration. The people responded positively, laughed often, and asked excellent questions. It became obvious that the Dominican nurses are critical to meeting the primary health care needs of the Dominican population, especially those who live in the rural areas along the Dominican–Haitian border. When asked how could they change the current health care system, one auxiliary nurse replied that there needs to be more emphasis on preventative medicine and health education for the people, especially those who live in the campos (rural areas). One licenciada stated, "It is impossible to change the system, because it is so political. The people and patients need to be educated about taking care of themselves and their families." The nurses realize the need to empower the rural population through education and self-care practices in order to strengthen the health and well-being of their families. They also realize that despite advances in technology and economical and social policies, the impact of these advances will have minimal effect on the health outcomes in the region most in need.

The partnership between nurse and host partners is often dependent on the leadership and vision of the organization. The sustainability is often dependent on the organization's ability to "groom" new leaders who will assume the ideals, mission, and sensitivity to the culture norms and practices established by the original organization partners (Leffers & Mitchell, 2011). At times, changes in leadership may change organizational goals, vision, and relationships with the host partners. This often is influenced by the expertise and particular interest of the new leadership group. This is also true of the host partners. Changes in leadership and new direction may lead to a different focus and goals. It highlights the importance in developing short-term and long-term goals as well as multiple areas of joint endeavors within local communities, public hospitals, and academic settings. These relationships can continue to foster joint projects in service learning, nursing practice, and research. For example, the faculty began to explore opportunities to build relationships with the health care providers at a senior center, head start program, and nutrition center. In addition, the need to learn about sustainable solutions to increasing the income of the farmers through agricultural projects, empowering women through creating head start programs for their children, and providing low-interest business loans led faculty to an adjacent community where a community organizer had worked with the community to develop and implement a number of programs.

CHANGING THE FOCUS FROM SHORT-TERM CLINICAL VISITS TO THE COMMUNITY HEALTH NURSING EXPERIENCE

With the increasing interest of student nurses in international programs, the internationalizing of the university curriculum, the changing demographics of the U.S. population, and the need for a global perspective and approach to health care, the faculty began to select a number of senior baccalaureate nursing students to participate on a volunteer medical mission to the Dominican Republic with a nonprofit organization. Initially the faculty from the college of nursing provided supervision and guidance for the immersion experience, but no formal curriculum was established until 2009. During the years prior to formalizing the curriculum, the faculty mentors further developed relationships with potential partners such as community organizers, hospital staff, and local agencies in the host setting. At the university, efforts addressed the need to understand cultural differences and improve the language skills of the faculty and students who participate. Concerns for safety, priorities for experiential learning, and intercultural communication and the development and maintenance of these relationships were foundational in developing the curriculum and service-learning program.

Each year improvements were made to strengthen the program. It became clear to us that the best service partnership for the nursing students would be to work with the community groups where we had developed such strong personal relationships. In this way, the students would practice in a community health nursing student role, learn important lessons about the Dominican people and culture, and provide essential services requested by the community partners. After we made connections with the University of Santa Domingo nursing and public health faculty, we determined that it would be a richer experience for the students to move from our participation with the U.S.-based nursing NGO and launch our own partnership between the university and the community partners in the DR. When the nursing NGO decided to move to another, distant location in the DR, we believed that our commitment to the rural community and our community partners must be maintained.

During the 2009 to 2010 academic year, four pretrip seminars to prepare students for the intense learning experience were added. The four seminars focused on Dominican history, politics, language, and culture and on the health care system. While seminar attendance was voluntary, the students' commitment to completing educational assignments varied. In-country faculty continued to build their partnerships with public health and community programs for sustainable projects for student engagement. In the evaluation of the program, faculty realized the need for further curriculum development, including goals and objectives and mandatory attendance at all seminars in order to participate in the "in-country" experience.

During the 2010 to 2011 academic year, the faculty developed the program goals and objectives to align with the university's mission for internationalization and globalization of the university's learning environment for students.

Mezirow and Taylor's (2009) Transformational Learning Theory was used as the conceptual framework for the development of the program. Mezirow describes transformative learning as a process whereby individuals engage in critical reflection to develop new perspectives, skills, and behaviors. The core elements include the individual experience, critical reflection, dialogue, a holistic orientation, an awareness of context, and an authentic practice. From this perspective, learning is based on prior experiences and involves critical self-reflection and challenging our own deeply held beliefs, feelings, and actions. By linking the reflection process to intended learning objectives and goals, students can then begin to articulate learning about personal and professional growth, cultural differences, and global engagement (Mezirow & Taylor, 2009; Riner, 2011).

Riner's (2011) framework for globally engaged nursing education is consistent with the description of the development of the program. Riner's framework includes the institutional and program mission and goals, program characteristics (pre-experience, on-site, and post-experience), global health core content, learner characteristics, reflection, and perspective transformation.

Institutional and Program Mission and Goals

The university's mission and goals for transformation supported the changes necessary in the development of the international service-learning program for students in the college of nursing. Two of the university's major transformational goals for the 21st century are

(1) to internationalize and globalize the University by preparing students to live and work in an increasingly globalized economy and by expanding the scope of our international research and education partnerships, increasing the number of

graduates fluent in languages and encouraging more students to study abroad and (2) [to] build a community that values and embraces equity and diversity by assisting students to develop the ability to communicate, understand and engage productively with people of diverse cultures, ethnicities, religions, lifestyles and values. (Dooley, 2011)

With this mission and financial support for student travel, the faculty developed the program's goals and objectives with an emphasis on service learning and public health.

Global Health Core Content

From Riner's (2011) framework, the global health core content recommends four areas of learning to promote student development of attitudes, knowledge, and skills for engagement in global health. The four areas of learning are global learning, international service learning and social consciousness, global cultural competence development, and country-specific knowledge. In the development of this international service learning experience in the DR, the university faculty emphasized the country-specific knowledge, service learning elements, basic Spanish-language acquisition and integration of cultural competence perspectives in preparation for the trip. These areas of learning were also integrated throughout the experience.

Program Characteristics (Pre-Experience, On-Site, and Post-Experience)

Once developed as an official university program, it was offered as a three-credit independent study with credit toward culture and/or diversity cluster requirements and was planned to evolve from a voluntary service program to a service learning and cultural immersion experience. The pre-immersion experience included mandatory attendance at four 2-hour seminars and one day-long orientation seminar. The seminars included what Riner (2011) calls the global health core content with a major focus on country-specific knowledge, elements of international service learning, and social consciousness. To meet the program objectives, the students had assigned readings, a book critique and presentation, and creation of health educational projects based on the host country's needs. Examples of books used for the critiques are *In the Time of the Butterflies* (Alvarez, 1994), *The Feast of the Goat* (Llosa, 2002), *The Brief Wondrous Life of Oscar Wao* (Diaz, 2008), *The Farming of Bones* (Danticat, 1998), *How the Garcia Girls Lost Their Accent* (Alvarez, 1991), and others.

The 2-week, on-site experience took place during winter break in the rural southwest area of the Dominican Republic. Initially, the students and faculty stayed at a retreat center at western side of town where two meals, Dominican-style, daily, as well as laundry services and sleeping quarters for students and other organization participants, were provided. At that time, students participated in a service learning experience with a nonprofit organization delivering health care to the rural areas of the country.

In collaboration with a Dominican nurse from the public hospital, faculty developed sites for students and partnered with community agencies. Instead of living in a separate center on the outskirts of town, students would live in homes provided by local nurses in the community. The focus of the work would be learning activities at four different sites: (1) prenatal and well-child clinics at the public hospital, (2) adult day health program, (3) "head start" program, and (4) rural clinics. At these sites the students would perform nursing assessments and health teaching with interpreters and present their health education projects. In addition to their daily service learning activities, students participated in debriefing seminars with faculty guidance and completed daily journaling while in country, reflecting on daily encounters and on the day's experience (Curtin, Martins, Schwartz-Barcott, DiMaria, & Soler-Ogando, 2013).

The post-experience component of the trip included two seminars, the first held 2 weeks posttrip, to give students a chance to acclimate to the United States and to reflect

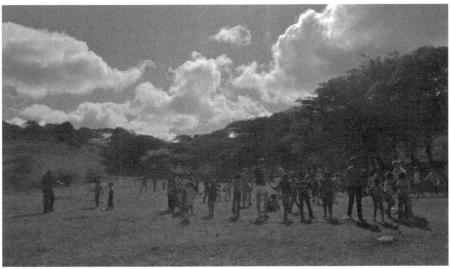

University of Rhode Island College of Nursing students with local children.   *Credit*: A. Curtin and D. Martins

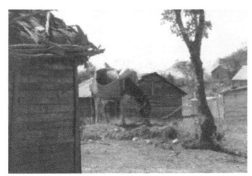

Rural scene.   *Credit*: J. Leffers

on their experience. During the first meeting, faculty facilitated the discussion to assist students in processing their emotions and evaluate and reflect on the experience. Additionally, students submitted their journals for review and completed posttrip evaluations. A second seminar included the students and other group participants (nurses, nurse practitioners, and interpreters) who shared their experiences, and provided feedback to the nonprofit organization about their on-site experience.

In order to allow the students to see a village that contrasted the rural villages on the Haitian border that were experiencing more severe shortages of water and food, a partnership with a community organizer in another community nearby was developed. This community organizer had helped mobilize the local women to replant cash crops after fields were burned for short-term crops (beans to avocado and coconuts). Additionally, she helped the women to be in charge of their education, water system, health care, and agriculture. The group is called Women in United Development (Mujeres Unidas en Desarollo [MUD]). This village also created a small peanut factory run by the women to develop a nutrient enriched peanut butter (Nutri-Forte) for the children experiencing malnutrition. Through the work of this program, the students learned about sustainability, community partnership for development, and global nutritional outreach strategies.

ETHICAL CONSIDERATIONS FOR NURSING PRACTICE IN THE DOMINICAN REPUBLIC

As the program was built, the most compelling issue for us was nursing ethics. The faculty's longstanding personal relationships with community members, built over many years, provided great insight into the Dominican culture. This was reinforced back at home, where the percentage of Dominican immigrants to the state is among the highest in the United States. This cultural insight reinforced our desire to focus on several factors:

- Focus our service toward specific expressed needs of the community members
- Ensure that issues of mutual respect are always most important
- Provide opportunities for nursing students to learn about community health nursing from the perspective of our Dominican partners
- Provide clinical experiences where nursing students practice within their student role

In our many years of global health nursing experience, we have encountered well-intended nurses whose participation raises ethical concerns about global health nursing. Unfortunately, due to the often overwhelming health needs of the host country people, nurses are tempted to practice at a level above their own nursing license. Taking on roles of prescribing medications when one is not certified to do so not only is unethical but also can cause serious harm to patients.

In addition, as a guest in the host country it is imperative to demonstrate respect for privacy, dignity, and culture. Taking or posting photographs without consent can be offensive and inappropriate, especially if the photographs are displayed without context. The participant's presentation of his or her international experience to others should be reviewed by a colleague from the host country if possible. This will provide a more accurate interpretation and depictions of the ideas and thoughts being presented.

Cultural immersion experiences for nurses and nursing students can be highly beneficial for learning about culture, health, and global public health. In order to provide ethical service to host country partners, awareness of and respect for cultural and religious practices in the host setting are crucial.

CONCLUSION

We strongly believe that in order to provide nursing students with an opportunity for cultural immersion with a service learning focus, the most effective approach is one that emphasizes strong relationships in the community, prioritizes experiences through an ethics lens, and provides services that meet the expressed needs of the community partners. While not every nursing service-learning program is able to build relationships over a 20-year period, our experiences highlight the advantages of a long-term commitment to international partnerships.

REFLECTIVE QUESTIONS

1. What are the critical factors necessary in an academic partnership in a distant country?
2. Describe factors for nursing practice across international borders.
3. The role of guest in a host country raises ethical questions. Consider dilemmas that arise when a nurse guest is faced with serious health problems in the host setting and wants to practice within the scope of his or her nursing license. Consider how to best address these dilemmas.

REFERENCES

Alvarez, J. (1991). *How the Garcia girls lost their accents*. Chapel Hill, NC: Algonquin.

Alvarez, J. (1994). *In the time of the butterflies*. Chapel Hill, NC: Algonquin.

Central Intelligence Agency (CIA). (2013). World Factbook. Central America and the Caribbean: Dominican Republic. https://www.cia.gov/library/publications/the-world-factbook/geos/dr.html

Chapin Metz, H. (2001). *Dominican Republic and Haiti. Country studies* (3rd ed). Washington, DC: Federal Research Division, Library of Congress.

Curtin, A., Martins, D., Schwartz-Barcott, D., DiMaria, L., & Soler-Ogando, B. (2013). Development and evaluation of an international service learning program for nursing students. *Public Health Nurse, 30*(6), 548–556.

Danticat, E. (1998). *The farming of bones.* Danticat, Edwidge: Soho Press.

Diaz, J. (2008). *The brief wondrous life of Oscar Wao.* New York, NY: Riverhead Trade.

Dooley, D. (2011). Transformational goals for the 21st century. The president's 21st century fund for excellence. www.uri.edu/president/Transformational%20Goals.pdf

Leffers, J., & Mitchell, E. (2011). Conceptual model for partnership and sustainability in global health. *Public Health Nursing, 28*(1), 91–102.

Llosa, M. V. (2002). *The feast of the goat.* New York, NY: Picador.

Mezirow, J., & Taylor, E. (2009). *Transformative learning in practice: Insights from community, work-place and higher education.* San Francisco, CA: Jossey-Bass.

Pan American Development Foundation (PADF). (2010). *The Haitian–Dominican borderlands. Opportunities and challenges post-earthquake. Final report of the program. 2003–2010.* Washington, DC: PADF.

Pan American Health Organization (PAHO). (2001). Regional Core Health Data System: Country profile: Dominican Republic. www1.paho.org/english/sha/prfdor.htm

Riner, M. (2011). Globally engaged nursing education: An academic program framework. *Nursing Outlook, 59,* 308–317.

World Health Organization (WHO). (2009). Country cooperation strategy at a glance. www.who.int/countryfocus/cooperation_strategy/ccsbrief_dom_09_en.pdf

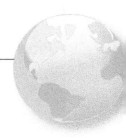

CHAPTER 4

Host Partner Factors for Partnership and Sustainability

Nancy Hoffart
Jenny Vacek
Myrna A. A. Doumit
Judy Liesveld
Debra Brady

An abundance of literature published in recent years provides rich evidence that global nursing partnerships are increasing to advance nursing education, the nursing profession, and health care delivery worldwide. There are examples of partnerships between higher income countries (HICs) (Casey, 1999; Ganske, Zerull, Guinn, Dowling, & Tagnesi, 2007) and among low- and middle-income countries (LMICs) (Uys & Middleton, 2011). In this chapter, however, we focus on partnerships between LMICs and HICs. We use the term *host* or *host partner* to refer to the developing country that is the setting for the work being performed. We use the term *nurse partner* or *visiting partner* to refer to the nurses/others from HICs.

We present information about three types of international partnerships. The first type is partnerships that focus on academic education, prelicensure as well as advanced degree programs. In this type of partnership the visiting nurse typically serves as faculty for students from the visiting country or from the host country. The second type is partnerships that focus on advances in professional nursing, which provide professional development for nurse leaders and clinicians in specific settings and capacity-building measures for the profession in the host country. The nurse partner usually will serve as a consultant or as faculty for staff development programs. The third type is partnerships that provide direct clinical care or improve a specific aspect of health care in a developing country; the visiting nurse generally is involved in direct care or service.

A limitation in understanding the host partner perspective is that many of the reports are written by the nurse partner, with little or no authorship participation by the host partner. For example, in the literature on nursing education partnerships less than 50% of the primary or co-authors were from the host country (Kulbok, Mitchell, Glick, & Greiner, 2012). This raises questions about the validity of the reported host partner factors. Continued underrepresentation of the host partner's voice will impair mutuality, respect, program outcomes, and sustainability. Indeed, the final outcome for the global partnership is sustaining a long-term global partnership (Finkelman & Kenner, 2008). We have included the voice of the host as much as possible by relying primarily, although not exclusively, on reports that included one or more authors from the host partner.

CONCEPTUAL MODEL

The Leffers and Mitchell Conceptual Model for Partnership and Sustainability in Global Health (2011) is used as the framework to facilitate the reader's understanding of the host partner's context and expectations of the nurse partner. The model maintains that "engagement and partnership must precede any planning and intervention in order to create sustainable interventions" (p. 91). In this chapter we address host partner factors exclusively. Leffers and Mitchell explain that host partner factors include "the influence of the social, economic, political, and environmental status of the host country" (p. 95).

EDUCATIONAL PARTNERSHIPS

Purposes

Nurses from Western countries have long been acknowledged as leaders in global nursing because of the level of their nursing knowledge development, advancement in medical technology, and educational models (Xu, 2012). With an overarching goal to improve national health outcomes, host partners such as governmental agencies, medical and nursing leaders, and academic organizations seek assistance from Western nurse educators to work on academic education projects. Assistance has varied depending on the host's specific educational needs or goals. The following host partner needs were identified in the literature:

- Educate nurses to practice at the level of international standards (Berland, Richards, & Lund, 2010; Parfitt, Mughal, & Thomas, 2008; Plager & Razaonandrianina, 2009; Wollin & Fairweather, 2012).
- Improve the social status of nursing as a profession (Lasater, Upvall, Nielsen, Prak, & Ptachcinski, 2012; Parfitt et al., 2008) and eliminate the adverse social stigma of selecting nursing as a career (Berland et al., 2010).
- Acquire current knowledge and innovations in the science of nursing (Xu, 2012).
- Facilitate faculty development and leadership (Evans, Razia, & Cook, 2013; Lasater et al., 2012; Xu, 2012; Zheng, Hinshaw, Yu, Guo, & Oakley, 2001).
- Increase visibility and prestige of the host educational institution (Xu, 2012).
- Develop nursing curriculum (George & Meadows-Oliver, 2013; Xu, 2012), both postsecondary (Lasater et al., 2012; Xu, 2012), and graduate level (Plager & Razaonandrianina, 2009).
- Integrate specialty content into current nursing curriculum, such as palliative care (Malloy et al., 2011) and dementia care (Zheng et al., 2001).
- Alleviate shortages of nurses by increasing the nursing workforce (Evans et al., 2013; Kemp & Tindiweegi, 2001; Plager & Razaonandrianina, 2009).
- Use nurse partner faculty to teach host nursing students (Berland et al., 2010; Kemp & Tindiweegi, 2001; Wollin & Fairweather, 2012).

Regardless of the specific educational needs of the host country, the goal is a two-way exchange of knowledge and understanding between host and nurse partner that results in improved public health outcomes.

Social and Cultural Factors

Cultural respect is of ultimate importance, yet it is sometimes disregarded (Shah, Robinson, & Al Enezi, 2001). The visitor should respect the values of the host country and not impose his or her own value system. Cultural awareness, including religious practices, is a key theme in the literature. Host partners expect their counterparts to learn about their culture and to practice cultural humility (Foster, 2009). Evans et al. (2013) described the effect of the Muslim and Hindu communities' belief systems on nursing shortages in India. Until recently, nursing was stigmatized as a low-status profession because female nurses were required to touch strangers, work outside the home, handle bodily fluids, and interact with the male gender (Evans et al., 2013). Crow and Thuc (2011) stated that males in Vietnam would never work in labor and delivery, give postpartum care, or practice as a lactation consultant.

Xu (2012) posed questions that the host partner would expect the visiting nurse partner to ask of himself or herself: What are my cultural assumptions that can affect this partnership? What cultural sensitivity is needed to adapt to the culture in the host country? What are the moral and ethical responsibilities to the host partner? Is it appropriate for the host partner to impose what he or she thinks is culturally appropriate on the nurse partner? Xu suggested using a cultural broker or other representative to facilitate relations between those from differing cultures.

Culture of Education

Expectations of the host included that the nurse partner must have an understanding of the culture of education (Xu, 2012). Xu gave an example of how the application of nursing theory perspectives may not be cross-culturally relevant. In China, Dorothy Orem's Self-Care Deficit Theory is inconsistent with the Asian belief system that dependence during illness and recovery is acceptable. Cultural values that are contrary to Western nursing's emphasis on critical thinking are evident in the literature. For example, in Bangladesh the tradition of subservience to authority figures and elders creates challenges for nurses to develop critical thinking skills (Berland et al., 2010).

The host partner should be alert for differences in teaching styles. For instance, in India didactic teaching is a predominant strategy. Experiential learning such as problem identification, reflection, and action planning were found to be foreign concepts (Evans et al., 2013). Cook, Sheerin, Bancel, and Gomes (2012) described how nurse educators in Central and Eastern Europe favored one student poster presentation at a time, whereas nurse educators in Western countries displayed student posters all together in a setting that emphasized informal dialogue. In Bangladesh, education focuses on memorization and rote learning (Berland et al., 2010).

Communication is imperative for successful nurse partnerships. Lasater et al. (2012) found that key strategies to strengthen communication between partners included preparation prior to arrival, openness to learning in the host environment, and flexibility. Leininger (1998) provided an important caution to the visitor in regard to communication. She noted that in many non-Western countries, cultural deference to visiting faculty is a normative rule and practice. Host partners may remain polite and communicate only "safe" statements in the face of ideas and practices that do not fit their culture. In some settings the need to "save face" means that they will not engage in public debate. Only after a trusting relationship has been established with the nurse partner can open communication occur.

Worldwide, English is among the most commonly used second languages, yet partnerships in many LMICs may be affected due to limitations with English fluency. The type and extent of difficulty encountered may vary by country. For example, some from Asian countries may have difficulty speaking English even though their reading and listening skills are strong. In some countries translators are needed to facilitate communication (Crow & Thuc, 2011; Wros & Archer, 2010). The majority of nursing resources, such as Internet-based materials, audiovisual teaching materials, and textbooks, are written in English (Berland et al., 2010), which may limit accessibility by some nurse participants; they may also present content that is not culturally relevant. When communication occurs through the Internet, careful attention to netiquette is essential. Finally, being unaware of language nuances can be problematic for the nurse partners. For instance, in China the statement "We will consider it" is a culturally accepted way of saying *no* (Xu, 2012).

Historical and Political Factors

The nurse partner must understand that historical and political forces impact current health care challenges and issues. Lasater et al. (2012) described the years 1975 to 1979 in Cambodia, when the Khmer Rouge regime eliminated a generation of health care leaders, leaving few nurses with the education required to move into faculty positions—thus the country currently has a shortage of nurses. Parfitt et al. (2008) described the historical influence of the Soviet Union on the Tajikistan Republic's health care system until its independence in 1991. Health care under the Soviet system was mechanistic, emphasized treatment of medical conditions by physicians, and showed little understanding of the importance of nursing care. Nurses were regarded as technical assistants to physicians, which influences nursing practice to this day. In India, to avoid the stigmatization of nursing in Muslim and Hindu societies, colonial British missionaries attempted to establish nursing schools and recruit poor women or widows from predominantly Christian communities (Evans et al., 2013). This historical movement, along with other complex factors, contributes to the large supply of nurses in India today. These examples show that history and politics can affect the nursing profession in quite different ways in different countries. The examples reinforce the need for nurse partners to seek understanding of such factors prior to their visit to the host country and through dialogue when on site.

An interesting political factor that may be found at both national and local levels in some host countries is the role of physicians in the governance of nursing education and practice. In the United States nursing has for decades held responsibility and accountability for its education and practice. But the same is not yet the case in all countries. Some examples indicate that physicians play crucial roles in nursing partnerships (Arnold et al., 1998; Bernel, Church, Arevian, & Schensul, 1995; Donahue, Wilimas, Urbina, Grimaldi, & Ribeiro, 2002; Zheng et al., 2001). Nurse partners must be open to these situations, recognizing that they present an opportunity to collaborate with the host to address both structural and workforce development so that in time nurses can assume the appropriate level of authority for the nursing profession within the host country.

Economic and Environmental Factors

Educational institutions in host countries often lack resources, such as instructional supplies, suitable space, and educational equipment for classroom and clinical learning (Berland et al., 2010). This can create a theory–practice gap in student learning. For example, host country students may be taught a certain process or skill but because of limited resources or facilities never experience or witness the actual practice (Evans et al., 2013). Nurse partners who are teaching in the host country must be flexible regarding the technology available for instruction. In addition, donated equipment or materials must be culturally appropriate for the host country if they are to be useful.

Considerations for Students

When nursing student visits and exchange programs are planned efforts must be taken to ensure that expectations of both partners (host and nurse) are congruent (Leffers & Mitchell, 2011). Emphasis should focus on preparing students on both sides of the exchange for cultural differences and variations needed for learning in an unfamiliar environment (Kulbok et al., 2012). The focus of the international exchange must embody goals and values of both partners to avoid academic tourism (Cook et al., 2012).

Host partners expect proper student selection and orientation for the host setting. Recommended criteria for selection include cultural sensitivity, interpersonal skills, flexibility, and maturity (Memmott et al., 2010). Leffers and Plotnick (2011) suggested the following criteria for successful student experiences:

- Strong infrastructure for the nurse–host partnership
- Identified outcome indicators for both the host partner and visiting students
- Institutional requirements for safety, health, and liability
- Post-experience reflection and follow-up for sustainability

Frequently reported outcomes for the nurse partner's students have been development of empathy, self-awareness, self-confidence, adaptability, cultural sensitivity, growth in coping mechanisms, and understanding of different nursing practices (Button, Green, Tengnah, Johansson, & Baker, 2005; Edmonds, 2012; Wros & Archer, 2010).

Considerations for Partnering

The host partner expects that the educational partnership will contribute over time to improvements in its nation's public health. They expect cultural bridging to identify mutual goals and anticipate respect and adaptability from the nurse partner (Shah et al., 2001). Ethnocentrism of the nurse partners and their tendency to replicate their own educational programs must be recognized (Cook et al., 2012). To minimize this risk, the nurse partner must set aside ethnocentrism and engage with the host, learning from and with them over the course of the project. Shah et al. purported that nurse partner faculty take on the role of facilitators in the partnering process. For success, the project should be by and from the host partner. The host partner anticipates that the nurse partner understands the major health issues and history of the country (Xu, 2012). Leffers and Mitchell (2011) identified that host partners expect their visitors to be flexible, open to others' perspectives, willing to share leadership, and ready to take personal risks to advocate for social justice and achieve morally sound outcomes.

PARTNERSHIPS TO ADVANCE THE NURSING PROFESSION

Nurses around the world are confronting concerns associated with the delivery of nursing care, recognition of nursing's contributions to health care outcomes, and the strength of the profession in general (Canadian Nurses Association, 2006; Donkor & Andrews, 2011; George & Lovering, 2013; Hennessy, Hicks, Hilan, & Kawonal, 2006). International partnerships are a means of sharing information about professional nursing practice and approaches for advancing the profession within LMICs. These experiences provide opportunities for nurse partners to enhance their knowledge of the global community and develop professionally and personally. This type of partnership forges connections among nurses from different cultural backgrounds, thereby increasing the opportunities to learn, value, and empower other cultures. In this section we review how host factors influence international nursing partnerships focused on advancing the nursing profession.

Purposes

The nursing profession in Western countries is perceived as having relatively high status and exhibits educational and leadership sophistication, specialization and subspecialization, and a diversity of practice models. Continuing education programs, models of leadership development, and the influence of professional societies on nursing practice and status are well established. Nursing departments in health care institutions are typically empowered with decision-making authority commensurate with the centrality of their role to health care. These structures and processes position Western nurse partners to offer expertise and strategies to help nursing in LMICs advance professionally so that their citizens can benefit from their knowledge and skills. Assistance varies depending on the specific professionalizing needs of the host partner. The following were identified as needs and goals of nursing in LMICs:

- Continuing education and training for nurses to practice at a level consistent with international standards (Bernal et al., 1995; Collins, 2011; Halabi, Majali, Carlsson, & Bergbom, 2011; Lasater et al., 2012; Parfitt et al., 2008)
- Professional development in hospital-based nursing staff (Bentson, Latayan, Olander, & Rocco, 2005; Kemp & Tindiweegi, 2001)
- Leadership development for top-level nurse leaders (Parfitt et al., 2008; Spicer et al., 2010)
- Integration of specialty knowledge into current clinical practice (Caniza et al., 2007; Donahue et al., 2002; Girot & Enders, 2004; Pieper & Caliri, 2002; Reed, 2011)
- Advice on capacity building for the nursing profession at national levels (Bernal et al., 1995; Parfitt et al., 2008; Swenson, Salmon, Wold, & Sibley, 2005)
- Establishment of dialogue among nurses globally (Driever, Perfiljeva, Callister, & McGivern, 2005; Swenson et al., 2005)

A variety of mechanisms are used for this type of partnership. Twinning, a collaborative relationship between two organizations, has been used to link nurses from a partner hospital to nurses at a host hospital (Bentson et al., 2005; Brown, Rickard, Mustriwati, & Seilor, 2013; Jiang, Erickson, Ditomassi, & Adams, 2012). Schools of nursing also have developed twinning relationships to address care needs in particular nurse specialties (Girot & Enders, 2004; Pieper & Caliri, 2002). Twinning usually involves exchange opportunities for nurses from both organizations, with assessment of needs, individual and group staff development, and completion of projects to address the identified needs. Leinonen (2006) reported on outcomes of the international nurse exchange programs that the nursing department at Mayo Clinic has had with hospitals around the world. The programs have fostered global exchange of practice knowledge to enhance quality of care, enhance cultural competence, and reinforce that nurses around the world value human caring.

Another mechanism is links between professional associations, such as the sister chapter partnership between a Wisconsin chapter of the Association for Professionals in Infection Control and Epidemiology and a similar association in Nairobi (McKinley et al., 2013) or the many partnerships the Canadian Nurses Association (2006) has established with nurses around the world. Many others are sponsored through entities such as the World Health Organization, international aid associations within HICs, and nongovernmental organizations (NGOs) (Brown et al., 2013; Caniza et al., 2007; Donkor & Andrews, 2011; Parfitt et al., 2008).

Social and Cultural Factors

As with educational partnerships, many sociocultural dimensions in the host country influence the status and practice of nursing. These include predominant religions, cultural beliefs about health, and gender roles. Nurse partners who understand these dimensions will be better able to work with the host partner to determine a road map for nursing advancement (Hamlin & Brown, 2011). Demographic factors may impact efforts to advance the profession—for example, in some LMICs, the number of physicians exceeds the number of nurses (Ammar, 2009; Berland et al., 2010). Nursing status may be due to the low level of nursing education, such as in Armenia, where nurses may have only completed high school (Bentson et al., 2005). Low status generally is associated with poor pay and lack of respect from physicians and the public (Bentson et al., 2005; Berland et al., 2010).

The social stigma associated with giving personal care to patients is a significant barrier to the advancement of the profession in many LMICs. Reed (2011) noted that Cambodian families, rather than nurses, give the personal care to their hospitalized loved ones. Similarly, after dissolution of the former Soviet system in Tajikistan, nurses were not involved in providing personal care to patients and instead focus primarily on administering drugs and injections. They lack leadership, decision-making, and problem-solving skills. In Brazil, nurses who specialize in obstetrics follow a medical model and focus on assisting the obstetrician; they also spend considerable time on administrative duties to support the institution, leaving less time for direct patient care (Girot & Enders, 2004).

Communication factors like those discussed in the Educational Partnerships section of this chapter also influence partnerships to advance the profession. The exchange program described by Leinonen (2006) assesses the English-language proficiency of nurse visitors through TOEFL examination or telephone conversation prior to the trip. When a minimum level of communication is not demonstrated through these means, the visitor is accompanied by a translator. Likewise, when the hospital's nurses travel abroad, their preparation includes learning about verbal and nonverbal communication patterns, exchange of gifts, and strategies for presenting through an interpreter.

Historical and Political Factors

The same types of historical and political factors that affect educational partnerships again affect partnerships to advance the profession. Health policies and structures at the national or regional level determine where and in what roles nurses can practice. For example, in countries that emerged from the former Soviet Union, the physician-dominated health structure kept nurses in physician assistant roles. Partnership projects have aimed at increasing nurses' independent functioning, but the processes have involved physicians in recognition of their historical role vis-à-vis nursing (Bernal et al., 1995; Driever et al., 2005; Parfitt et al., 2008).

It is vital for the nurse partner to understand the regulation of nursing in the host country and the dynamics between health professions so that advancement of nursing practice can be planned in a judicial manner without creating additional problems for host-country nurses. For example, in Lebanon, where the number of physicians is almost double the number of nurses, it would be very difficult to advocate for the nurse practitioner role (Mouro, 2012). In other countries nurses are needed to practice in advanced roles because of the high demand for specialized care, such as nurse anesthesia (Collins, 2011) and nurse midwifery (Girot & Enders, 2004).

Economic and Environmental Factors

Economic factors in a host setting determine the future work environment of nurses and how much money can be invested in supporting the nursing profession. Nurse partners must work with host partners to develop plans that match the financial resources of the host country. For example, China has a large nursing workforce, but is facing a critical nursing shortage because Chinese nurses are being recruited by HIC. Nurse migration is an issue worldwide that affects the nurse workforce and professional status of nurses globally. It is worth noting that Sigma Theta Tau International (2005) recognized international nurse migration as a serious issue affecting nursing worldwide. The International Council of Nursing (ICN) has asserted that nurses in all countries have the right to migrate as a function of choice and recognizes the potential benefits of nurse migration. However, international nurse migration can affect health care quality in regions or countries in negative ways by seriously depleting the nursing workforce in the home country (ICN, 2007). Jiang et al. (2012) described a twinning relationship between a Chinese and an American teaching hospital that would help the Chinese hospital enhance the role, presence, and overall impact of nursing, and presumably increase retention of their nurses in China.

Factors in the work environment for nurses in many host countries, such as scheduling, shift rotation, and relations with physicians, control the level of nurse job satisfaction and retention (Yaktin, Azoury, & Doumit, 2003). Equipment that nurses use to provide care may be old, out-of-date, or not even existent in the host setting (Bentson et al., 2005; Reed, 2011). Even things as basic as linens, clean water, and electricity may be in short supply (Foster, 2009). Therefore, it is imperative that careful assessment be made of the physical and practice environment to ensure that planning for professional development activities matches the context in which the host partners work.

Arnold and colleagues (1998) described another aspect of the host environment that nurse partners may determine a barrier to advancement efforts: the milieu and involvement of patients in care. They reported the absence of values such as patient rights, privacy, and informed consent in the health care system of countries formerly within the Soviet Union. Additionally, hospitals and clinics were cold, dark, and dreary. Foster (2009) reported that similar deficits in the clinical setting coupled with an unrelenting workload contributed to compassion fatigue among nurses. Nurse partners who are inculcated with the patient-centered care approach will find such settings very challenging.

Considerations for Partnering

Nursing practice in one country cannot be copied in total to another, nor can the structure of the profession. Nurse partners must be open to learn the cultural, political, economic, and environmental contexts of the host partner. Preparation will help prevent nurse partners from having incomplete or shallow knowledge about the host country and culture and preclude adverse outcomes (Currier, 2001; Leininger, 1998). Mutual preparation by the partners can include introductory meetings and communications to share institutional and contextual information, clarify goals, establish criteria and roles for those involved from both partners, determine the partnership activities, and establish how ongoing communication and monitoring will occur (Bentson et al., 2005; Jiang et al., 2012; Leinonen, 2006). It also is important to assess the predisposing, enabling, and reinforcing factors that will contribute (or not) to the success of the partnership. Predisposing factors are those that provide the reason for making a change, such as knowledge, attitudes, cultural beliefs, and readiness to change. Enabling factors are the available resources, supportive policies, assistance, and services that are present and allow the host to act on his or her predispositions. After a change has been initiated, the reinforcing factors encourage persistence through rewards or incentives (Glanz & Rimer, 2005).

International partnerships to develop the profession provide an arena for nurses from many countries to have open discussion about nursing practice. Through these partnerships nurses increase their understanding of global health care issues and nursing concerns. At the same time the opportunity helps them establish relationships with various cultures and expands opportunities to learn, empower, and value other cultures (Scholes & Moore, 2000). It is essential to emphasize that the exchange of nursing knowledge and practice patterns is mutually beneficial.

PARTNERSHIPS FOR PROVIDING CLINICAL CARE

The third type of partnership is aimed at providing clinical and preventive care for a specific population or group of citizens. This category overlaps in some ways with educational partnerships that include a clinical or service-learning component. Using the lens of providing clinical services to a population offers further understanding and appreciation for how host factors impact an international partnership. In reviewing the literature on clinical care partnerships we found no examples that involved nurses exclusively. Rather, nursing is one discipline of the interprofessional team; in some cases we draw from medical literature.

Purposes

The United Nations Millennium Development Goals 2000–2015 (MDG) (www.undp.org/mdg/goallist.shtml) provide a broad context within which clinical care partnerships with LMICs can occur. This, however, is not always the case. Many clinical care programs in

LMICs are designed to meet the interests of the visiting partner and may involve little mutuality with the host during the planning or service delivery phase. Nurse partners can use the MDG as a framework for proactive planning with the host to ensure that when the visitors leave, whether the service delivery has been long or short, the host is in a better position to achieve the MDG than before the service was provided.

1. Eradicate extreme poverty and hunger
2. Achieve universal primary education
3. Promote gender equality and empower women
4. Reduce child mortality
5. Improve maternal health
6. Combat HIV/AIDS, malaria, and other diseases
7. Ensure environmental sustainability
8. Develop a global partnership for development

The following are examples of specific programs that link with the MDG:

- Professional development on women's health topics (Nicholas et al., 2009; Vitols, du Plessis, & Ng'andu, 2007)
- Developing and delivering primary care (Sherr et al., 2013; Sloand & Groves, 2005)
- Prevention of communicable diseases through immunization (Andrus, Jauregui, De Oliveira, & Matus, 2011)

These examples illustrate several fundamental elements. Partnerships that fulfill the meaning of "partner" and are strong enough to address persistent health needs can take years to develop (Vitols et al., 2007). To address the intractability of the problems targeted by the MDG, the partnership should include efforts and activities to strengthen the local, regional, or national health care system (Sherr et al., 2013). Sloand and Groves (2005) showed that building the service on a partnership model that has been successful in other settings can enhance the effectiveness of a new project with different partners. Another feature of successful and sustainable clinical care projects is to collaborate with initiatives already underway in the host setting (Andrus et al., 2011). Nurses from HIC who have enthusiasm for developing a short-term project in an LMIC can use the above approaches to convert a one-time effort into a partnership that has higher potential for sustained impact for both host and visitor.

Social and Cultural Factors

Each clinical care partnership will encounter social and cultural factors unique to their locale, but two examples show how important it is to understand these influences. One of the social factors is demographics. Leng and colleagues (2010) reported a partnership with a health care institution in China to develop a geriatrics program. The need for this program was driven by changing demographic and social factors. China has the largest aging population in the world: In 2008 1.65 million Chinese were older than 65 years of age. This is coupled with migration of many working-age adults from rural to urban settings to seek employment, which has disrupted the traditional practice of children caring for their aging parents. Another demographic factor in China is the "inverted pyramid" phenomenon, or "4-2-1," whereby prior limits on family size leads to a three-generation family composed of one child who is responsible for caring for two parents and four elderly grandparents.

Gender issues can have a striking influence on clinical care partnerships. Nicholas et al. (2009) reported on opportunities for American nurses to contribute to HIV/AIDS care in sub-Saharan Africa. In these countries, women's health status is negatively affected by the absence of women's rights, gender inequality, sexual violence, and economic disempowerment as a result of unemployment and discrimination. The high incidence of HIV/AIDS in women is devastating to families and communities and to the health care system. Vitols et al. (2007) reported that the prevalence of HIV/AIDS is high among nurses in sub-Saharan countries. In addition to transmission through sexual violence, HIV/AIDS is an occupational hazard because of the high number of patients with the disease. And although nurses may have knowledge about HIV/AIDS, generally they have received little training in prevention and clinical management. They often have inadequate knowledge and protection from exposure in the work setting.

Historical and Political Factors

Many clinical partnerships are developed to help countries recovering from political disturbances, war, or natural disasters. Patients who present for care in these circumstances usually have significant illnesses, so the clinical work is heavy and challenging (Henderson, 2007). Sometimes the health workforce has left the country or been devastated during the conflict. Before leaving the host setting the visiting partner may be expected to train individuals who have little or no health background to provide care needed by the patients. For visiting partners who work in areas where conflicts are still occurring, security concerns can arise.

National, regional, and local politics have the potential to influence the efficacy of clinical service partnerships, especially when all levels of government have a role in health care policy and regulation. Gill et al. (2013) discussed the poorly articulated goals and lack of coordination among aid agencies, governmental agencies, NGOs, funders, and the private sector in efforts to reduce childhood mortality from pneumonia and diarrhea. Sherr and colleagues (2013) noted that it can be difficult to determine what level of government (district, provincial, or national) is responsible for a particular scope of services.

Economic and Environmental Factors

When reporting on factors that influence the availability of drug therapy for children, MacLeod, Finch, Macharia, and Anabwani (2013) explained that even in LMICs there are discrepancies in care: children in rural regions, who have less education and who are poorer, tend to be marginalized. Thus, a nurse partner may encounter health disparities when engaged in a partnership service with a host agency.

Anecdotal stories from anesthesiologists who spent time providing care in war-torn and low- and middle-income countries confirm the severe limitations on care when resources are constrained (Henderson, 2007). Small tasks become big challenges when the proper resources are not available. Even though many countries receive donated equipment, often it cannot be used in the setting because it doesn't fit the context. Visiting partners may experience stress and guilt because they are unable to meet the standard of care they expect of themselves. Foster (2009) described the difficulties encountered in a project to improve maternity care at a public hospital in the Dominican Republic because there was an "absolute lack of resources."

Knowledge Resource Factors

Knowledge is a critical resource in providing effective health care that can also be in limited supply in LMICs. Standardized treatment guidelines often aren't available, need to be translated, or need to be adapted to the host culture and available resources (MacLeod et al., 2013). Santesso and Tugwell (2006) linked the difficulty in knowledge translation with a variety of political factors such as conflicts between governmental officials and clinicians about the use of new practices. At the institutional level habits, traditions, and superstitions serve as barriers to knowledge translation. These factors may create difficulty for nurse partners engaged in clinical initiatives, making it problematic for them to deliver care based on current best practices.

Closely linked with the lack of standardized treatment guidelines are data inadequacies. Data collection systems in LMICs typically are weak, capacity for data analysis is limited, and systems to monitor and evaluate the services also serve as impediments to clinical practice upgrades (Andrus et al., 2011; Epelman & Magrath, 2013; Gill et al., 2013; Sherr et al., 2013). For the visiting partner, this may make it difficult to determine the priorities for care and to assess the impact of the services provided.

Considerations for Partnering

Kraeker and Chandler (2013) conducted a qualitative study to determine the perceptions of nine local health care professionals (host partners) associated with a medical school in Namibia that received many visitors. The interviewees had previous contact ranging from a few months to several years with visiting partners. They reported that visiting students and teachers often showed a lack of concern about the local culture, which rendered the clinical services they provided ineffective. Partners were described by the host professionals as attempting to impose their own visions of care. While they brought good ideas, the ideas were rarely relevant to the context. A second area of concern was that visiting partners often tried to carry out projects without seeking input from the hosts, which led to duplication, frustration, and wasted time. Educational models frequently did not fit the context and did not involve the host participants. Nonetheless, the host partners yearned to improve the process of the visits, feeling that if the partnership between the visitors and hosts became equal, they stood to gain more than they would lose.

In contrast, a report by Sloand and Groves (2005) provided an example of equality between the nurse and host partners and of the positive benefits that accrued. Theirs is an ongoing project in which an interprofessional team uses a community primary care service model to deliver 1 week of care each year in Haiti. The host champion is the pastor of a local church who selects the villages that will be served. The visiting partners who provide the primary care work with local nurses, translators, and lay village leaders who advise, communicate to the population to be served, set the fee structure, staff clinic registration, and work alongside the visiting professionals. These hosts also provide information to the visitors about usual treatments for indigenous diseases, management options for local diseases, and the local health care system. The translators "translated both words and the deeper meanings of those words" (p. 48). For the community care services Haitian school teachers and an order of sisters help the visiting partners understand the community health needs and assist in providing community education.

CONCLUSION

In the most successful international nursing initiatives the nurse and host partners do not singularly teach, translate, or give (Freire, 1993). On the contrary, the essence of the collaborative process is about exchange of nursing knowledge to build a dynamic, mutually beneficial, and sustainable nursing exchange. Baumann's (2012) editorial about dilemmas in international partnerships further reinforces this position. He wrote, "Efforts to improve nursing and the health and quality of life of people in various places in many parts of the world cannot be done without engaging in cultural and political change. . . . Governments may have little ability or be unwilling to provide universal access to quality healthcare. . . . The nature and manner of the assistance to be provided should be guided by the recipients of the project. . . . Nurses need to maintain the attitude that they are the guests and students of the local history and ways" (p. 182).

As the examples presented in this chapter show, no two host countries or settings will be alike. Each country has a different set of sociocultural factors, its own history and politics, and unique economic and environmental factors that will affect the partnering effort. Both partners have a role in identifying the factors in the host setting that will influence their project and its outcomes. The nurse partner will be well served by using the three elements of a framework proposed by Hunt and colleagues (2012) for those doing humanitarian work in LMICs—"The Ethics of Engaged Presence":

1. Recognize his or her shared humanity with those in need of assistance.
2. Acknowledge the limits of his or her ability to assist and the risks that are associated with helping.
3. Provide competent, practical assistance.

By adopting this ethical stance, the nurse partner will both learn and contribute.

REFERENCES

Ammar, W. (2009). *Health beyond politics*. Beirut, Lebanon: World Health Organization.

Andrus, J. K., Jauregui, B., De Oliveira, L. H., & Matus, C. R. (2011). Challenges to building capacity for evidence-based new vaccine policy in developing countries. *Health Affairs, 30*(6), 1104–1112. doi: 10.1377/hlthaff.2011.0361

Arnold, L., Bakhtarina, I., Brooks, A. M., Coulter, S., Hurt, L., Lewis, C., . . . Younger, J. (1998). Nursing in the newly independent states of the former Soviet Union: An international partnership for nursing development. *Journal of Obstetric, Gynecologic and Neonatal Nursing, 27*(2), 203–208.

Baumann, S. L. (2012). Dilemmas of international collaborative nursing partnerships. *Nursing Science Quarterly, 25*(2), 182–183. doi: 10.1177/0894318412437954

Bentson, J., Latayan, M. B., Olander, L., & Rocco, J. (2005). A nursing partnership: The forces of magnetism guiding evidence-based practice in the Republic of Armenia. *Journal of Continuing Education in Nursing, 36*(4), 175–179.

Berland, A., Richards J., & Lund, K. D. (2010). A Canada–Bangladesh partnership for nurse education: Case study. *International Nursing Review, 57*, 352–358.

Bernal, H., Church, O. M., Arevian, M., & Schensul, S. L. (1995). Community health nursing in a former Soviet Union republic: A case study of change in Armenia. *Nursing Outlook, 43*(2), 78–83.

Brown, D., Rickard, G., Mustriwati, K. A., & Seiler, J. (2013). International partnerships and the development of a sister hospital programme. *International Nursing Review, 60*, 45–51.

Button, L., Green, B., Tengnah, C., Johansson, I., & Baker, C. (2005). The impact of international placements on nurses' personal and professional lives: Literature review. *Journal of Advanced Nursing, 50*(3), 315–324.

Canadian Nurses Association. (2006). Celebrating international nursing partnerships. *Canadian Nurse, 102*(6), 15–17.

Caniza, M. A., Maron, G., McCullers, J., Clara, W. A., Cedillos, R., Duenas, L., . . . Tuomanen, E. I. (2007). Planning and implementation of an infection control training program for healthcare providers in Latin America. *Infection Control and Hospital Epidemiology, 28*(12), 1328–1333. doi: 10.1086/521655

Casey, D. J. (1999). Professional links: An international program for nursing knowledge exchange. *Journal of Pediatric Nursing, 14*(3), 143–149.

Collins, S. B. (2011). Model for a reproducible curriculum infrastructure to provide international nurse anesthesia continuing education. *AANA Journal, 79*(6), 491–496.

Cook, S. S., Sheerin, F., Bancel, S., & Gomes, J. C. R. (2012). Curriculum meeting points: A transcultural and transformative initiative in nursing education. *Nurse Education in Practice, 12*, 304–309.

Crow, G., & Thuc, L. B. (2011). Leading an international nursing partnership: The Vietnam nurse project. *Nursing Administration Quarterly, 35*(3), 204–211.

Currier, P. A. (2001). An Azorean–American nursing accord of cooperation and exchange: Nurturing the process. *Journal of Multicultural Nursing & Health, 7*(2), 23–28.

Donahue, N., Wilimas, J., Urbina, C., de Grimaldi, G., & Ribeiro, R. (2002). International hematology-oncology nursing education in Latin America. *Journal of Pediatric Oncology Nursing, 19*(3), 79–83. doi: 10.1053/jpon.2002.123448

Donkor, N. T., & Andrews, L. D. (2011). 21st century nursing practice in Ghana: Challenges and opportunities. *International Nursing Review, 58*, 218–224.

Driever, M. J., Perfiljeva, G., Callister, L. C., & McGivern, S. (2005). Creating a context for professional dialogue between U.S. and Russian nurses: Design of an international conference. *Journal of Continuing Education in Nursing, 36*(4), 168–174.

Edmonds, M. L. (2012). An integrative literature review of study abroad programs for nursing students. *Nursing Education Perspectives, 33*(1), 30–34.

Epelman, S., & Magrath, I. (2013). Planning cancer control: The view of an NGO. *The Lancet Oncology, 14*(5), 388–390. doi: 10.1016/S1470-2045(13)70090-1

Evans, C., Razia, R., & Cook, E. (2013). Building nurse education capacity in India: Insights from a faculty development programme in Andhra Pradesh. *BMC Nursing. 12*(8), 1–8. doi: 10.1186/1472-6955-12-8

Finkelman, A., & Kenner, C. (2008). Educational and service partnerships: An example of global flattening. *Journal of Professional Nursing, 24*, 59–65.

Foster, J. (2009). Cultural humility and the importance of long-term relationships in international partnerships. *Journal of Obstetric, Gynecologic and Neonatal Nursing, 38*(1), 100–107.

Freire, P. (1993). *Pedagogy of the oppressed.* New York, NY: Continuum.

Ganske, K., Zerull, L., Guinn, C., Dowling, G., & Tagnesi, K. (2007). Reaching across the pond: A global exchange between health systems. *International Nursing Review, 54*, 295–300.

George, V., & Lovering, S. (2013). Transforming the context of care through shared leadership and partnership: An international CNO perspective. *Nursing Administration Quarterly, 37*(1), 52–59. doi: 10.1097/NAQ.0b013e3182751732

George, E. K., & Meadows-Oliver, M. (2013). Searching for collaboration in international nursing partnerships: A literature review. *International Nursing Review, 60*(1), 31–36. doi: 10.1111/j.1466-7657.2012.01034.x

Gill, C. J., Young, M., Schroder, K., Carvajal-Velez, M. A., McNabb, M., Aboubaker, S., . . . Bhutta, Z. A. (2013). Bottlenecks, barriers and solutions: Results from multicountry consultations focused on reduction of childhood pneumonia and diarrhoea deaths. *The Lancet, 381*, 1487–1498. doi: http://dx.doi.org.ezproxy.lau.edu.lb:2048/10.1016/S0140-6736(13)60314-1

Girot, E. A., & Enders, B. C. (2004). International educational partnership for practice: Brazil and the United Kingdom. *Journal of Advanced Nursing, 46*(2), 144–151.

Glanz, K., & Rimer, B. (2005). *Theory at a glance: A guide for health promotion practice* (2nd ed.). Publication Number: T052. NIH Number: 05-3896. U.S. Department of Health and Human Services. National Institutes of Health. Bethesda, MD: National Cancer Institute. www.cancer.gov/cancertopics/cancerlibrary/theory.pdf

Halabi, J. O., Majali, S., Carlsson, L., & Bergbom, I. (2011). A model for international nursing collaboration. *Journal of Continuing Education in Nursing, 42*(4), 154–163. doi: 10.3928/00220124-20101001-01

Hamlin, L., & Brown, D. (2011). Changing perioperative practice in an Indonesian hospital. *AORN Journal, 94*(4), 403–408. doi: 10.1016/j.aorn.2011.05.012

Henderson, K. (2007). Lessons from working overseas. *Anaesthesia, 62* (Suppl. 1), 113–117.

Hennessy, D., Hicks, C., Hilan, A., & Kawonal, J. (2006). The training and development needs of nurses in Indonesia. *Human Resources for Health, 4*(10). www.human-resources-health.com/content/4/1/10 doi:10.1186/1478-4491-4-10

Hunt, M. R., Schwartz, L., Sinding, C., & Elit, L. (2012). The ethics of engaged presence: A framework for health professionals in humanitarian assistance and development work. *Developing World Bioethics, 1471*–8847. doi: 10.1111/dweb.12013

International Council of Nurses. (2007). *Position statement: Nurse retention and migration.* Geneva, Switzerland: Author. www.icn.ch/publications/position-statements

Jiang, H., Erickson, J. I., Ditomassi, M., & Adams, J. M. (2012). Promoting a culture of international professional practice for nursing through a twinning relationship. *Journal of Nursing Administration, 42*(2), 117–122. doi: 10.1097/NNA.0b013e318243384e

Kemp, J., & Tindiweegi, J. (2001). Nurse education in Mbarara, Uganda. *Journal of Advanced Nursing, 33*(1), 8–12.

Kraeker, C., & Chandler, C. (2013). "We learn from them, they learn from us": Global health experiences and host perceptions of visiting health care professionals. *Academic Medicine, 88*(4), 1–5. doi: 10.1097/ACM.0b013e3182857b8a

Kulbok, P. A., Mitchell, E. M., Glick, D. F., & Greiner, D. (2012). International experiences in nursing education: A review of the literature. *International Journal of Nursing Educational Scholarship, 9*(1), Article 7. doi: 10.1515/1548-923X.2365

Lasater, K., Upvall, M., Nielsen, A., Prak, M., & Ptachcinski, R. (2012). Global partnerships for professional development: A Cambodian exemplar. *Journal of Professional Nursing, 28*(1), 62–68. doi: 10.1016/j.profnurs.2011.10.002

Leffers, J., & Mitchell, E. (2011). Conceptual model for partnership and sustainability in global health. *Public Health Nursing, 28*(1), 91–102. doi: 10.1111/j.1525-1446.2010.00892.x

Leffers, J., & Plotnick, J. (2011). *Volunteering at home and abroad: The essential guide for nurses.* Indianapolis, IN: Sigma Theta Tau International.

Leininger, M. (1998). Nursing education exchanges: Concerns and benefits. *Journal of Transcultural Nursing, 9*, 57–63.

Leinonen, S. J. (2006). International nursing exchange programs. *Journal of Continuing Education in Nursing, 37*(1), 16–20.

Leng, S. X., Tian, X., Liu, X., Lazarus, G., Bellantoni, M., Greenough, W., . . . Durso, S. C. (2010). An international model for geriatrics program development in China: The Johns Hopkins–Peking Union Medical College experience. *Journal of the American Geriatrics Society, 58*, 1376–1381. doi: 10.1111/j.1532-5415.2010.02927.x

MacLeod, S. M., Finch, J. K., Macharia, W. M., & Anabwani, G. M. (2013). Better drug therapy for the children of Africa: Current impediments to success and potential strategies for improvement. *Pediatric Drugs, 15*, 259–269. doi: 10.1007/s40272-013-0015-7

Malloy, P., Paice, J. A., Ferrell, B. R., Ali, Z., Munyoro, E., Coyne, P., & Smith, T. (2011). Advancing palliative care in Kenya. *Cancer Nursing, 34*(1), 10–13. doi: 10.1097/NCC.0b013e3181ea73dd

McKinley, L., Auel, C., Bahr, M., Hutchings, A., Leary, M., Moskal, N., . . . Rosemeyer, S. (2013). Building global partnerships in infection prevention: A report from APIC Badger and the Nairobi Infection Control Nurses Chapter. *American Journal of Infection Control, 41*, 281–282. doi: 10.1016/j.apic.2012.03.024

Memmott, R. J., Coverston, C. R., Heise, B. A., Williams, M., Maughan, E. D., Kohl J., & Palmer, S. (2010). Practical considerations in establishing sustainable international nursing experiences. *Nursing Education Perspectives, 31*(5), 298–302.

Mouro, G. (2012, November). Lebanese hospitals in 2020: Shaping the future of nursing, nurse retention strategies. Beirut, Lebanon: Arab Hospitals Federation, Med Health 2012.

Nicholas, P. K., Adejumo, O., Nokes, K. M., Ncama, B. P., Bhengu, B. R., Elston, E., & Nicholas, T. P. (2009). Fulbright Scholar opportunities for global health and women's health care in HIV/AIDS in sub-Saharan Africa. *Applied Nursing Research, 22*, 73–77. doi: 10.1016/j.apnr/2008.09.006

Parfitt, B., Mughal M., & Thomas, H. (2008). Working together: A nursing development project in Tajikistan. *International Nursing Review, 55*, 205–211.

Pieper, B., & Caliri, M. H. L. (2002). An international partnership: Impacting wound care in Brazil. *Journal of Wound, Ostomy and Continence Nursing, 29*(6), 287–294.

Plager, K., & Razaonandrianina, J. (2009). Madagascar nursing needs assessment: Education and development of the profession. *International Nursing Review, 56*, 58–64. doi: 10.1111/j.1466-7657.2008.00696.x

Reed, K. S. (2011). Introduction of rehabilitation nursing concepts in Cambodia. *Rehabilitation Nursing, 36*(5), 186–190.

Santesso, N., & Tugwell, P. (2006). Knowledge translation in developing countries. *Journal of Continuing Education in the Health Professions, 26*, 87–96. doi: 10.1002/chp.55

Scholes, J., & Moore, D. (2000). Clinical exchange: One model to achieve culturally sensitive care. *Nursing Inquiry, 7*(1), 61–71.

Shah, M. A., Robinson, T. C., & Al Enezi, N. (2001). International allied health education and cross-cultural perspectives. *Journal of Allied Health, 31*(3), 165–170.

Sherr, K., Cuembelo, F., Michel, C., Gimbel, S., Micek, M., Kariaganis, M., . . . Gloyd, S. (2013). Strengthening integrated primary health care in Sofala, Mozambique. *BMC Health Services Research, 13*(Suppl. 2), 54. www.biomedcentral.com/1472-6963/13/S2/S4. doi:10.1186/1472-6963-13-S2-S4

Sigma Theta Tau International. (2005). International nurse migration. www.nursingsociety.org/aboutus/PositionPapers/Pages/position_resource_papers.aspx

Sloand, E., & Groves, S. (2005). A community-oriented primary care nursing model in an international setting that emphasizes partnerships. *Journal of the American Academy of Nurse Practitioners, 17*(2), 47–50.

Spicer, J. G., Guo, Y., Liu, H., Hirsch, J., Zhao, H., Ma, W., & Holzemer, W. (2010). Collaborative nursing leadership project in the People's Republic of China. *International Nursing Review, 57*, 180–187.

Swenson, M. J., Salmon, M. E., Wold, J., & Sibley, L. (2005). Addressing the challenges of the global nursing community. *International Nursing Review, 52*, 173–179.

Uys, L. R., & Middleton, L. (2011). Internationalizing university schools of nursing in South Africa through a community of practice. *International Nursing Review, 58*, 115–122.

Vitols, M. P., du Plessis, E., & Ng'andu, O. (2007). Mitigating the plight of HIV-infected and -affected nurses in Zambia. *International Nursing Review, 54*, 375–382.

Wollin, J. A., & Fairweather, C. T. (2012). Nursing education: A case study of a bachelor of science nursing programme in Abu Dhabi, United Arab Emirates. *Journal of Nursing Management, 20*, 20–27. doi: 10.1111/j.1365-2834.2011.01298.x

Wros, P., & Archer, S. (2010). Comparing learning outcomes of international and local community partnerships for undergraduate nursing students. *Journal of Community Health Nursing, 27*, 216–225. doi: 10.1080/07370016.2010.515461

Xu, Y. (2012). International nursing exchange and collaboration with China: A perspective from the south and the east. *Nursing Forum, 47*(4), 236–244. doi: 10.1111/j.1744-6198.2012.00280.x

Yaktin, U. S., Azoury, N. B., & Doumit, M. A. A. (2003). Personal characteristics and job satisfaction among nurses in Lebanon. *Journal of Nursing Administration, 22*(7/8), 384–390.

Zheng, X. X., Hinshaw, A. S., Yu, M. Y., Guo, G. F., & Oakley, D. J. (2001). Building international partnerships. *International Nursing Review, 48*, 117–121.

Considering Host Partner Factors in Developing a Nursing Program in Lebanon

Nancy Hoffart
Jenny Vacek
Myrna A. A. Doumit
Judy Liesveld
Debra Brady

This case reports on the educational partnership between the Alice Ramez Chagoury School of Nursing (ARCSON), the Lebanese American University (LAU), and the University of New Mexico College of Nursing (UNMCON). The ARCSON-UNMCON partnership incorporated three of the purposes we presented in Chapter 4: (1) develop a pre-licensure curriculum, (2) use an innovative curriculum model, and (3) provide faculty development. In this case study we illustrate how some of the host factors discussed in Chapter 4, at the national and university levels, influenced our educational partnership.

CONTEXT: LEBANON

Lebanon is a small country on the eastern shore of the Mediterranean Sea. It occupies only 10,452 km^2 (4,015 mi^2), yet it has varied geography and a beautiful natural environment, with 225 km of Mediterranean coastline, rugged mountain peaks as high as 3,088 m (10,131 ft), and the fertile Bekaa Valley. The Lebanese population is estimated to be 4.2 million, although an official Lebanese census has not been taken in decades. Lebanese citizens fall into primarily four religious groups: Christians, Druze, Shia Muslim, and Sunni Muslim; this mix of religions makes it unique within the Middle East. There are also close to 0.5 million Palestinian refugees, who have been displaced from their homeland for three generations. Lebanon is also receiving a significant influx of refugees from the Syrian civil war, estimated to be over 1 million at the time of this writing. Regardless of their background, the Lebanese are warm and welcoming to visitors and are proud of their traditional hospitality.

Education is a high priority in the country, and the literacy rate is over 87%. Arabic is the official language, and many Lebanese speak two or more secondary languages—French and English are the most common. The elementary, intermediate, and secondary school system is modeled on the European model, with schools offering their curriculums in either French or English. On passing a national Baccalaureate II examination (equivalent to the International Baccalaureate) students can apply for admission to university and enroll as sophomores.

In the 2013 UN Human Development Report, Lebanon was ranked number 72 and fell into the category "high human development," with reported gross national income per capita of $12,364 (www.undp.org/content/dam/undp). Economically it is considered a developing country and receives aid from many high-income countries to support improvements in infrastructure and services in several sectors (e.g., health, education, environment, and energy). There are wide disparities in income among Lebanon's residents, with high unemployment and pockets of citizens who live in abject poverty. Employment in the country is largely service-based, and remittances from abroad are an important contribution to the economic base. Tourism and banking are two of the main service sectors.

Lebanon's built environment is somewhat haphazard. Damaged and abandoned buildings serve as reminders of the long civil war from 1975 to 1990. The population density and lack of public transportation options leads to crowded and chaotic roads. The electrical and communication technology grids reflect little planning, but entrepreneurs have created an informal grid. Periodic electricity and Internet service interruptions are experienced throughout the country. Lebanon's location in the Middle East puts it into the UTC+2 (Coordinated Universal Time) zone.

Lebanon has been the crossroads for many great civilizations, including the Phoenicians, Romans, and Ottomans. The ruins of these civilizations, often built one on top of the other, can be found throughout the country. Lebanon was established as an independent democratic republic in 1943. It has a parliamentary form of government with representation based on confession (religious group). The country is affected by the political unrest within the Middle East. Tensions among some Lebanese religious sects that are tied to politically active groups in the region create uncertainty and wariness; over the years these tensions have led to disruptions and bombings with resultant internal and international repercussions. After a bombing in 1983 killed more than 200 American soldiers, the U.S. State Department banned all American travel to Lebanon. The travel ban was lifted in 1997, but even now travel warnings remain in effect for the country. Nonetheless, many expatriates reside in Lebanon, and the country receives international tourists and business travelers.

Lebanese citizens have access to health care through a wide array of hospitals and ambulatory settings; payment for care is through a mix of private and governmental insurance. Most hospitals are privately owned as family businesses, and there are several academic medical centers. Many NGOs have been established to address specific health needs and offer preventive services. Citizens can access care ranging from primary preventive care to tertiary care, although links among the services along the continuum of care are not well developed. The least developed type of service is community-based care. Data on the incidence and prevalence of disease is not readily available, although the Ministry of Health and a few specialty health associations periodically collect and disseminate health statistics.

The Lebanese environment for nursing education and practice can be confusing to an outsider. The number of physicians in the country is approximately double the number of nurses, which is currently 10,518 (bachelor of science in nursing [BSN] graduates number 4,965) (www.orderofnurses.org.lb). Graduates of three types of nursing programs are eligible to sit for the RN licensure examination: high school–level programs, technical school certificate level, and BSN degree (Huijer, Noureddine, & Dumit, 2005). The examination, or colloquium, is an oral examination administered through the Lebanese ministry of higher education. Colloquium questions are written by faculty from the various nursing programs, and nursing faculty from the schools serve as the examiners. Consequently, nursing program faculty are aware of the topics covered so that they can ensure that this content is included in their respective curricula.

Lebanese American University

LAU is a New York State–chartered higher education institution located in Lebanon. LAU has a rich history from its beginning in 1835 as the first school for girls in the Middle East (www.lau.edu.lb/about/history). In the ensuing decades the school underwent much growth and many changes, converting to coeducation and developing multiple campuses (one in Beirut, Lebanon's largest city, and the other in Byblos, one of the oldest continuously occupied cities in the world and the place where the Phoenician alphabet, the precursor to the modern alphabet, originated [www.middleeast.com/byblos.htm]).

At the university level, LAU is open to all religions and citizens of the country and the Middle East. It has become the largest and one of the leading private universities in Lebanon, with enrollment in its seven schools exceeding 8,000 undergraduate and graduate students. All instruction is in English and built on a strong liberal arts and science foundation. Professional schools are expected to follow American standards and are encouraged to seek accreditation through American accrediting bodies. In 2010 it received accreditation through the New England Association of Schools and Colleges, substantiating its commitment to meeting high educational standards. Several programs offered by the university aim to instill in the youth of Lebanon a vision of peace within the region and prepare them with skills in negotiation, mediation, and conflict resolution. One of the hallmarks of this effort is the Model United Nations program, which brings middle- and high-school students to campus to learn skills that will prepare them for future civic engagement.

LAU is a private institution, with revenues generated primarily through tuition. Through prudent fiscal management it provides a wide array of academic services to students, generous financial assistance, and many extracurricular programs. Faculty and staff salaries are highly competitive in the region. An example of the expansion of facilities is the recent opening of a new, state-of-the-art building to house the schools of nursing, medicine, and pharmacy. When ARCSON was established, a 10-year budget was approved that included funds for securing needed consultation.

The Alice Ramez Chagoury School of Nursing, the newest school at LAU, admitted its first class into the bachelor of science in nursing (BSN) program in fall 2010. ARCSON is located on LAU's Byblos campus. It is a small school, with six faculty (excluding the dean), who are young (mean age is 34 years). Like the rest of the university, the ARCSON faculty, staff, and students reflect the diversity in the country, coming from different regions and religions. The school's emphasis on human diversity and cultural sensitivity reinforces the university's focus on inclusivity. Other than the assistant dean, faculty members' teaching experience before starting at LAU ranged from 0 to 2 years. Being able to help establish a new school at a reputable university was one factor that most of them considered in seeking a position at ARCSON. All faculty are Lebanese, yet each has studied or lived in the United States: two completed internships in the United States as part of their MSN degree; three earned nursing PhDs at American universities, and one worked in the United States for 3 years. They all also studied at another American university in Lebanon. ARCSON earned accreditation through the Collegiate Commission on Nursing Education in 2013.

THE CONSULTATION AGREEMENT

ARCSON, the host, began operational planning for the BSN program in September 2009, when the founding dean arrived in Lebanon from the United States. When the BSN program was being planned, she decided to use *The Essentials of Baccalaureate Education for Professional Nursing Practice* (AACN, 2006) as the guide for curriculum content, as well as to adopt the concept-based curriculum (CBC) model. She wrote the broad outline for the curriculum, which was approved in spring 2010 through the university's new program approval process. ARCSON's first class of 13 students was admitted to the school in fall 2010 to begin their science prerequisites and liberal arts courses. Hiring of full-time nursing faculty began in February 2011, when an individual with strong nursing education experience was hired to serve as assistant dean. At the same time, two faculty members sponsored by LAU to complete their PhD studies were teaching on a part-time basis. Additional full-time faculty were hired in fall 2011 and fall 2012.

The UNMCON, a leader in development of the CBC in nursing, was invited by the dean to serve as a consultant for curriculum development. Telephone consultations with a CBC faculty champion at the UNMCON, study of CBC publications (Giddens & Brady, 2007; Giddens et al., 2008; Heims & Boyd, 1990; Lasater & Nielsen, 2009; Lee-Hsieh, Kao, Kuo, & Tseng, 2003; Schreier, Peery, & McLean, 2009), and review of UNMCON's website were helpful in creating the framework for the curriculum. Further consultation, however, was deemed necessary to select concepts that would form the matrix for the BSN curriculum, develop the courses, level concepts across the curriculum, develop teaching and evaluation strategies for the CBC, and provide related faculty development. The UNMCON champion suggested that a team of faculty who had expertise across nursing specialties might be an appropriate approach for providing ongoing consultation to the ARCSON faculty. This approach was agreed on, and in May 2011 a formal agreement was negotiated between the two universities.

The consultation activities included in the final agreement were conference calls, webinars, and e-mails between consultants (nurse partners) and host faculty, feedback on drafts of host curriculum materials by consultants, host-partner meetings when faculty from both attended the same professional conference, ARCSON faculty visits to UNM, and consultant visits to LAU. Five UNMCON faculty, the nurse partners, were selected to serve on the consultation team based on their expertise with the CBC and their interest in the project. The agreement was written for 1 year, with the option to renew on an annual basis. The agreement was renewed once. For UNMCON the CBC consultation was a revenue-generating activity and part of the college's faculty practice plan.

UNMCON adopted a concept-based BSN curriculum secondary to concerns that nursing curricula in general have reached the point of content saturation and that the traditional mode of teaching (e.g., lectures) was impairing students' ability to absorb the knowledge and think critically (Giddens & Brady, 2007; Giddens et al., 2008). The curriculum includes health and illness constructs, which address the biophysical needs of the client, and professional nursing constructs, which focus on professional skills needed by the practicing nurse. Concept instruction includes use of exemplars based on disease incidence and prevalence and to address all levels of health promotion, life-span needs and problems, and application to various health care settings. Integrative learning strategies have been implemented in addition to traditional lecture-style presentations.

HOST FACTORS AND THEIR INFLUENCE ON THE PARTNERSHIP

Historical and Political Factors

A factor related to the political situation in Lebanon had the most significant impact on our partnership. When the consultation agreement was negotiated with the UNMCON the plan specifically included UNMCON faculty travel to Lebanon to provide on-site consultation. A number of drafts of the agreement were exchanged between the two universities' contract offices. The final version of the agreement received approval at that level. Nonetheless, when the partners began to initiate plans for the first UNMCON consultants to come to Lebanon, their travel was forbidden by their university because of the U.S. State Department advisory against travel to Lebanon. This came as a shock and disappointment to both partner and host. It meant that the host partner would not be able to serve as host in the traditional sense of the word, and partner faculty who looked forward to traveling to Lebanon did not have the opportunity. More important, it meant the consultants would not gain a full understanding of the context for their assistance. Several attempts were made by the UNMCON team to secure university approval for travel to Lebanon, but the decision was firm. In the long run, it was this political factor that limited the potential outcomes for the consultation, maximization of benefit for both partners, and particularly the sustainability of the partnership.

In an effort to lessen the negative impact of this change, the consultation team offered more flexibility for LAU faculty visits to UNM. They were open to having more faculty come to UNM in the first year of the agreement than was originally planned. This would help ensure that ARCSON faculty would have in-person contact with the consultants during the first year of consultation, rather than contact only through videoconferences and e-mail. In essence, during the first year of the agreement, UNMCON became the "host" for five faculty and the dean. One group (dean and assistant dean) and one group (four faculty) traveled to UNM in the summer and over semester break, respectively. Each group participated in 4 days of intensive learning. The sixth faculty member visited during semester break of year 2 of the project. It was fortunate that the LAU academic calendar starts about 1 month later than the UNM calendar, for if our academic calendars were simultaneous, classroom and clinical observations would not have been possible during these visits. Table 4.1 identifies the elements of the consultation that were achieved in a 2-year period, even though the UNMCON faculty were not able to travel to Lebanon.

During each visit the host faculty met with the consultants for group and individual sessions and observed classes where concept-based instructional approaches were being used. Time was spent touring their clinical and simulation laboratories and visits were made to hospital and community clinical sites. When possible, ARCSON faculty had opportunities to interact or observe UNM classes that were comparable to the courses they taught at LAU. This enabled the ARCSON faculty to interact with students to learn their perspective and understanding of the concept-based approach. The consultant team generously shared documents that helped ARCSON faculty understand how the concept-based model was translated into instructional and assessment tools. The UNMCON faculty also did what the ARCSON faculty had expected to do when the partners visited Lebanon— the UNM faculty introduced ARCSON faculty to New Mexican cuisine at restaurants and American West cuisine in their homes. Of course, shopping excursions were included in

TABLE 4.1 Consultation Activities by Year

Agreement year	Consultation activities
Year 1	Monthly video conference calls between the host faculty and the partner consultation team, focusing generally on faculty development
	ARCSON dean and assistant dean to UNMCON for 4-day intensive consultation with the nurse partner team
	Meeting at National League for Nursing annual conference between host assistant dean with two members of the nurse partner consultation team
	All ARCSON faculty sent drafts of materials (e.g., concept templates, course syllabi, active learning strategies) for review and feedback by UNMCON consultants
	Four ARCSON faculty to UNMCON for 4-day intensive consultation with the nurse partner team
	Several individual videoconferences, e-mail exchanges, or Skype calls between one host faculty and one partner faculty
Year 2	Consultation and review of documents by e-mail between ARCSON faculty and UNMCON partner faculty on multiple occasions
	4-day intensive consultation site visit to UNMCON by one ARCSON faculty
	Several individual videoconferences, e-mail exchanges, and Skype calls between one host faculty and one partner faculty

the evenings. These activities helped foster personal ties between the partners and laid the groundwork for more relaxed interactions during later videoconferences and technology mediated communications.

Because UNMCON faculty could not travel to Lebanon, when ARCSON faculty visited UNM they gave presentations that would help the partners better understand the host setting. During the first visit to UNMCON a presentation about Lebanon and LAU was given, with many photos to help the consultants develop an image of Lebanon. During the second visit one presentation was about nursing practice in Lebanon and progress in development of ARCSON. As well, during both visits ARCSON faculty shared recent findings from their research, which helped the partners understand some of the cultural influences on health care in Lebanon. In the final visit, 1 year after the second visit, an update on ARCSON progress was presented. These presentations were welcomed by the consultants and other UNMCON faculty who attended. Gifts were exchanged also, including Lebanon's traditional baklava and desk boxes illustrating the Phoenician alphabet and UNM memorabilia.

Social and Cultural Factors

Launching the partnership went smoothly. Host faculty literacy in English minimized the communication challenges that are encountered in many international partnerships. The faculty's familiarity with American model education from their own studies at American universities meant there was no need to use consultation time to explain such things as the liberal arts foundation for a professional curriculum, course credit and semester structures, and other higher education models that might be unfamiliar to faculty in other low- and middle-income countries.

Economic and Environmental Factors

One environmental factor that had to be considered in our partnership was the 9-hour time difference—New Mexico is in the UTC-7 time zone. Videoconferences were scheduled for 5 p.m. in Lebanon, 8 a.m. in New Mexico—so as the host faculty were ending their day, the nurse partners were beginning theirs. Generally, the conferences were productive, though during a few videoconferences productive time was lost due to connectivity problems. After some early difficulties in connecting we learned to plan a pretest; the information technology departments at both institutions were key in supporting this aspect of our partnership. At the time of one planned videoconference we learned that Lebanon and New Mexico do not switch to daylight savings time on the same date. By the time we discovered this, it was too late to correct the problem, so the call had to be rescheduled. The difference in time zones had implications for alertness and productivity when ARCSON faculty traveled to UNM. Efforts were made to accommodate the expected jet lag in the preplanned schedule of activities.

Factors related to the nursing practice environment that had to be considered were the availability of data on disease incidence and prevalence and the structure of the colloquium examination. The CBC model used by UNMCON identifies two to three exemplars for each concept taught. Students are expected to transfer knowledge of the concept from these exemplars to other health conditions or professional situations. The health and illness exemplars that are taught are chosen because of their high incidence and prevalence in New Mexico. ARCSON faculty felt this approach would not work in Lebanon for two reasons. First, there is limited availability of incidence and prevalence data. Second, the colloquium is more likely to require students to answer based on memorization of facts than on application of concepts through critical thinking. The faculty did not want to put students at a disadvantage when sitting for the colloquium. Faculty decided to use several exemplars for each health and illness concept. Selection of exemplars was based on their own recent practice, curricula of other nursing programs in Lebanon, data that were available, and knowledge of the topics typically addressed in the colloquium.

CONCLUSION

The consultation between ARCSON and UNMCON was important for ARCSON in achieving its vision of being a leading school within the Middle East. UNMCON faculty had expertise and confidence in the CBC model and experience in serving as consultants and providing CBC-related faculty development to other schools. Their inability to travel to Lebanon, however, was a significant barrier for developing a sustained partnership. While ARCSON faculty gained valuable insights about nursing education and practice as well as health care in New Mexico, the UNMCON partners were not able to experience the context for the curriculum they were helping ARCSON faculty to develop. Our case, however, illustrates that all is not lost even when a major barrier is encountered. The flexibility that both partners showed resulted in the ARCSON faculty having the knowledge necessary to fully develop and implement a CBC.

REFLECTIVE QUESTIONS

1. How could the nurse partner have better prepared his or her faculty for the host partner's expectations (i.e., culture, history, sociopolitical factors of Lebanon)?
2. How could the host have provided more direct experience with the context, other than the presentations during trips to UNMCON?
3. How could we have anticipated earlier in the planning the impact of the travel warning for the partnership?
4. What are effective strategies for closure of the immediate project that address lessons learned from the international exchange?
5. What strategies could be used to facilitate sustaining a long-term partnership between LAU and UNM?
   a. Nursing and nursing education in Lebanon
   b. Higher education in Lebanon

REFERENCES

American Association of Colleges of Nursing. (2006). *Essentials of baccalaureate education for professional nursing practice*. Washington, DC: Author.

Giddens, J. F., & Brady, D. P. (2007). Rescuing nursing education from content saturation: The case for a concept-based curriculum. *Journal of Nursing Education, 46*(2), 65–69.

Giddens, J., Brady, D., Brown, P., Wright, M., Smith, D., & Harris, J. (2008). A new curriculum for a new era of nursing education. *Nursing Education Perspectives, 29*(4), 200–204.

Heims, M. L., & Boyd, S. T. (1990). Concept-based learning activities in clinical nursing education, *Journal of Nursing Education, 29*(6), 249–254.

Huijer, H. A.-S., Noureddine, S., & Dumit, N. (2005). Nursing in Lebanon. *Applied Nursing Research, 18*, 63–64. doi: 10.1016/j.apnr.2005.02.003

Lasater, K., & Nielsen, A. (2009). The influence of concept-based learning activities on students' clinical judgment development. *Journal of Nursing Education, 48*(8), 441–448.

Lee-Hsieh, J., Kao, C., Kuo, C., & Tseng. H.-F. (2003). Clinical nursing competence of RN-to-BSN students in a nursing concept-based curriculum in Taiwan. *Journal of Nursing Education, 42*(12), 536–545.

Schreier, A. M., Peery, A. I., & McLean, C. B. (2009). An integrative curriculum for accelerated nursing education programs. *Journal of Nursing Education, 48*(5), 282–285.

United Nations Development Programme. (2013). *Human development report, the rise of the south: Human progress in a diverse world*. New York, NY: Author. http://hdr.undp.org/en

CHAPTER 5

Resources for Global Health Partnerships

Jeanne M. Leffers

Resources are essential for any health program to succeed and are key components of partnership and sustainability (Leffers & Mitchell, 2011). Because of the rise in mortality rates in many countries, reduction of life expectancy in many low-income countries, an increase in global pandemics, and the recent crisis in the global economy, resource needs to meet the global health agenda have risen sharply. In the field of global health, programs most often develop in low- and middle-income countries (LMICs), where there are limited resources (George & Meadows-Oliver, 2013). Increasingly, funds move from higher income countries to LMICs (Ravishanker et al., 2009). Funding, however, is not the sole source of support necessary for successful global health programs. Resources can be considered to be human, material, or financial in nature. Reports indicate that a shortage of human (particularly nurses), material, and financial resources adversely affect the ability of nurses to meet their professional expectations to promote and restore population health (Costa Mendes et al., 2013). Nurses are often involved directly with each of these types of resources.

HUMAN RESOURCES FOR HEALTH

According to the World Health Report, the World Health Organization (WHO) estimated that there is a shortage of more than 7 million health workers needed for the provision of essential health services such as immunizations, maternal health services, and access to prevention and treatment strategies for common deadly epidemic diseases (WHO, 2013a). This shortage is compounded by several factors. The nursing shortage in LMICs is profound (Frenk et al., 2010), with a need for more than 600,000 nurses in sub-Saharan Africa (International Council of Nurses, 2006). First, most of the trained workforce is located in cities with inadequate staffing in rural areas. Second, in addition to the demand for maternal child health and infectious disease health services, the growth of chronic health conditions worldwide increases the need for health workers. In many countries, health care workers have not been adequately trained to meet the needs of the ageing population and chronically ill. Further, the global migration of highly trained health workers in LMIC locations moves the highly trained local health providers to countries that offer higher salaries and better working conditions (Chen et al., 2004; Kingma, 2007). The resultant loss of highly educated and skilled health workers in LMICs has led to the development of international strategies to address human resources for health (Global Health Workforce Alliance, 2013).

Nurse migration, particularly from LMICs to higher income countries where there is the prospect of higher income, professional development, and improved quality of life, has been one response to the global nursing shortage. While this practice can benefit the individual nurse, the flow of nurses from LMICs can have negative effects on the country that supplies the nurses (Kingma, 2001). As a result of the increasing migration of nurses, the International Council of Nurses (ICN) created a position statement that addresses the loss of skilled workers from LMICs and resultant negative consequences for health and the nursing profession as well as the possible negative impacts on the nurse who migrates. These issues include negative work contact conditions, discriminatory treatment of immigrant nurses, differences of education and the effects on practice in host country, and inequities in benefits provided by the hiring institution (ICN, 2007).

HRH Programs

WHO Global Forums for Human Resources for Health (HRH) that have been held in Kampala, Uganda, in 2008, in Bangkok, Thailand, in 2011, and in Recife, Brazil, in 2013 were developed to address the serious problems of workforce shortages, global migration, and inadequate education and training programs in LMICs. Each forum drew more than 1,000 participants from countries around the world to share strategies to meet this problem. To learn more about the conferences, objectives, and outcomes, visit www.who.int/workforcealliance/forum/en. Through these conferences, targeted strategies and actions were developed to help address these serious issues.

An outstanding example of a program to address the issue of human resources for health is the Rwanda HRH program (www.hrhconsortium.moh.gov.rw). In Case Study 8.2, "Rwanda Human Resources for Health Program," this program is highlighted. This is a 7-year partnership between the government of Rwanda; medical, health management, dental, and nursing programs in Rwanda; the U.S. government; the Global Fund to Fight AIDS, Tuberculosis, and Malaria; and 14 U.S. medical, nursing, and public health schools. In Rwanda, the HRH program operates in three educational institutions, four referral hospitals, and, begun in late 2012, seven district hospital schools for nursing and midwifery. The collaborative program focuses on the critical shortage of skilled health care workers, the need to improve the quality of health care worker education, and the inadequate infrastructure and equipment available in health facilities. By bringing select health professionals from the United States to Rwanda to partner with Rwandan health care workers in locations throughout the country, the goal is to build capacity in Rwanda for education, practice, and health care management (Human Resources for Health, 2013).

The WHO maintains more than 800 collaborating centers worldwide. In the United States there are seven located in nursing schools and colleges (WHO, 2013a). The WHO Collaborating Centre for Nurse Human Resource Development and Patient Safety at the University of Miami focuses on strengthening nursing education in the Americas, promoting patient safety, and developing the nursing workforce in the Americas and Africa (University of Miami, 2013). Other examples as well as issues related to the need for skilled health professionals can be found in the HRH Open Access journal available at www.human-resources-health.com.

Nurses' Role for Human Resources for Health

Nurses are reported to provide 90% of health care services worldwide, but severe shortages exist in many parts of the world (Davis, 2012). Increasingly nurses from higher income countries volunteer or work with organizations in LMICs. As participants in global health programs, nurses can support but should not replace the health care workers in the host country. Those nurses who participate in the direct care of patients in the host country must partner with local health care workers to build capacity in the host country. This requires that the visiting nurses share expertise with and learn from their host country partners through collaboration and support. It is essential for visiting nurses to understand how their organization or sponsoring program collaborates with the local health care system.

There are many programs, often called medical missions, that provide direct care in under-served areas of the world. Without collaboration with local health care partners, that care can actually be harmful to the local setting (Cohen, 2006; Levi, 2009). As guests in the host country, the nurse partner or visiting team must provide care that is culturally appropri-ate, that is ethically responsible, and that is sustainable after the visitors depart. In some cases, a partnering organization depends on a large number of nurse volunteers who par-ticipate for short periods of time. In the Chapter 2 case study "Building and Sustaining an Academic Partnership in Haiti," the examples show that if nurses participate as part of an ongoing partnership, follow protocols established by the host country partners, work col-laboratively with host country health professionals, and support the long-term goals of the program, they can provide culturally sound and ethically appropriate direct care services in the host country.

A further ethical consideration is the need to balance between the needs of the visiting nurse or nursing student as learner and the essential service to the host partner. Crump and Sugarman (2008) argue that short-term trainee field experiences in resource limited settings pose ethical concerns. These include the limitations of language, cultural knowledge and communication capabilities of visiting trainees, time demand and burden on host partner staff and institutions, and the results as manifested in patient care. For true partnership to occur, learning should be reciprocal and the demands of either partner should not unduly burden the other. When nursing students who travel to a host country for service and for learning actually burden the services of the host country, the ethically imperative balance and partnership are absent.

FINANCIAL RESOURCES FOR GLOBAL HEALTH

Globally, the costs for health care have been rising for decades. In the United States in 2010, total health expenditures were $2.6 trillion—18% of the gross domestic product. The per capita expenditure on health was $8,402 (CDC, 2013). In comparison, Uganda's per capita expenditure on health reported by the World Bank for 2012 was $45USD (Trading Econom-ics, 2013). While most of the global health focus for nursing has been in LMICs, the need for financial support for global health projects is evident. Financial support for global health comes from government aid agencies, donors, corporate social responsibility programs, charities, and private foundations (see Table 5.1). Most frequently, global health nursing projects are funded through the sponsoring organization or agency. Sometimes these are large international programs such as the WHO, foundations such as the Bill & Melinda Gates Foundation, and corporate programs such as the Merck program to address oncho-cerciasis (river blindness).

To achieve the goals for the development of HRH (in this case health professionals including nursing), funding from the U.S. government, the Global Fund to Fight AIDS, Tuberculosis, and Malaria, and other sources provides the financial support to ensure proj-ect success. A second example is the collaborative learning initiative funded at Makerere University in Uganda by the Bill & Melinda Gates Foundation. Developed through a $4.97 million grant, the partnership linked the schools of public health, nursing, and medicine at Johns Hopkins University in the United States and Makerere University in Uganda to strengthen educational, research, and service capacity at Makerere to improve health out-comes across Uganda (Johns Hopkins, 2011). One significant outcome of this partnership for nursing was the collaborative scholarship with almost all the College of Health Sciences Department of Nursing faculty members to conduct research and disseminate the findings in nearly a dozen publications. Many of these publications were presented in the Volume 11 supplement to the BMC International Health and Human Rights Open Access journal (www.biomedcentral.com/1472-698X/11?issue=S1).

Programs with nurse participation are generally financed through grants, foundations, or small nongovernmental organizations (NGOs). Nurses frequently serve as primary investigators for research or program grants for collaborative partnerships in global health

TABLE 5.1 Global Health Funding Sources

Organization	Location	Focus	Grants/Funds	Health focus	Partners
Bill & Melinda Gates Foundation	United States	Global development and global health U.S. programs	Poverty and hunger globally Science and technology for global health	HIV, malaria, TB, pneumonia, neglected infectious diseases Polio nutrition vaccines	
PEPFAR	United States	HIV/AIDS	Government funding	Provision of ART to those infected with HIV, along with counseling and support	Global Fund to Fight AIDS, Tuberculosis, and Malaria and the United Nations Program on AIDS (UNAIDS), as well as the Peace Corps and local faith-based organizations
GAVI (Global Alliance for Vaccines and Immunization)		Access to immunizations			WHO, UNICEF, the World Bank, the Bill & Melinda Gates Foundation, donor governments, developing countries, international development and finance organizations, and the pharmaceutical industry
Global Fund to Fight AIDs, Malaria, and Tuberculosis	Geneva, Switzerland	Programs to address AIDs, malaria, and tuberculosis	Operates at a funding level, and attracts, manages, and disperses funding to fight these three diseases	Programs to address AIDs, malaria, and tuberculosis	Public/Private partnership (PPP) at the country level with a wide diversity of implementing government bodies and international development partners (including United Nations agencies and donors), national civil society organizations (including local media, professional associations, and faith-based institutions), the private sector, and communities living with or affected by the diseases

World Bank	United States	Five institutions as one group Goals to reduce poverty and advance prosperity	Provides low-interest loans and grants	Health systems, reproductive health, and health economics	PPP practitioners, PPP units, policymakers, and specialists in PPPs, line ministries, as well as with parliamentarians, local governments, civil society organizations, banks, private sector developers, and users of infrastructure services
Clinton Foundation	United States	Global Health Economic development Childhood obesity Climate change Health and wellness		HIV/AIDs, tuberculosis and malaria Human resources for health, global health partnership	Clinton Health Access Initiative; Clinton Health in Haiti Other global health partners

settings and in this way contribute financial resources for the partnership. Frequently the funding is limited to particular activities based on the guidelines of the sponsoring organization. Since many LMICs require material resources as well as financial funding for the program, nurses might be involved in assisting program organizers gain funding that supports infrastructure, supplies, and materials. The Chapter 9 case study, "Conducting Nursing Research in Uganda," offers an example of how grant funding was able to build capacity as well as leave concrete contributions.

In some cases, nurses must pay their own personal expenses to participate in programs sponsored by nongovernmental organizations. This might include a program fee, transportation, housing, and food. Depending on the NGO and its sources of funds, participants might actually be required to subsidize part of the program through the fee that they pay to participate.

MATERIAL RESOURCES FOR GLOBAL HEALTH

Material resources for health can be defined as the resources that are present in a physical form, generally created by humans, that sustain health. They can be basic conditions for health, such as access to clean water, energy sources, and basic sanitation. Additionally, they can be materials used directly for health care, such as medical equipment, books or library resources, educational materials for health providers or patients, and pharmaceuticals. The former basic conditions for health often create the opportunity for health, while the latter support health care delivery. Nurses must be part of any global health program. Without material resources, the health of the population served is reduced (Alley et al., 2009; Kamadieu et al., 2011).

Basic Resources for Healthy Living

Nurses working in global settings often find that the host country population has limited access to clean water or basic sanitation (WHO, 2013b). More than 1.1 billion people worldwide lack access to safe water, causing health problems such as more than 1.6 million deaths from diarrheal diseases, particularly among children, and infection with intestinal parasites that cause blindness and vision impairment.

For the more than 2.6 billion people lacking adequate sanitation and without an adequate latrine available, the frequent infections from waterborne agents contribute to morbidity and mortality. More than 1.5 million cases of hepatitis A can be attributed to lack of sanitation (WHO, 2013b). The United Nations Millennium Development Goal 7 (MDG 7) seeks to achieve 88.5 % access to clean water and 75% basic sanitation coverage by 2015. If the targets for this goal are met, it is estimated that more than 470,000 lives would be saved and that people could gain 320 million productive working days each year (WHO, 2013b). The target for access to clean water has been met (UNICEF, 2013), but great disparities exist between LMICs. Information about access to clean water and basic sanitation can be found at www.who.int/water_sanitation_health/mdg1/en or at the nonprofit http://water.org/water-crisis/water-facts/water.

In addition to the health risks related to the lack of sanitation and clean water, the negative impact on women and children is enormous. Women and children spend hours each day fetching clean water, carrying large jerry cans of water from distribution sites that can be many miles from home. For women who are the caregivers in the family, this impacts the entire family, rendering them unable to participate in income-generating work, while children are often unable to attend school to further their education. These additional distal factors increase other health problems as well. By meeting the target for MDG 7, more children would be able to attend school, while more women could generate income for their families and spend more time as caregivers to their family members.

For billions of people worldwide, there is no reliable source of energy to meet their needs for cooking, heating, or maintaining safety during the hours of darkness. Nurses can be involved with collaborative project teams that address energy needs. Nursing students at Valparaiso University in Indiana have partnered with engineering, business, and health professional students since 2007 for health promotion in Nicaragua. While engineers have worked on projects to address sustainable wind turbines and piped water to the community, the nursing students assessed health needs. Their focus was on the safety of cooking stoves to reduce respiratory illness due to smoke in the living quarters. In response to the re-engineering of the cook stoves to reduce wood consumption and improve ventilation, the local women reported a reduction in respiratory complaints (Leffers & Plotnick, 2011; Snyder, Wingstrom, Crave, Simonpetri, & Lundy, 2013; Snyder, Wingstrom, & Zeman, 2012). The collaborative Water for Waslala project between engineering and nursing students at Villanova University began in 2002 (Leffers & Plotnick, 2011; Water for Waslala, 2013). This collaboration in the community has led to the program partnership for community health workers that is described in the Chapter 11 case study "Interprofessional Partnerships With a Telehealth Project in Waslala, Nicaragua."

Furthermore, with the growth of cell phone technology that is transforming communication globally, most people in the world have limited access to electricity for charging their telephones. The case studies in Chapters 9 and 11 offer information on the use of cell phones to advance health, demonstrating how technology can advance health in LMICs.

Health Material Resources

Nurses commonly identify medical supplies as essential resources for their work in global settings. Due to the high costs of supplies in most LMICs, the availability of medical equipment for screening and treatment of patients is limited or absent. Hospitals often lack sufficient basic supplies, such as thermometers, sphygmomanometers, glucometers, and equipment necessary for urinary catheterization, wound care, intravenous infusion, oxygen administration, intubation, and other emergency supplies. Patients often are required to pay out of pocket for laboratory testing, medications, and other equipment. Consequently, nurses often serve as procurers and providers of medical supplies for the programs where they serve. This raises several ethical concerns (Levi, 2009). First, when visiting partners are the source of donated material medical supplies, a void occurs once those supplies are consumed and must be constantly renewed by other visiting nurses or health professionals. Second, donations of supplies from higher income countries must be able to be monitored for effectiveness and be able to be repaired easily in the host country in order to provide a usable and sustainable resource. In the case of medications, it is imperative that donated medications be appropriate for the host country population and that they be within their expiration date. Furthermore, many host partners develop their own protocols and formularies in order to ensure that host country patients are not prescribed medications for use in noncommunicable diseases that cannot be sustained over time. Third, while the proper use of medical supplies is paramount to responsible care, the proper disposal is of equal importance. Health Care Without Harm is the leading organization that addresses environmentally responsible health care. Through the work of leading scientists, health professionals, and advocates, they address waste management of toxic materials such as mercury, PVC and phthalates, flame retardants, electronics, cleaners, pesticides, pharmaceuticals used in hospital and health care settings, healthy food systems, green buildings and energy use, green purchasing, climate, and health all as part of their focus on environment and health (www.noharm.org). One example of irresponsible donations is the overuse of small plastic bags for dispensing small supplies of medications in what are often referred to as medical missions. Not only are there problems with proper identification of the medication, instructions for use, and proper disposal but also in many countries plastic is burned, releasing carcinogens into the air. While the MDG 7 targets specifically water and basic sanitation, an important aspect of environmental sustainability is the assurance that health care practices do not harm the health of the population.

Many global programs have policies regarding donations and supplies. For example, Health Volunteers Overseas, a private nonprofit U.S.–based program "dedicated to improving the availability and quality of health care in developing countries through the training and education of local health care providers," states on its website:

> Volunteers are encouraged to make maximum use of locally available equipment and supplies in order to foster long-term sustainability. If donations of equipment, medications or other supplies are deemed essential to accomplish the educational goals of the project, these donations should be appropriate to the needs of the site and meet international donation standards as established by WHO or other similar organizations. (Health Volunteers Overseas, 2013)

Other programs that provide direct service are likely to monitor and manage the supplies through a central office, and nurses should ensure that any donations that they consider bringing with them meet the requirements of the partner organization and the needs of the host country partners. Additionally, organizations can make use of programs such as Global Links (www.globallinks.org), where much needed supplies can be recovered in higher income countries and adapted for reuse in LMICs.

Teaching Materials

Nurse partners who collaborate with nurses and health professionals across international borders are frequently most helpful as educators who share materials for nurse or patient education in order to build capacity of host partners. These can range from assistance in developing curriculum plans in academic settings to short professional development modules for nursing staff. Nurses from countries with more abundant resources available for health often bring teaching materials from their home country but also, through the use of the Internet to access resources and nursing literature as well as for document preparation, can collaborate with host country nurses to ensure that teaching materials are culturally appropriate and fit the needs of nursing education in the host country. To promote sustainability, having an electronic version is advantageous, because revisions can be made easily, shared electronically, and reprinted as needed.

As part of the capacity building and empowerment agenda, it is recommended that guest nurse partners not only access existing electronic materials, toolkits, and curriculum resources for their use, but also share these with their global partners to build programs in the host country. Various organizations in higher income countries sponsor resource sites that can be most helpful to nurses across the globe. Some of these are listed below. If these resources are shared with global health partners, the partners are then able to create their own evidence-based educational models.

CONCLUSION

As noted in the Conceptual Model for Partnership and Sustainability in Global Health, resources are essential to the development and maintenance of partnerships as well as the sustainability of global health programs. In the absence of strategies that address global health inequities at the system level that limit resources in LMICs, nurses can aid access to resources as well as assist in their judicious and responsible use. Whenever possible, the use of readily available, sustainable, and culturally appropriate resources is strongly preferred.

RESOURCES FOR MATERIAL RESOURCES FOR HEALTH

American Academy of Pediatrics Section on International Child Health (www2.aap.org/sections/ich/toolkit.htm, www2.aap.org/sections/ich)
American Association of Colleges of Nursing (for curriculum materials) (www.aacn.nche.edu)

Canadian Association of Schools of Nursing (www.casn.ca/en)

Global Health Delivery Online (www.ghdonline.org/dashboard and www.ghdonline.org/cases)

Global Health Media Project (designed to provide educational materials for use by health workers globally) (http://globalhealthmedia.org)

Health Volunteers Overseas (HVO) Volunteer Toolkit (www.hvousa.org/volunteerToolkit/index.shtml)

International Council of Nurses (ICN) (www.icn.ch)

Medical Aid Films (produced in UK for health workers with a particular focus on the needs or women and children) (http://medicalaidfilms.org/our-films)

National League for Nursing (educational and leadership resources) (www.nln.org/facultyprograms/index.htm)

Royal College of Nursing (UK) (resources for professional development) (www.rcn.org.uk/development)

University of Washington Health Sciences Library. Global Health Toolkit (http://hsl.uw.edu/toolkits/global-health)

REFERENCES

Alley, D. E., Soldo, B. J., Pagan, J. A., McCabe, J., deBlois, M., Field, . . . Cannuscio, C. (2009). Material resources and population health: Disadvantages in health care, housing, and food among adults over 50 years of age. *American Journal of Public Health* Supplement 3, 2009, 99, No. S3g.

CDC. (2013). Health expenditures fast stats. www.cdc.gov/nchs/fastats/hexpense.htm

Chen, L., Evans, T., Anand, S., Bouffard, J. I., Brown, H., Chowdhury, . . . Wibulpolpresert, S. (2004). Human resources for health: Overcoming the crisis. *The Lancet, 364* (9449), 1984–1990.

Cohen, J. (2006). New world of global health. *Science, 311*, 162–167.

Costa Mendes, I. A., Marchi-Alves, L. M., Mazzo, A., Nogueira, M. S., Trevizan, M. A., Godoy, S., & Arena Ventura, C. A. (2013). Healthcare context and nursing workforce in a main city of Angola. *International Nursing Review, 60*(1), 37–44. http://dx.doi.org.libproxy.umassd.edu/10.1111/j.1466-7657.2012.01039.x

Crump, J., & Sugarman, J. (2008). Ethical considerations for short-term trainees in global health. *JAMA, 300*(12), 1456–1458. doi: 10.1001/jama.300.12.1456

Davis, S. (2012). Why nurses are the unsung heroes of global health. *Huffington Post Impact*. www.huffingtonpost.com/sheila-davis-dnp-anpbc-faan/international-nurses-week_b_1499802.html

Frenk, J., Chen, L., Bhutta, Z., Cohen, J., Crisp, N., Evans, T., . . . Zurayk, H. (2010). Health professionals for a new century: Transforming education to strengthen health systems in an independent world. *The Lancet, 376*, 1923–1958.

George, E. K., & Meadows-Oliver, M. (2013). Searching for collaboration in international nursing partnerships: A literature review. *International Nursing Review, 60*(1), 31–36.

Global Health Workforce Alliance. (2013). The human resources for health crisis. www.who.int/workforcealliance/about/hrh_crisis/en/index.html

Health Volunteers Overseas. (2013). Mission, vision and values. www.hvousa.org/whoWeAre/mission.shtml

Human Resources for Health. (2013). Republic of Rwanda. http://hrhconsortium.moh.gov.rw

International Council of Nurses (ICN). (2006). *The global nursing shortage: Priority areas for intervention*. Geneva: International Council of Nurses. www.icn.ch/images/stories/documents/publications/GNRI/The_Global_Nursing_Shortage-Priority_Areas_for_Intervention.pdf

International Council of Nurses (ICN). (2007). *Position statement: Nurse retention and migration*. www.icn.ch/images/stories/documents/publications/position_statements/C06_Nurse_Retention_Migration.pdf

Johns Hopkins. (2011). *Johns Hopkins and Uganda's Makerere University complete collaborative learning initiative.* Johns Hopkins Bloomberg School of Public Health. www.jhsph.edu/news/news-releases/2011/peters-bmc-series.html

Kamadieu, R., Assegid, K., Naouri, B., Mizra, I. R., Hirsi, A., Mohammed, A., . . . Mulugeta, A. (2011). Measles control and elimination in Somalia: The good, the bad, and the ugly. *Journal of Infectious Diseases, 204* (Suppl. 1), S312–S317.

Kingma, M. (2001). Nursing migration: Global treasure hunt, or disaster-in-the-making? *Nursing Inquiry 89*(4), 205–212.

Kingma, M. (2007). Nurses on the move: A global overview. *Health Services Research, 42*(3 Pt 2), 1281–1298. doi: 10.1111/j.1475-6773.2007.00711.x

Leffers, J., & Mitchell, E. (2011). Conceptual model for partnership and sustainability in global health. *Public Health Nursing, 28*(1), 91–102. doi: 10.1111/j.1525-1446.2010.00892.x

Leffers, J., & Plotnick, J. (2011). *Volunteering at home and abroad.* Indianapolis, IN: Sigma Theta Tau.

Levi, A. (2009). The ethics of nursing student international clinical experiences. *JOGNN, 38,* 94–99. doi: 10.1111/j.1552-6909.2008.00314.x

Ravishanker, N., Gubbins, P., Cooley, R. J., Leach-Kemon, K., Michaud, C. M., Jamison, D. T., & Murray, C. J. L. (2009). Financing of global health: Tracking development assistance for health from 1990 to 2007. *The Lancet, 373*(9681), 2113–2124. doi:10.1016/S0140-6736(09)60881-3

Snyder, P., Wingstrom, C., & Zeman, C. (2012). *Beyond the volcanoes: A community partnership for health in rural Nicaragua.* Celebration of undergraduate scholarship. Paper 121. http://scholar.valpo.edu/cus/121

Snyder, P., Wingstrom, C., Crave, C., Simonpietri, C., & Lundy, C. (2013). *Beyond the volcanoes: A community partnership for health in rural Nicaragua.* Celebration of Undergraduate Scholarship. Paper 221. http://scholar.valpo.edu/cus/221

Trading Economics. (2013). Health care expenditures in Uganda. www.tradingeconomics.com/uganda/health-expenditure-per-capita-us-dollar-wb-data.html

UNICEF. (2013). Progress on drinking water and sanitation: 2012 update. UNICEF and WHO. http://www.childinfo.org/files/JMP2013Final_Eng.pdf

University of Miami. (2013). WHO Collaborating Centre for Nursing Human Resources Development and Patient Safety. University of Miami School of Nursing and Health Sciences. www.miami.edu/sonhs/index.php/sonhs/centers/pahowho_collaborating_center

Water for Waslala. (2013). www.waterforwaslala.org

World Health Organization. (2013a). Global health workforce shortage. http://www.who.int/mediacentre/news/releases/2013/health-workforce-shortage/en/index.html?utm_content=buffer50126&utm_source=buffer&utm_medium=twitter&utm_campaign=Buffer

World Health Organization. (2013b). Health through safe drinking water and basic sanitation. www.who.int/water_sanitation_health/mdg1/en

Educating the Educators: The International Nurse Faculty Partnership Initiative, Regis College Haiti Project

Cherlie Magny-Normilus
Alexis Lawton

Haiti's nursing corps has not had the means to provide advanced education to its nursing faculty and nurses, particularly in the face of technological change revolutionizing the delivery of health care. The International Nurse Faculty Partnership Initiative (INFPI) or Regis College Haiti Project (RCHP) developed and carries out a unique model to equip the educators and build up the human infrastructure of nursing and nursing education in Haiti.

CONTEXT: HAITI

The Republic of Haiti, locally called *Ayiti,* is located southeast of Florida to the east of Cuba. It shares the island of Hispaniola with the Dominican Republic and occupies the western third of the island. Its name is from the indigenous Taíno language and means "land of high mountains" (Central Intelligence Agency, 2013). Access to health service varies from next to nothing for those living in rural regions across Haiti to better availability in the capital, Port-au-Prince. Even prior to the devastating earthquake of 2010, the health care system in Haiti has struggled with a severe shortage of health care workers, poor infrastructure, and routine lack of care. Haiti has the highest rates of maternal and infant mortality. The health crisis is rooted in extreme poverty, inadequate sanitation, contaminated water, infectious disease, and malnutrition. The January 12, 2010, 7.0-magnitude earthquake, which killed as many as 200,000 people—leaving more than 2 million Haitians homeless and more than 3 million in need of emergency aid—has made health care delivery even more challenging. Haiti's nursing corps has never had the means to provide advanced education to nursing educators and nurses, particularly in the face of technology change revolutionizing the delivery of health care. The earthquake worsened this situation and struck a further blow to Haiti's human capital in nursing.

The nursing shortage is a global issue. The World Health Organization (WHO) and the International Council of Nurses (ICN) issued a report linking the global nursing shortage with poorer health outcomes (Lane, Antunes, Kingma, & Weller, 2010). However, the shortage approaches the crisis level in developing countries such as Haiti. The earthquake worsened the nursing shortage in Haiti by instantly taking the lives of numerous student nurses and nursing faculty and reducing schools to rubble. Now Haiti's nursing workforce, which consists of 1 nurse per 10,000 people, is dramatically below the WHO's recommendation of 25 nurses per 10,000 persons.

The Health Agenda for the Americas (PAHO) speaks to five challenges of workforce development:

- Define and implement evidence-based policies to develop the health workforce
- Address inequities in the distribution of health personnel
- Develop initiatives to promote retention of educated and trained health workers
- Improve health worker capacity
- Link training institutions with health services for collaboration (PAHO, 2013)

These are necessary goals for improving Haiti's health care system, and a struggling but valiant group of nursing professionals in Haiti has embraced them.

BACKGROUND FOR THE HAITI PROJECT

The INFPI started in May 2006 when Regis College honorary degree recipient and cofounder of the Boston-based organization Partners in Health (PIH) Ophelia Dahl met Dr. Antoinette Hays, then dean of the Regis College School of Nursing Science and Health Professions and now president of Regis College in Weston, Massachusetts. PIH founders Dr. Paul Farmer and Ophelia Dahl proposed performing an evaluation of the status of nursing within the country of Haiti. The results of this evaluation, which Regis College School of Nursing conducted in 2007, show that Haiti's nurses strongly desire to improve nursing education throughout Haiti but also to strengthen this through educational opportunities for nursing faculty. PIH's sister organization in Haiti, Zanmi Lasante, is a well-known NGO in Haiti, and Regis College is a well-known school of nursing throughout New England as well as within the Haitian community in Boston. The growing conviction was that the Regis College School of Nursing Science and Health Professions would be an optimal partner for advancing nursing education in Haiti (www.regiscollege.edu/about_regis/haiti_project.cfm).

Through PIH's sponsorship and collaboration with government officials and nursing leaders in Haiti, Regis's dean of the School of Nursing Science and Health Professions, a Regis faculty member, and a Haitian graduate of the master of science nurse practitioner program at Regis conducted a needs assessment of the nursing education programs in fall 2007. The assessment of nursing education in Haiti demonstrated that a targeted effort to advance the level of education of Haitian nursing faculty is vital, and the Regis leadership specifically targeted the goal of advancing nurse faculty from the current equivalency of an associate's degree to a master's degree in nursing. In 2008 the director of nursing in the Haitian Ministry of Health and the dean of the school of nursing in Port-Au-Prince visited Regis College, and the alliance between the Ministry of Health, PIH, and Regis College was formed shortly thereafter.

The January 12, 2010, earthquake initially placed those plans on hold—Haiti's primary responsibility was to respond to the emergency needs. The destruction of the national school of nursing, including the loss of many nursing faculty and students, furthered the goal of building collaboration for nursing education. Regis administrators viewed this partnership as an aspect of their educational mission and kept in close contact with their Haitian colleagues during this difficult time. A team from Regis College traveled to Haiti in June 2010, a few months after the devastating earthquake, to reconfirm this partnership. Even then, it was clear that the education of Haitian nursing faculty remained a top priority among the Haitians. During the June 2010 trip and throughout 2011, the new joint Regis–Haitian nursing leaders team consulted to begin working out the practical means by which the mutual goal of educating Haitian educators in nursing could be achieved. Together this team began cutting through the red tape and the institutional silos that kept nursing education and nursing disparate and uneven across Haiti.

Working tirelessly through meetings with friends and colleagues, the joint team continued the conversation about why this project was needed and sought funding. Our passion for Haiti and the project itself kept us going. The success of the Regis College "upward mobility" track educating American nurses at the master's level suggested it as a model that could work for Haiti. After months of conversations and outreach, two private donors in the Boston area stepped in to sponsor and make this project a reality.

In June 2012, the Regis College campus welcomed its first cohort of 12 Haitian nurse faculty for their summer session of intensive teaching and learning. Following this, the RCHP was recognized as a superior program to help rebuild the human infrastructure and workforce of Haiti. As a result, the project received further funding by the Clinton–Bush Haiti Fund. It is important to note that Regis College nursing faculty have given their services, and the college its physical and spiritual resources, as part of the funding of this program, in which the interrelationship of nursing professionals from nation to nation has been a deep source of mutual exchange and passion within the RCHP.

PROGRAM OF STUDY FOR RCHP

The program of study, modeled on Regis College's "Upward Mobility" program, enables enrollees to earn a bachelor's degree en route to a master's degree. The INFPI endeavors to promote a master's level of education for faculty, and at minimum a bachelor's level for practicing nurses in Haiti. The curriculum for this program is specifically designed to address the most pressing health care needs in the nation—namely, strategies for preventing and treating HIV/AIDS and preventing maternal and infant mortality.

The project delivers its educational courses presented on site in an intensive format to 12 nursing faculty from Haiti. Fall- and spring-semester courses are offered in a hybrid or online format in Haiti facilitated by Regis nurse faculty. A key component of the program is a 6-week summer residency by the Haitian faculty on the Regis College campus in Weston. Through this structure, the first cohort of graduates will receive their degrees in 2½ years.

Regis College has committed to provide ongoing consultation with Haitian nurse faculty program graduates, who will then continue with the implementation and expansion of the faculty education program model to other Haitian nurse educators. Beginning with 12 nurse faculty, the RCHP could eventually impact as many as 1,600 nurse educators and nurses in Haiti. Along the way, the INFPI of the RCHP is collecting data on the number of baccalaureate-prepared graduates who provide care on the front lines, as well as on the impact of their work in serving the people of Haiti.

Aims

1. Increase the numbers of qualified nurse faculty throughout Haiti
2. Expand the number of qualified nurses providing direct care throughout Haiti by increasing access to qualified educators across the country
3. Improve access to quality health care for the people of Haiti
4. Prepare Haitian nursing faculty to assume leadership roles in diverse health care settings and/or academic institutions of higher learning in Haiti

Implementation

INFPI is built on the established relationships that exist between Regis College School of Nursing Science and Health Professions and the Ministry of Health in Haiti, and it is fortified by the mutual association with PIH. A team at Regis College that includes Dr. Nancy Street, executive director; Cherlie Magny-Normilus, director of Advocacy and Policy; Alexis Lawton, director of Communications; and Dr. Antoinette Hays, president of Regis College as project lead advisor, coordinates the program. Regis College faculty members partner with nursing faculty members in Haiti to deliver the educational program throughout the calendar year using the Regis College campus, locations in Haiti, and Internet technology to facilitate the program.

Year 1 of the project included the enrollment of 12 Haitian nursing faculty in the Upward Mobility master's in nursing curriculum, in the leadership in education program track of the graduate school of nursing program. Initial course offerings are provided to our Haitian colleagues at our campus at Regis College, allowing for a complete orientation of these new students to the programs and resources offered by the college.

- Enrollment begins with Haitian nurse faculty attending the 6-week summer residency program, an intense course schedule with shortened timelines.
- The fall semester entails Regis faculty teaching in Haiti, complemented by online course enrollment, using laptops provided to those nursing faculty enrolled in the program.
- Spring semester offers on-site Regis faculty consultations in Haiti as well as online courses to the faculty in Haiti. Further travel between the programs will be arranged as needed.

Year 2 will follow a similar format with the expectation that faculty attend academic courses on the Regis campus during the summer session. Hands-on teaching and nursing care highlight this second summer session program with the hope of maximizing Haitian faculty's time in clinical practicum in the Boston area to see advances in both nursing education and care. In turn, the winter session in Haiti provides additional opportunity to develop an understanding of the issues facing a developing nation suffering from abject poverty and the resulting health conditions, including infectious disease, malnutrition, and diarrheal diseases.

CONCLUSION: LOOKING AHEAD FOR THE REGIS COLLEGE HAITI PROJECT

The long-term goal for RCHP is the complete adoption of this program of study by the University of Haiti faculty over the next 7 years. Each graduate of the Regis College Haiti Project will be prepared to teach at both the baccalaureate and graduate levels of nursing and will be engaged in active educational mentoring over the next 7 years with Regis College nursing faculty. We anticipate a total of 36 Haitian nursing faculty members' completing the requirements for a master's degree in nursing education and leadership over the next 4 years and expect to be able to continue the program by passing it on to other nurses in Haiti. Partnerships to advance nursing education and leadership in host settings illustrate the sustainability of building human resources for health.

REFLECTIVE QUESTIONS

1. Reflecting on your experiences with local or international programs, in what ways will capacity building with partners strengthen human resources for health?
2. Discuss how financial resources are linked to human resources in order to build programs such as the RCHP. Does any program that you work with address human, financial, or material resources for health?
3. What is the relationship between nursing leadership and strengthening nursing education in low- and middle-income countries?

REFERENCES

Central Intelligence Agency (CIA). (2013). Central American and the Caribbean: Haiti. https://www.cia.gov/library/publications/the-world-factbook/geos/ha.html

Lane, C., Antunes, A. F., Kingma, M., & Weller, B. (2010). The nursing community, macroeconomic and public finance policies: Towards a better understanding. World Health Organization & International Council of Nurses. www.icn.ch/images/stories/documents/pillars/sew/ICHRN/Policy_and_Research_Papers/The%20nursing%20community%20macroeconomic%20and%20public%20finance%20policies_towards%20a%20better%20understanding_2010.pdf

PAHO. (2013). Health Agenda for the Americas 2008–2017. www.paho.org/hq/index.php?option=com_content&view=article&id=1976%3Ahealth-agenda-for-the-americas2008 2017&catid=1546%3Akmckey-paho-publications&lang=en

Toward a Sustainable Model of International Public Health Nursing Education

Sarah E. Abrams

The purposes of study abroad in nursing are many, but among them are immersion in another culture, understanding of global health issues, and creation of an opportunity for direct application of skills that are difficult to practice in the United States. The Peace Corps provided that first opportunity for me many years ago, and it had been my goal to have senior nursing students from the University of Vermont (UVM) learn something about global health work. While this is fine as an objective, achieving a successful experience in another country requires planning, development of relationships, understanding of the environment and culture in which students and faculty will work and, overall, a good bit of luck. The subsequent years have affirmed these as necessary, but insufficient, conditions and provided new lessons about working with partners who have disparate values and objectives, the work necessary to ensure sustainability, and the importance of understanding travelers' first experiences in an unfamiliar culture.

CONTEXT UGANDA: GETTING TO KAMULI FROM VERMONT

The work that is now entering its fifth year started serendipitously. In early 2009, I received a call from one of the infectious disease physicians in our college of medicine asking if I would be interested in going to Uganda. I did not know this doctor, but I was intrigued. We met that same day in a short meeting in which I learned of the intent of our medical school to affiliate with Makerere University for a student rotation in tropical medicine/ infectious disease. Another university already had been successfully running such a program for some time, and my colleagues had the opportunity to develop a similar venture. What made this doctor ask me was that directors of the Makerere University program had asked specifically if there was an opportunity to create a similar program in nursing. Two physicians and I traveled to Kampala, Uganda, to explore the prospects. We returned with a plan and a proposal for funding to send students and faculty to Uganda in a pilot project. Unfortunately, our grant application was not selected for funding, although the review committee was interested in the proposal on a conceptual level.

Because of that connection, however, I was introduced to a local alumnus of UVM who was running a program of educational and practical support for 52 children in Kamuli, Uganda. The 52 Kids Foundation had been in operation only a few years, but had already provided the basic necessities—housing, meals, clothing, medical care, and adult supervision—for selected children in the area, most of whom were orphaned as a result of their parents' AIDS infections. As my colleague and I talked about the potential of creating a partnership between UVM's Department of Nursing and the Foundation, we found common ground in our belief that whatever program we created had to be sustainable and empowering to the Ugandans he was trying to help. I learned that the 52 Kids Foundation had worked with a local NGO in identifying the children and extended families who needed the most help, and in creating systems by which donors and volunteers could make a difference. I thought the prospects seemed promising, but I needed to be "on the ground" in the region to ascertain the feasibility of bringing a group of nursing students to Kamuli.

For that first trip to Uganda, I traveled as part of a team of five from Vermont to explore options for collaboration there. Our team included my physician colleague, a family practice physician, a newly admitted medical student, and an undergraduate interested in African studies and, potentially, a career in global health care. Only two members of the team had been to Africa before.

Kamuli is a district in southeastern Uganda, about 4 hours northeast of Kampala, Uganda's capital city. Estimates of the population of the Kamuli District vary widely but exceed, at this time, half a million individuals. Kamuli Town is the largest urban area of the district, but is really a small town comprised of dirt roads and small businesses built around a road that connects Kamuli with Jinja to the south. During our 2 weeks, we learned about the work of the Kamuli Area People's Independent Development Association (KAPIDA), the NGO that had supplied the names of children in need of assistance. We toured hospitals, clinics, and schools; we also spent time in villages meeting residents and doing some of the development work KAPIDA had begun. Nutrition, hygiene, and safety in the villages surrounding Kamuli Town were the main concerns of our KAPIDA hosts.

PLANNING AND SETTING THE STAGE FOR UGANDA PARTNERSHIP

Following the first trip to Kamuli, I knew that we had enough "organizational chemistry" to run the first public health nursing course in Uganda. The intangible chemistry was felt in the compatibility of missions and a feeling of mutual respect for our respective roles. The Kamuli Mission Hospital Training School for Midwifery and Comprehensive Nursing had leaders with vision, even though they had few resources. The Mission Hospital had a medical director who saw potential in collaboration. KAPIDA was already engaged in work to improve health and the economic status of families in several villages in the district. The 52 Kids Foundation gave us an opportunity to work with children and adolescents as they were being educated. On a microcosmic level, there were complex relationships among the people in the NGOs and in the town governance that boded well for strong partnerships.

Standards, Theories, and Values

The Public Health Core Functions and Essential Services (CDC, 2013; Public Health Functions Steering Committee, 1994) provided the boundaries of work (see Table 5.2) we would undertake. Obviously in a 3-week period we would only touch on one or two of the essentials, but my vision was that over time we would build on our own work and on that of KAPIDA, 52 Kids, and the Ugandan Ministry of Health as reflected in the district health offices. As the project evolved, I began to realize that I needed to know more about community development and to find out whether that work had relevance for our health interventions. A summer intensive course helped with the language of the discipline and provided fresh insights into collaborations between community development and public health work. Table 5.3 shows the values Vincent (2009, p. 60) described as foundational to community development work. They are consistent to a large extent with values underpinning public health and with community-based participatory action research, both of which emphasize mutual ownership of the work and shared products (Faridi, Grunbaum, Gray, Franks, & Simoes, 2007). Students learned about the Quad Council Competencies (2011), the Scope and Standards of Public Health Nursing (ANA, 2007), and the Public Health Intervention Wheel (Keller, Strohschein, Lia-Hoagberg, & Schaffer, 2004; MDH, 2001) as bases for their practice both in the United States and in Uganda.

TABLE 5.2 The Essential Services of Public Health

- Monitor health status to identify community health problems
- Diagnose and investigate health problems and hazards
- Inform, educate, and empower people
- Mobilize community partnerships
- Develop policies and plans
- Enforce laws and regulations
- Link people to needed services
- Assure a competent health care workforce
- Evaluate effectiveness, accessibility, and quality of services
- Research for new insights and innovative solutions to problems

Source: Public Health Functions Steering Committee (1994).

TABLE 5.3 Values and Beliefs Supporting Community Development

People have the right to
- Participate in decisions that affect them
- Strive to create the environment they desire
- Make informed decisions and modify or reject externally imposed conditions
- Maximize human interaction to increase chances of success
- Create community dialogue to work on common goals
- Own the process through participation in strategic planning
- Cultivate their ability to independently and effectively deal with community issues

Adapted from Vincent (2009), p. 60.

Educational Collaboration

The course was easy to plan—UVM's Nursing Department already had a model of immersion education and service learning in Bangladesh, taught by Dr. Hendrika J. Maltby. We decided to use the same syllabus and assignments, altering our approach in terms of the specific needs of each country. We also set out to study what happened to students during the cross-cultural immersion and public health nursing experience, based on her early observations in Bangladesh. Together, we crafted a proposal for joint research; the study was approved by the UVM Human Subjects Protections Office's institutional review board (IRB). We will complete the study in the winter of 2014. Since the first trip, students have been required to write daily reflective journals. Our annual analysis of student reflections has provided an opportunity to develop strategies to help students cope with new stressors. The assignment helps them integrate emotions with events and question their assumptions, and the product provides them with a permanent memory book about this life-altering trip. Before departure, students are prepared with a bit of history, basic cultural information, geography, and a multitude of pictures as well as all the mandatory information from our faculty-led programs abroad (FLPA).

The Educational Program

The objectives of the public health nursing course are set by the faculty of the Department of Nursing with guidance from those of us prepared in public health nursing. The course has several formats, but the objectives are the same whether geared for on-campus traditional baccalaureate students, RN to BS students who learn online and with individually designed public health field work, master's entry students, or students who travel with faculty for a more global application. By the end of each course, students are expected to

1. Examine historical, environmental, social, and political forces that impact the health of populations
2. Describe the purposes of epidemiology and its importance in caring for populations
3. Compare and contrast community and public health nursing models, theories, and standards of practice
4. Employ the nursing process—incorporating research and theory—in health promotion, disease prevention, and protection strategies with populations
5. Demonstrate integration of previous knowledge and experiences in caring for populations
6. Apply the concepts of community partnerships to provide a holistic approach to enhance health and quality of life of the population
7. Analyze the complexity of the roles of the nurse in community and public health through a variety of experiences in the community across the continuum of primary, secondary, and tertiary prevention
8. Use the ANA Standards of Nursing Practice and Code for Nurses to guide practice

The course involves 126 hours of clinical work and 45 hours of classroom learning.

Application of population-focused nursing actions in the unfamiliar environment of Uganda represents a real challenge due to language barriers, dissimilarities in health status and systems of care, cultural expectations, and the stress of travel halfway around the world. Objectives are met through listening, observing, and comparing. A typical day begins at 7 a.m. with breakfast followed by class and then hospital experience in maternity, pediatrics, antenatal clinic, and male or female inpatient wards. Students cannot do a great deal of direct care since they are unable to communicate effectively with most patients, but they do learn and coach women through labor and delivery, assess infants, administer medications and treatments to children, do rounds with the medical officer or doctor, and provide antenatal and postnatal care to women who come for HIV testing, immunizations, and well-baby checks. They may also work at a health district office and do community outreach to pregnant women. We are fortunate to have a nurse midwife who is also a health center administrator teach our students about immunizations and procedures at the clinics. Before arrival we make contact through the 52 Kids Foundation and KAPIDA with the Kamuli District health officer and with hospital administrators and other officials. Because we always work with Ugandan nurses, UVM faculty have not needed to apply for Ugandan nursing licenses, but we did originally verify our credentials and obtain official authorization to practice. Students are always supervised by UVM faculty as well as appropriately licensed Ugandan nurses, physicians, and health officers. Nursing faculty from the Kamuli Mission Hospital School of Midwifery and Comprehensive Nursing help teach our students in the classroom, in the hospital wards, and occasionally in the villages.

In the afternoon, there is time for debriefing and lunch followed by a short nap before the group heads to the villages where our focus goes far upstream. By this we mean that we examine the root causes of health problems by a focus on prevention. Upstream factors include socioeconomic, environmental, and political conditions that predispose individuals and population groups to excess risk of disease and disability

In the beginning, students learn what other groups have done before them, seeing kitchen gardens previous students have planted, latrines and garbage pits they have dug, fuel efficient stoves they have helped communities build, and hand-washing stations and plate stands that students have built. This public health approach helps our students identify key connections between basic sanitation and health. Within the first week, students begin to teach hand hygiene, toothbrushing, how to decrease flies around the latrines, how to control mosquitoes and jiggers (sand fleas), and help the poorest families with "gifts" of soap, paraffin, salt, sugar, and seedlings at the end of each project. The funds to support the interventions come from the students' program fees and sometimes from me. The cost is small, the payoff big. We have washed clothes, smeared houses with a dung-and-clay mixture to decrease jigger infestations, purchased insecticide for children with badly infested feet and then treated them, debrided necrotic skin, and purchased shoes for children who could not walk due to infestation. Nursing students help carry water and teach children how to keep the pump and the jerry cans clean to decrease the risk of food contamination. They make sure that as many children as possible sleep under bed nets treated with insecticide, and that the nets are securely hung and draped so that they actually provide protection. They learn to look for the early and later manifestations of anemia and kwashiorkor, or protein-calorie malnutrition. With the guidance of knowledgeable KAPIDA workers, students learned to make nutritious porridge to increase protein intake among children younger than 5 (and others) and work with whole groups of village women who learn to make this communally by sharing locally grown grains and seeds. All these actions demonstrate that healthier living begins with clean water, nutritious food, good hygiene and sanitation, and willingness to labor together to accomplish what each family cannot do alone. None of this involves complex program planning, but there is significant coordination involved. Having the students *do*, rather than watch, is more meaningful to students than any of the classroom work. Each day we tackle problems that our colleagues at home also address: domestic violence, occupational safety, and the burden of chronic disease, the impact of climate change, the accessibility and affordability of health care, among others. I teach while we work, and I pitch in whenever the students will make room for me. Working right alongside villagers removes us from the health care tourist role. We do not practice what some refer to as "duffle bag" medicine—we live their life as much as we can. (The term refers to popular approaches by those living in higher income countries to host small clinics and provide basic medications and medical care without appropriate partnership or concern for continuity and sustainability.) Our efforts to experience the life of those with whom we work fosters understanding of life in low- and middle-income countries, the impact of scarce resources, and our impact as guests in another country. We buy local; we eat what is available. Small things demonstrate commitment and willingness to learn from our partners, and give us opportunities to eat and play together. Of course we enjoy clean housing and ample food each night, but even in the guest house we learn to cope with power outages that exceed 50%, cold showers—if any—with limited water, and hot nights under mosquito netting.

Our days end in a communal late supper and reflective discussion. Most nights we are joined by the 52 Kids staff and a few of the older children who have helped in the villages. KAPIDA directors come once in a while. Sometimes there are impromptu language classes, but more often we talk about what we have in common and what is strange to us or to the Ugandans. Students gradually drift away to study for the next morning's class, to write in their journals or simply to go to sleep. The work is tiring for everyone.

Back home, one faculty member who accompanied us was asked the question that was on many faculty members' minds: Is a 3-week period sufficient, and do they really get a good education there? Our visitor responded, "Better."

FACULTY LESSONS LEARNED

Planning is important. Each year, months are devoted to preparation—from meeting university requirements to writing letters requesting permission to come. Budgeting takes weeks, and the program fee must be set 5 months in advance of departure. But even with all the preparation, there are things to be learned on the ground, in country. Table 5.4 lists some of the factors that influence the success of an international health project. The lessons we learned are relevant.

Lesson 1: Planning Is Not Always Enough

The logistics of the first trip were reasonably planned—we had a place to stay on arrival, transportation to Kamuli, housing in the town close to the school and hospital, people who were expecting us, and clearances with police and governmental officials to visit and work in local health agencies. The partners all had a copy of the syllabus with a daily plan for

TABLE 5.4 Facilitators and Barriers to Partnerships in International Health Work

Identification of "the boss"
Clarity of intent
Mutuality of purpose
Strength of commitment
Addition of players
Distractions and detractors

classes, hospital practice, and public health work in one of the district health clinics and in the villages. We had left time for work with the children of 52 Kids who were on summer vacation during our stay. I had even arranged for a colleague from Kenya, a nurse midwife, to stop by and help us during our first week in Kamuli. KAPIDA and 52 Kids Foundation staff had arranged a series of meetings with village leaders and residents; we did the tours of family compounds that had been improved by the addition of deep latrines, hand-washing stations, kitchen gardens, and fuel-efficient stoves. We ate with villagers and played with their children. We toured the hospital and had tea with faculty and administrators of the nursing school. Each year we have extended our circle of acquaintances a bit farther. Students were sometimes impatient to begin the actual work of nursing and helping provide the things families needed. I had to explain the need for us to see, assess, and to begin new relationships before work could take place.

Among the challenges we faced during the first course was the realization that the Ugandans had completely different ideas about our purposes. Despite correspondence among the key players and my assumption that we shared a common language, the reality of a full-fledged course in which students were expected to achieve certain competencies and have particular educational experiences had not sunk in. Time and goals were understood from two perspectives. As one community leader was fond of reminding us, "You Americans are richer than us in many things, but there is one thing in which we are richer than you. Time."

Underscoring this point, our American students wanted their usual structured day, a habit of much hospital education in nursing. They responded variably to surprises, and were frustrated with the schedule changes and the differences between the hosts' and the visitors' time orientation. Beyond that, there were major adaptations demanded of students. Children die far more often in developing nations than they do in the United States. Although I had warned students with stories and pictures, the experience of death, particularly that of young children, was a phenomenon students had not encountered as novice nurses. Ugandans seemed puzzled by their response to situations that are daily occurrences in rural villages. Both the Ugandan nurse educators and I came to appreciate the trauma of coming face to face for the first time with the effects of poverty and endemic disease.

Lesson 2: We Are Not Tourists

Before we leave the United States, students are required to read a number of articles to help them get into the right mindset. One is a classic article called *Duffle Bag Medicine* (Roberts, 2006). We talk about not just dropping in, dropping off, and leaving the country without ensuring that the work we do is what is needed, what is wanted, and what is sustainable. Cultural humility and willingness to learn from our hosts are attributes I look for in students and in colleagues who want to share the experience.

In the months between selection of students to go to Uganda and arrival in Kamuli, I think I do a thorough job of letting the nursing students know what would be expected in terms of practice, study and behavior in social situations. One the more distressing experiences for me as leader of the group occurred not in the first year but with the second group of students. Midway through the 3 weeks of this compressed course, I realized that students needed a break—time away from the demands of always being watched. Being watched is an inevitable side effect of working in a community where diversity in race and culture is uncommon. The phenomenon of being remarkable is so common in Uganda that there are T-shirts attesting to it: "My name is not Muzungu," they say. Muzungu is a Swahili term for White person.

We achieved some anonymity during an overnight trip to Jinja, the nearest city at the head of the Nile, one of Uganda's main tourist areas. In Jinja, students seemed to shed their professional roles and their culturally sensitive behaviors as easily as they threw off their flip-flop sandals. They acted, in most cases, like privileged tourists in Uganda for the purpose of buying souvenirs. From my perspective, they took on the attributes of "ugly Americans" who made poor representatives of the university and of the profession.

There is a time during an immersion experience when a break is ideally situated. Traveling in a group of 12, including faculty and a teaching assistant, is grueling. Everything takes time, from ordering meals to assigning rooms, to changing money. Nerves become frayed and internal conflicts arise. Having seen this now several times over, I believe that it is a normal part of the process and have planned a regular break midway through our stay.

As noted earlier, in a rural town like Kamuli where Caucasians are still rare, we were constantly under scrutiny. There was undoubtedly judgment on the part of some Ugandans, but more often there was simple curiosity. Still, students felt they were always "under the microscope." They came to resent this, quietly, but in ways that can be destructive to the work and their own psychological well-being. This became manifest in their irritability, and in their journals. Some students complained that the Ugandans did not contribute enough work, that they sat and watched and made jokes about us. Another group waited until we had left Kamuli but told other Westerners about their annoyance with the Ugandans. It was unprofessional at best, and it was disheartening that they had interpreted their experience in that way. Patience and understanding are essential for anyone leading students or even groups of professionals who are unfamiliar with working in foreign countries.

In places like Jinja where tourists from all over the world congregate, it is easy to fall into bad habits. Ugandans fulfill service roles, and tourists are their bread and butter. To see students change from service learners to privileged Americans in the space of an hour was distressing.

A 24-hour period of tourism can interrupt a trip, but the tourist approach to public health work is antithetical to effective action. Since the initial year, we have worked hard to have students examine their assumptions about the experience. During the first year, a small group of students became frustrated with the multiple changes to a day's schedule and their perception that their learning needs were not a priority for the Ugandans, a not wholly inaccurate evaluation. The students behaved badly, rudely addressing one of the leaders of the community and refusing to accept a ride back to town despite the distance of the journey and the intense heat of the afternoon. A series of mishaps had caused the day's disorganization, along with miscommunications and inattention to the goals of our public health work. Both NGOs were involved, but we were left out of the equation, as were the villagers who had been expecting us.

At the end of the day, students were short-tempered and snubbed not only their village hosts but also the KAPIDA personnel who were late arriving to take us back to town. The students' failure to observe social courtesies of Ugandan life conveyed their message of displeasure in tone of voice and body language as much as by refusing food and transportation. Our hosts are astute observers of our behavior as well, and they are keenly aware when something is amiss. Most importantly, it sent an unintended message that the villagers were not respected. Grateful for a ride back to town, I was sitting in the truck when this group of four students refused to get in. I heard their quiet but condescending remarks, and I was angry. One of the KAPIDA directors calmed me by reminding me that, indeed, they were *students* whose behavior was inappropriate but would be best dealt with when I was no longer annoyed. The advice was right, of course. When I sat with the students later that evening, my question was simple, "How do you think the Ugandans here regard us?" We were nearing the end of our stay in Kamuli. Opening the floodgates both to their frustrations and their perceptions gave us all the perspective that we needed to come to terms with our position in that community. The students examined themselves a bit and were contrite. Relationships were restored to equilibrium in the remaining days and drew praise from our hosts. Each subsequent year has yielded a deepening understanding of all parties' mutual responsibility for making the partnership work.

Lesson 3: Competing Interests Among Partners

The 52 Kids Foundation developed with the assistance of KAPIDA, and KAPIDA has derived important financial support from the 52 Kids. From the perspective of an outsider, I see this symbiotic relationship as mutually beneficial and necessary to our work. Could we work without either? This is a question of urgent importance as we enter our fifth year of collaboration. Over the years, there have been some rough spots in the relations between the two entities. Both have important goals; both organizations articulate values and visions that are consistent with our interests in working in a sustainable manner to improve health in rural Uganda. At the same time, they sometimes have competing interests and often separate priorities. Legitimately, the two directors demonstrate some self-interest with respect to what they get out of their mutual relationship or the partnership with UVM. It has been essential to learn to recognize where interests converge and where they must differ based on the different purposes of each organization.

Negotiating disparate interests is frequently a function of public health work; rarely, if ever, are partners of one vision. I am not naive about this, for as the designer of this educational experience for UVM nursing students, I represent another set of interests. The course demands positive interaction with the partners to ensure the best experience for the students. My own interest in working with communities in the Kamuli District of Uganda adds another dimension of complexity; there I represent myself as a public health practitioner, and as sensitive as I may try to be to the desires and goals of my collaborators, our work has to work for me, too.

To maximize the potential for each partner organization to meet the objectives of its unique mission there must be acknowledgment of (a) the value of those objectives, (b) the right of each partner organization to put its needs first, and (c) the need to explore together how best to maximize interorganizational synergy. On more than one occasion, we have had discussions about what to do and how to get it done. These are probably best done in advance, but more often sessions are in response to failures to coordinate, frustrations with the process, lost opportunities, or even interpersonal conflict.

Among the foundational tenets of community-based participatory action (and research) is social justice; such action is meant to overcome social inequities and to involve those communities affected by specific problems in developing solutions that are meaningful and

TABLE 5.5 Evolving Purposes of the Project

2009	Enter into relationship with Makerere University for the education of UVM medical and nursing students
2010	Work with the 52 Kids Foundation to provide services to AIDS orphans aged 7 to 18 and their guardian families in Kamuli, Uganda
2011	Provide cross-cultural and hands-on public health nursing experience for senior UVM students in a Ugandan community
2012	Combination of 2010–2011, but increasing focus on rural health and building community relationships
2013	Development of independent relationships and extension of services to areas related to health (e.g., community development, economic security)

TABLE 5.6 Building a Sustainable Program

Openness to new possibilities
Health fundamental to economic development
Partners come from unexpected places
Economic development essential for long-term success
Local leadership and commitment
Dissonances inevitable

beneficial to them. Working with partners across cultures and with different aims complicates matters—particularly when partners do not share the same assumptions. Neither is at fault; a long history of power relationships conditions their responses. I was proud when the director of KAPIDA quietly observed on our last night in Kamuli, "We like working with you, it's different than with [omitted]. . . . You listen to us." There was more, of course, but it was clear that we had conveyed respect and honored the right of the residents of Kamuli District to determine their own destiny.

UPCOMING CHALLENGES

Table 5.5 summarizes the evolving focus of the UVM public health nursing course in Kamuli.

As we move into the next phase of development, we hope to grow our program so that there are students from UVM present several times a year, perhaps even year-round. The limitations of the baccalaureate nursing program are such that students can only participate at specific times, but physical therapy students, medical laboratory technology students, students of agriculture, engineering, global and regional studies, and others have expressed interest in participating. We are proceeding with caution. It would be easy to overwhelm the fragile system in which we are working (see Table 5.6). We ask the following questions as we move forward:

- Whose interests will come first?
- What can students and faculty from each of the disciplines contribute to the health and well-being of the Ugandans in Kamuli?
- How much money is needed to support locally identified projects?

If money can be obtained, with what strings might it come? My model of sustainability in global health work has been influenced by the nursing perspective of Leffers and Mitchell (2011) but incorporates a community development framework as articulated by a leader in that profession (Vincent, 2009). Until now, the effort has involved capacity-building and development of social capital. Our plan is to move steadily toward community outcomes. I share with these authors and with colleagues from UVM a desire for a balance between social, ecological, and economic influences to support health and hope that we will continue to champion viable, bearable, and equitable conditions for all members of the communities with which we work.

REFLECTIVE QUESTIONS

1. This case study describes the importance of planning and ongoing evaluation for academic partnerships in global health settings. How can you apply the successes and challenges shared in this case study to your academic partnership?
2. Discuss "the things unexpected" that were shared in this case study. Have you experienced similar surprises in your global health work?
3. How might you be viewed as a tourist when you are involved in global health work in another country? How can you plan for this aspect of your work?

REFERENCES

American Nurses Association. (2007). *Public health nursing scope and standards of practice.* Washington, DC: American Nurses Association.

CDC. (2013). Public health system and the 10 essential public health services. National Public Health Performance Standards. http://www.cdc.gov/nphpsp/essentialservices.html

Faridi, Z., Grunbaum, J. A., Gray, B. S., Franks, A., & Simoes, E. (2007). Community-based participatory research: Necessary next steps. *Preventing Chronic Disease* [serial online]. www.cdc.gov/pcd/issues/2007/jul/06_0182.htm

Keller, L. O., Strohschein, S., Lia-Hoagberg, B., & Schaffer, M. A. (2004). Population-based public health interventions: Practice-based and evidence-supported, part I. *Public Health Nursing, 21*(5), 453–468.

Leffers, J., & Mitchell, E. (2011). Conceptual model for partnership and sustainability in global health. *Public Health Nursing, 28*(1), 91–102.

Minnesota Department of Health. (2001). Public health interventions: Applications for public health nursing practice. http://www.health.state.mn.us/divs/opi/cd/phn/docs/0301wheel_manual.pdf

Public Health Functions Steering Committee. (1994). Essential public health services. Public Health in America. www.health.gov/phfunctions/public.htm

Quad Council of Public Health Nursing Organizations. (2011). Quad Council competencies for public health nurses. www.resourcenter.net/images/ACHNE/Files/QuadCouncilCompetenciesForPublicHealthNurses_Summer2011.pdf

Roberts, M. (2006, April 5). A piece of my mind: Duffle bag medicine. *Journal of the American Medical Association, 295*(13), 1491–1492.

Vincent, J. W. (2009). Community development practice. In R. Phillips & R. Pittman (Eds.), *An introduction to community development* (pp. 58–73). London, UK: Routledge.

CHAPTER 6

Capacity Building for Global Health Nursing

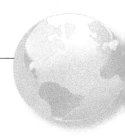

Marie J. Driever
Valentina Sarkisova
Natalia Serebrennikova
Barbara Mandleco
Janet L. Larson

Global nursing practice continues to increase as nurses develop collaborative relationships with colleagues across geographic and cultural borders for various projects and student learning experiences. Using capacity building as a search term in the PubMed database brings up numerous articles, demonstrating that this is a concept with a long history in discussions of international development and global efforts and has been used to guide these collaborative relationships. Therefore, the purpose of this chapter is to illustrate how capacity building can be used within the context of global health and nursing's potential and vital role in addressing health problems, issues, and concerns across national boundaries. Specifically, this chapter does the following:

- Reviews a current definition of capacity building
- Describes how capacity building relates to global health
- Proposes an updated definition of capacity building that better fits the new context of global health
- Explores dimensions of the collaborative relationship: counterparts and facilitation
- Explores capacity building for nursing research

CAPACITY BUILDING: A CURRENT DESCRIPTION

In a 2003 publication, Ogilvie et al. (2003) synthesized a definition of capacity building and cited the work of Morgan (1999). In doing this, they began with a definition of capacity as used by Morgan (1999, p. 37), who defined capacity as the "abilities, behaviors, relationships, and values that enable individuals, groups, and organizations at any level of society to carry out functions or tasks and to achieve their development objectives over time." Ogilvie et al. continue with Morgan's definition, noting that building capacity refers to "an intervention or activity by an organization or group in one country to help those in another to improve their ability to carry out certain functions or achieve certain objectives" (Morgan, 1999, p. 14). Further, Ogilvie et al. described building capacity as including micro- (individual), meso- (organizational), and macro- (systemic) level changes over time and requiring "long term changes in ways of relating that support systemic or structural change with some permanence or sustainability" (Angeles & Guerstein, 2000, p. 454). Finally, capacity building may be better described as a process rather than a single intervention or activity (Ogilvie et al., 2003). Thus, to summarize, capacity building refers to an intervention that partners from one country or organization use over time to aid partners from another country or organization in developing competence to achieve desired function and goals.

Definition of Global Health in the Current Context of Capacity Building

Globalization and the increasing interconnectedness it brings creates a context that must be considered when applying capacity building to global health efforts. In 1997, the Institute of Medicine (IOM) defined global health as "health problems, issues and concerns that transcend national boundaries, may be influenced by circumstances or experiences in other countries, and are best addressed by cooperative means and solution." However, a paradigm shift is inherent in changing the term *international* health to *global* health and suggests new coordination, resources, and solutions for worldwide health problems (Bunyavanich & Walkup, 2001). Importantly, global health supplies a context for capacity building through emphasizing the interconnectedness of activities within and between nations that create joint benefits of collaboration, since collaboration assumes shared contributions and mutual benefits. This paradigm shift in redefining global health also creates the basis for establishing partnerships between countries. These kinds of partnerships in nursing foster resource sharing to meet goals, which strengthens nursing in both countries. Such collaboration sets up partnerships based on and evolved from mutual learning and problem solving, the focus of a collaborative process. This shift guides and shapes an understanding of nursing's role in advancing global health (Jairath, 2007).

Revising the Definition of Capacity Building

In the current definition of capacity building, the notion of counterparts in one country helping counterparts or host partners in another country, even in a collaborative relationship, suggests some level of need or dependency by those in the host country. However, by emphasizing interconnectedness between both counterparts, the contributions of each partner are considered to be equal yet also needed. For example, when a group of U.S. researchers collaborated with the Russian Nurses' Association (RNA) to bring information about nursing research to Russian nurses, the U.S. researchers brought knowledge and experience of how to implement studies and use study results in clinical practice. Adding to this level of expertise of the U.S. partners, the Russian partners contributed goals for sharing this knowledge with Russian nurses and information about the needs, norms, and expectations which affected strategies necessary to meet the goals. It soon became evident that each partner's contribution needed to be melded together and equal to create a successful workshop.

Another addition to an updated definition of capacity building is to consider using facilitation as a major method for implementing a collaborative partnership, as it contributes a way of organizing communication. Facilitation also enables and eases the way to jointly undertake a global health project and is a process with a variety of strategies and techniques to guide and structure ongoing collaborative partnership communication. To maximize a collaborative partnership process during a global health project with a focus on capacity building, it is most helpful if both partners are mindful of and carefully plan their use of the facilitation process. In this way the partners build in a way of using various facilitation techniques to clarify their communications to both promote understanding and, importantly, set the stage for discussion of cultural nuances as well as concerns. Generally the partner from the donor country needs to bring knowledge and skills of the facilitation process and monitor that the process is promoting constructive communication. It is also helpful if the partner(s) from the host country brings knowledge and skill in facilitation to the interaction and is willing to use facilitation throughout the project.

This interconnectedness brings equal contributors to the collaborative relationship and increases nurses' interest in being involved in global health endeavors. However, there is a need to rethink and update the concept of capacity building as it underpins development, implementation, and evaluation of global health projects. The updated definition overtly and strongly refers to a collaborative process of two counterparts using a partnering relationship to share and exchange diverse knowledge, skills, and resources to facilitate creation of sustainable strategies, structures, and resources to achieve desired goals over time.

In this proposed revised definition, capacity building refers to a collaborative process of two counterparts using a partnering relationship for sharing and exchanging diverse knowledge, skills, and resources to facilitate one of the counterparts' creation of sustainable strategies, structures, and resources to achieve desired goals over time. This comprehensive definition maintains the core meaning of the counterpart in one country using interventions to help the counterpart in another country develop competence, but stresses and reframes the collaborative process as a partnering relationship using the facilitation process to emphasize sharing and exchanging knowledge and skills to create or modify structures and resources.

Exploration of Collaborative Relationship: Partners and Facilitation

In further examining this definition, particularly reframing the collaborative relationship and adding facilitation as a method to promote collaborative relationships, it is helpful to consider two aspects: (1) a model of counterparts proposed by DeSantis (1995) as a way to structure this relationship and (2) review of characteristics and strategies of facilitation used in implementing this process. In her model, DeSantis emphasizes the concept of counterparts, which can be used to structure the collaborative partnerships in capacity building endeavors. In this model, counterparts are persons designated from the donor or guest and recipient or host countries that represent the countries involved. The counterparts' relationship is seen as a continuum during which each brings necessary knowledge and skills across the life of the work (DeSantis, 1995). According to DeSantis there are four key components that are important when evaluating whether or not the partnerships are collaborative and equally balance interests of partners from both donor/guest and host countries (DeSantis, 1995):

1. Negate the need for the donor group over time. Considering that the updated definition of capacity building stresses a process of collaborative partnerships, it seems that no longer needing the donor can be continually renegotiated over time. Indeed, the conduct of research relates to collaborative endeavors which are likely to evolve over time and exemplify how the need and contributions of the donor group may also change over time.
2. Address the needs, available resources, and developing potential of the host country
3. Address the sociocultural, political, and economic factors in the collaborative planning process
4. Develop the potential and further skills of those involved from both countries

These counterpart components further delineate ways to consider and structure the collaborative partnership relationship so that it is workable and supportive of capacity building work.

Facilitation: Core to the Collaborative Partnering Process of Capacity Building

Facilitation is core to the collaborative partnering process in the updated capacity building definition and important because it brings elements to help partners maximize communication and other strategies for developing relationships over the life of the work. In the

TABLE 6.1 Definitions of Facilitation

Author	Definitions
Harvey et al., 2002	"The process of enabling (making easier) the implementation of evidence into practice" (p. 579)
Stetler et al., 2006	"A deliberate and valued process of interactive problem solving and support that occurs in the context of a recognized need for improvement and a supportive interpersonal relationship" (para. 4)

literature on promoting evidence in practice and quality improvement, there is a consistent theme of using facilitation as a core component when assisting nurses to apply evidence in their practice. In developing this updated definition of capacity building, an analysis of and studies reported about the definition of facilitation, its components, and ways to organize this process can be adapted to capacity building research.

Harvey et al. (2002) performed a concept analysis of facilitation in relation to successfully implementing evidence into practice. These authors proposed a working definition of facilitation as helping and enabling, which fits with the essence of capacity building. Within helping/enabling, the focus of facilitation can encompass a broad spectrum, ranging from helping to achieve a specific task to using methods that enable individuals and teams to review their attitude, habits, skills, and ways of thinking and working (Harvey et al., 2002). In addition, Dogherty et al. (2010) conducted a literature review of the definition and demonstrated how the role and function of facilitation evolved since Harvey's publication. This review confirmed two previous definitions and added another as noted in Table 6.1 (Dogherty et al., 2010, p. 80).

From this review of definitions, Dogherty et al. (2010, p. 76) summarized these findings:

1. Facilitation is viewed as an individual role as well as a process involving individuals and groups.
2. The process of facilitation involves supporting and enabling.
3. Project management and leadership are important components.
4. It is critical that facilitation be tailored to the local context.
5. There is a growing emphasis on evaluation, particularly linking outcomes to nursing actions.

This review of definitions of facilitation and key elements offers a way to conceptualize the capacity building partnership over time and organize communication and elements of work to be done to achieve desired goals and objectives.

Dogherty et al. (2010) also outlined a taxonomy of facilitation strategies that can be used singly and in various combinations over the course of capacity building work. In order to use facilitation strategies when building capacity, the strategies are considered along a spectrum as outlined in Table 6.2, which presents classes of facilitation strategies and select examples. These strategies also include additional elements identified in a study of facilitation on adaptation of guidelines and early implementation (Dogherty et al., 2012).

Two additional facilitation strategies are added to this taxonomy: sense making and using appreciative inquiry (AI). The first, sense making, developed by Parchman et al. (2013), stressed the helpfulness of strategies for teams as they make sense of or gain insight into the changes they make and are experiencing. Specific approaches to enable individuals and teams to make sense are part of relationship building and communication, and also increase awareness of the need for change. Enabling individuals and groups to increase the meaning of their experiences is also likely to help them understand changes encountered.

A second facilitation strategy relates to adding AI. Integrating AI into the facilitation process brings an energizing and "uniquely effective approach to nurturing organizational change" (Carter et al., 2007, p. 195). As a contrast to traditional approaches emphasizing

TABLE 6.2 Taxonomy of Facilitation Strategies

Relationship Building and Communication	Leadership and Project Management
Acknowledging success, recognizing and celebrating achievements	Thinking ahead in the process
Sense making	Taking on specific tasks
	Ensuring the group remains on task and things are not missed
Being available as needed	

Importance of the Local Context	Increased Awareness of the Need for Change
Use of appreciative inquiry	Creating an open, supportive, and trusting environment conducive to change
	Ongoing monitoring and evaluation
	Interpreting data and providing feedback about performance gaps

problems, AI focuses on meaningful and fundamental change that occurs through discovering and valuing the strengths, assets, vision, and ideals of individuals in an organization. According to Carter et al. (2007, p. 195), "by appreciating core strengths and values, people in an organization recognize those factors that give purpose and meaning" to their efforts. This approach focuses on the positive and builds on aspects those involved value. It also helps individuals find meaning in their work and changes they are encountering. In reflecting on using facilitation with the RNA to integrate nursing research as an organizational priority, the addition of AI as a strategy would have been helpful. Ongoing work with the RNA will incorporate this strategy.

However, using facilitation strategies has been helpful in aiding the RNA build nursing research as an organizational capacity and is used as an example of how facilitation is operationalized. Specifically, facilitation helped the RNA decide to prepare a grant in response to a call for proposals from the Bristol-Myers Squibb Foundation grants program, Bridging Cancer Care, to improve cancer care in Eastern Europe. This decision was based on a strong relationship and open communication that allowed discussion of options and ways of using those options in writing the grant. Facilitation techniques must also be used to introduce, convey, and reinforce new information needed for decisions about how to proceed. A key decision was to identify the focus of the proposal and a decision was made to use evidence to support assessment of and interventions for side effects and complications experienced by patients on chemotherapy. That the chief nurse from a regional oncology dispensary was acquainted with evidence-based guidelines developed by the U.S. Oncology Nursing Society (ONS) made this focus seem workable and also built on a strength. It took a great deal of trust and open communication to honestly develop the proposal and make sure these elements met grant program requirements. Much discussion was also necessary to develop a timeline and manage the work to get the proposal written by the submission date. Last, revisiting key concepts and approaches and talking about methods was needed several times in developing the monitoring and evaluation section of the proposal. There was a review of the kinds of changes implementation of the proposal would bring, particularly the implementation of the proposal's monitoring and evaluation plan. This example also illustrates the need to make sense of the work on an ongoing basis as the work proceeds. Collaboration while developing the proposal helped make the transition to implementation easier when the RNA received the grant.

CAPACITY BUILDING FOR NURSING RESEARCH, PRACTICE, EDUCATION, AND LEADERSHIP

A more specific context for capacity building, and a focus of discussion in the case study for this chapter, is applying this concept to developing nursing research capacity. Priest et al. (2007) noted that developing nursing research capacity is a key challenge facing the profession worldwide since overall there is a need for nursing to have a more prominent voice in health services and policy decision making, as previously noted through World Health Organization forums (Antrobus & Kitson, 1999; World Health Assembly, 2006). Throughout the world, nursing must respond to demands to increase the safety, effectiveness, and quality of patient care. Using evidence is required to respond to these demands and expectations. There is also need for innovative responses addressing existing and future health concerns and calling not only for more evidence, but also for new sources of evidence (WHO, 2002). In fact, Edwards (2008) has called for leveraging nursing research to transform health care systems. Thus, within nursing, there is a need to advance research, both by generating knowledge and applying that knowledge to everyday practice. Involvement in research will also help nurses communicate as equally knowledgeable professionals in team communication that is increasingly part of care provision as well as enhancing and promoting nursing as a profession.

For many countries, nursing's development as a profession and discipline has proceeded through a common pattern. This pattern involves nursing moving from functioning as a handmaiden to physicians to having both an independent and complementary function with physicians in caring for patients, families, and communities. This developmental pattern has influenced nursing education and required that it move into degree-granting institutions. However, the struggle to become part of the academic community has provided nursing with both the challenges and benefits of being a discipline that uses research to generate knowledge for professional practice. Even though the specific drivers and state of capacity building vary across countries, all of nursing is facing the need to advance research in both academic and practice arenas. With the global trend of nurses and all health professionals being expected to use evidence as a basis of their patient care, there is a demand for practicing nurses to both conduct and use research as part of their practice. With this demand comes the need for nurses to increase their nursing research knowledge and skill.

Whether developing nursing research capacity is built in academic or practice settings, there are common barriers and potential strategies to consider in developing research that must be tailored to the specific country in which they are used (Edwards et al., 2009). For example, the RNA is encountering challenges to obtain health ministry support in being able to require a baccalaureate degree as the entry practice level for certain nursing specialties. At this time, the RNA believes that the BSN degree should be required initially for select nursing specialists because there are not sufficient universities or sufficient state funds to educate the needed number of nurses at the baccalaureate level. University nursing programs are also limited and offer the High Nursing Education Program, which is required only for administrative and managerial positions. The High Nursing Education Program started in Russia in 1992; by 2013, 43 universities had established nursing departments offering this program. These programs were equivalent to master's level and nurses graduating received a university diploma on specialty management. Prerequisites for entering the program included a nursing school/college diploma and a successful score on an entrance exam. The length of this program is 5 years.

The High Nursing Education Program is designed to prepare nurse leaders and managers for clinical settings and does not include nursing research. Because there have been no nurses with the university, scientific, or PhD degree needed to teach at the university, there are no nursing faculty members in the university. Therefore, physicians have taken the lead for several decades to develop higher education nursing programs, even at the college level. In reality they provide leadership for all nursing education programs, including at the nursing school/college level. This has been the situation for many decades and has also served as career opportunities for physicians to teach nurses. This old and established tradition influences nursing now and creates a barrier to changing Russian nursing education.

Thus, while RNA efforts have increased the number of higher education programs, all established programs continue to be headed by physicians. Since graduates of these programs mostly work in managerial positions, they are more interested in economics than in practice, and in global hospital issues rather than in patient problems. The health care ministry also decided to allow only nurses with higher education to work as chief nurses, and within 10 years wanted all chief nurses to have achieved this level of education.

However, many graduates were not able to find chief nurse positions and so continued working as staff nurses, even though they were not happy with this situation. Recently, nurse leaders in Russia have become aware of trends in the nursing profession and nursing education in other countries and have begun thinking about expanding the educational requirement for nurses in Russia in order to establish a university degree as a requirement for entry into the profession. The state was also interested in decreasing the number of years nurses study at the university, and they were not pleased with many diploma graduates who do not use their education. So in 2012, a bachelor-level educational requirement was approved, and starting in 2013, bachelor programs will become a reality in Russia. A new graduate level educational standard must also be negotiated, developed, and approved. However, physicians remain in charge of these programs even though over the past 20 years the number of nursing faculty has increased. Even though the number of nurses who are faculty remains low, it is not helpful for those in chief nursing positions to leave hospitals and start teaching at the university. The RNA believes nurses must provide leadership for nursing education and research, so the struggle to make this a reality continues.

In light of its access to technological advances, and as a member of the International Council of Nurses (ICN), the RNA belongs to the global nursing community and strives to bring knowledge about new areas of nursing emphasis to Russian nurses. The RNA believes Russian nurses need to have an organized way of learning about nursing research to both understand how to meet new global expectations and improve Russian nurse contributions to the Russian health care system. The RNA also believes that developing the research capacity of Russian nurses will improve the status of nursing in Russia.

Research capacity building has some specific aspects that must be understood for use in research situations. A framework can be helpful to further explore the specific dimensions of research capacity development. Cooke (2005) proposed a framework to evaluate capacity building in health care. In this framework, she delineated six principles, which can also be used while building capacity in nursing research and other areas. These principles state that capacity building in research must do the following:

- Develop appropriate skills and confidence through training and creating opportunities to apply skills
- Ensure research that is "close to practice" in order for it to be useful
- Support linkages, partnerships, and collaborations that enhance research capacity building
- Develop and ensure appropriate dissemination to maximize impact
- Invest in infrastructure
- Build elements of continuity and sustainability

While these principles identify key dimensions to address for building capacity for research, they can also be generalized to more general capacity building, including developing leadership capacity as well as capacity in nursing practice and education.

The framework with six principles by Cooke (2005) described for building research capacity can be adapted to building capacity in nursing practice, education, and leadership. However, when applying capacity building within these contexts, globalization needs to be considered. As noted by Wright et al. (2005), the global economy changes rapidly and frequently affects the ability of health care to respond to a variety of needs. Wright et al. also reported on the development of a short-term education program for professional capacity development in nurses and midwives living in east-central Europe.

In the realm of education, the Hartford Foundation partnered with the American Association of Colleges of Nursing (2006) to develop the capacity of U.S. nursing faculty for building current knowledge and skill that effectively cares for the increasing geriatric population at all levels of the nursing curriculum. In addition, Frenk et al. (2010) reported on the work of a collaborative network with representatives from 20 countries that recommended emphasizing patient-centered care and transprofessional team–based care to educate health professionals for this new century.

The ICN has focused on developing the capacity of leadership at both global and national levels. The first Global Nursing Leadership Institute (GNLI) was initiated in 2009 and with its successful start continues to develop global leadership capacity (Blaney, 2012). Six diverse members of the 2010 GNLI, representing Australia, Bhutan, Lebanon, Lesotho, Thailand, and the United States, shared their reflections on the week-long institute, discussing their understanding of how issues within their respective countries were similar to or different from each other (Zittel et al. 2012). Their reflections demonstrate application of Cooke's (2005) framework within the leadership realm as opportunities for developing leadership skills were provided along with the support for developing linkages and collaboration. At the national level, the ICN provides the Leadership for Change (LFC) program with modules addressing topics such as the focus of leadership roles, effective organization and leadership, resource management, quality improvement, mentoring, succession planning, and team project planning (Anazor, 2012).

Thus, the interconnectedness inherent in collaborations across national boundaries or organizations demonstrates productive work to build capacity for improving practice, education, and leadership. Of note is one report by Hamer (2008) on a model to build capacity for implementing a nursing best practice guideline. Here, capacity building focuses on a process to develop education for the purpose of increasing nursing practice competence. The word "capacity" is, at times, used in place of competence, especially when describing educational programs. However, by focusing on competence the collaborative partnership process and the importance of relationships may diminish over time. The collaborative partnering process, the basis of Cooke's principles, is required for effective global capacity building projects in nursing practice, education, leadership, and/or research and is supported through research and subsequent development of the model for partnership and sustainability in global health (Leffers & Mitchell, 2011).

CONCLUSION

The focus of this chapter has been to revise a definition of capacity building and offer an introduction to a more specific application to research capacity building. In this proposed updated definition, capacity building refers to a collaborative process of two counterparts using a partnering relationship for sharing and exchanging diverse knowledge, skills, and resources to facilitate one counterpart's creation of sustainable strategies, structures, and resources to achieve desired goals over time. With this background on capacity building, a case study of organizational capacity building to integrate nursing research as an organizational priority will illustrate this definition and key principles.

REFERENCES

American Association of Colleges of Nursing and John A. Hartford Foundation. (2006). *Caring for an aging America: A guide of nursing faculty*. New York, NY: American College of Nursing. www.aacn.nche.edu/geriatric-nursing/monograph.pdf

Anazor, C. (2012). Preparing nurse leaders for global health reforms. *Nursing Management, 19*(4), 26–28.

Angeles, L., & Guerstein, P. (2000). Planning for participatory capacity development: The challenges of participation and North–South partnership is capacity-building projects. *Canadian Journal of Development Studies, XXI*, 447–478.

Antrobus, S., & Kitson, A. (1999). Nursing leadership influencing and shaping health policy and nursing practice. *Journal of Advanced Nursing, 29*(3), 746–753.

Blaney, P. (2012). Senior nursing leadership-capacity building at the global level. *International Nursing Review, 59*, 40–47.

Bunyavanich, S., & Walkup, R. B. (2001). U.S. public health leaders shift toward a new paradigm of global health. *American Journal of Public Health, 91*(10), 1556–1558.

Carter, C. A., Ruhe, M. C., Weyer, S., Litaker, D., Fry, R. E., & Strange, K. C. (2007). An appreciative inquiry approach to practice improvement and transformative change in health care settings. *Quality Management in Health Care, 16*(3), 194–204.

Cooke, J. (2005). A framework to evaluate research capacity building in health care. *BMC Family Practice, 6*(44).

DeSantis, L. (1995). A model for counterparts in international nursing. *International Journal of Nursing Studies, 32*(2), 198–209.

Dogherty, E. J., Harrison, M. B., Baker, C., & Graham, I. D. (2010). Facilitation as a role and process in achieving evidence-based practice in nursing: A focused review of concept and meaning. *Worldviews on Evidence-Based Nursing, 7*(2), 76–89.

Dogherty, E. J., Harrison, M. B., Baker, C., & Graham, I. D. (2012). Following a natural experiment of guidelines adaptation and early implementation: A mixed-methods study of facilitation. *Implementation Science, 7*, 9.

Edwards, N. (2008). Leveraging nursing research to transform healthcare systems. *Nursing Inquiry, 15*(2), 81–82.

Edwards, N. J., Mill, J., Kahwa, E., & Roelofs, S. (2009). Building capacity for nurse-led research. *International Review, 56*, 88–94.

Frenk, J., Chen, L., Bhutta, Z. A., Cohen, J., Crisp, N., Evans, T., . . . Zurayk, H. (2010). Health professional for a new century: Transforming education to strengthen health systems in an interdependent world. *Lancet, 376*, 1923–1958.

Hamer, B., (2008). A capacity-building model for implementing a nursing best practice. *Journal for Nurses in Staff Development, 24*(1), 36–42.

Harvey, G., Loftus-Hills, A., Rycroft-Malone, J., Titchen, A., Kitson, A., . . . Seers, K. (2002). Getting evidence into practice: The role and function of facilitation. *Journal of Advanced Nursing, 37*(6), 577–588.

Jairath, N. (2007). Global health: The role of nursing research. *Nursing Research, 56*(6), 367–368.

Leffers, J., & Mitchell, E. (2011). Conceptual model for partnership and sustainability in global health. *Public Health Nursing, 28*(1), 91–102.

Morgan, P. (1999). Some observations and lessons in capacity building. In R. Maconick & P. Morgan (Eds.), *Capacity-building supported by the United Nations: Some evaluations and some lessons.* New York, NY: United Nations.

Ogilvie, L., Allen, M., Laryea, J., & Opare, M. (2003). Building capacity through a collaborative international nursing project. *Journal of Nursing Scholarship, 35*(2), 113–118.

Parchman, M. L., Noel, P. H., Culler, S. D., Lanham, H. J., Leykum, L. K., Romero, R. L., & Palmer, R. F. (2013). A randomized trial of practice facilitation to improve the delivery of chronic illness care in primary care: Initial and sustained effects. *Implementation Science, 8*, 93.

Priest, H., Segrott, J., Bree, B., & Rout, A. (2007). Harnessing collaboration to build nursing research capacity: A research team journey. *Nurse Education Today, 27*, 577–587.

Stetler, C., Legro, M., Rycroft-Malone, J., Bowman, C., Curran, G., Guihan, M., . . . Wallace, C. (2006). Role of "external facilitation" in implementation of research findings: A qualitative evaluation of facilitation experiences in the Veterans Health Administration. *Implementation Science, 1*(23). doi:10.1186/1748-5908-1-2

World Health Assembly. (2006). WHA59.27 *Strengthening nursing and midwifery.* The Fifty-Ninth World Health Assembly, Geneva, Switzerland.

World Health Organization. (2002). *Human resources and national health systems: Shaping the agenda for action. Final report.* Geneva: World Health Organization. hppt://www.who.int/hrh/documents/en/nhs_shaping_agenda.pdf

Wright, S., Cloonan, P., Leonhardy, K., & Wright, G. (2005). An international programme in nursing and midwifery: Building capacity for the new millennium. *International Nursing Review, 52,* 18–23.

Zittel, B., Ezzeddine, S. H., Makatjane, M., Graham, I., Luangamornlert, S., & Pemo, T. (2012). Divergence and convergence in nursing and health care among six countries participating in ICN's 2010 Global Nursing Leadership Institute. *International Nursing Review, 59,* 48–54.

The Russian Nurses' Association Experience of Establishing Nursing Research as an Organizational Priority

Marie J. Driever
Valentina Sarkisova
Natalia Serebrennikova
Barbara Mandleco
Janet L. Larson

CONTEXT: RUSSIA

Russia, with its rich culture and history, is the largest of 21 republics making up the Commonwealth of Independent States, known as the Russian Federation. It occupies most of eastern Europe and north Asia, stretching from the Baltic Sea in the west to the Pacific Ocean in the east, and from the Arctic Ocean in the north to the Black Sea and the Caucasus in the south. It is bordered by Norway and Finland in the northwest; Estonia, Latvia, Belarus, Ukraine, Poland, and Lithuania in the west; Georgia and Azerbaijan in the southwest; and Kazakhstan, Mongolia, China, and North Korea along the southern border. Russia is the largest country in the world in territory and is ranked ninth in population—according to the latest statistics, 143 million. Moscow is the capital and largest city of Russia; St. Petersburg is the second-largest city.

Russian nursing has a history of being an assisting profession that helps physicians treat patients. The nursing diploma serves as the entry to the profession, and the length of the program is 3 years. Over the past 20 years, Russia has experienced a nursing shortage. On general units such as medicine or surgery, one nurse typically cares for 30 patients, a contemporary topic for health care reform. In addition, the ratio of nurses to physicians is 1:2. Having more physicians than nurses reinforces a situation whereby nurses are expected to primarily serve as assistants to physicians, thus having fewer opportunities to provide individualized patient care.

Russia has about 900,000 nurses, and the number of specialists with "vocational" education is around 1.3 million. This specialist group includes midwives, laboratory technicians, and feldshers (medical assistants) who, along with midwives, have extended education and can practice as midwives and nurses with more independence. Feldshers function like nurse practitioners in the United States, working independently in rural areas or in emergency services. The Russian Nurses' Association (RNA), the national nursing organization of Russia and located in St. Petersburg, was initially founded in 1992 and celebrated its 20th anniversary at an All-Russian Nursing Forum in October of 2012. The RNA, with 55 regional members, has been a member of the International Council of Nurses (ICN) since 2005.

NURSING RESEARCH: INITIAL EFFORTS IN RUSSIA

An American who is a Russian specialist invited two U.S. nurse colleagues to help him organize a conference on the Russian waterways. The reason for proposing the conference with a cruise venue was because a group of Russian nurses who attended presentations offered by U.S. nurses in Russia noted they did not have sufficient time to talk in more depth with the presenters or have their questions answered. Therefore, the opportunity for such interchanges began as a conference cruise (CC) on the Russian waterways between St. Petersburg and Moscow in 1997. The CC has been held every other year since then, providing opportunities for interaction and encouraging discussions and development of collegial relationships between Russian and U.S. nurses around conference content. To date, there have been eight CCs offered, and the resulting interactions and relationships have created opportunities for follow-up projects. One such project, the focus of this case study, illustrates a collaborative partnership process prompting the RNA to offer opportunities for nurses to learn about and begin using nursing research for improving patient care. Thus, this case study provides a description of the collaborative journey from 2005 to 2013 and the process of helping Russian nurses learn about nursing research and aiding the RNA in creating opportunities for these nurses to use research in understanding and improving their practice.

The 2005 U.S.–RNA CC afforded an opportunity to develop a relationship between two U.S. nurse researchers and a regional leader of the RNA. After hearing two presentations on nursing research during a CC, this regional leader, the president of the Arkhangelsk Regional Nurses' Association, invited the U.S. researchers to bring nursing research education to Russia. Consequently, the cruise venue provided time after the presentations for the two U.S. nurse researchers and the president of the Arkhangelsk Nurses' Association, on behalf of the RNA, to begin developing a collaborative relationship and planning a research workshop for nurses living in the Arkhangelsk area. Considering the distance between Russia and the United States, and Archangelsk's location in the far north of Russia, a practical initial decision was to provide a 5-day workshop. These planners identified the purpose of the workshop as offering an introduction to nursing research focusing on what nurses study and what methods they use conducting research. During initial planning while on the CC, broad outlines and the 5-day workshop objectives agreed on included:

- Sharing a vision for nursing research and its potential to improve nursing care
- Exploring clinical research methodologies
- Sharing a vision for using research to improve nursing practice in participants' institutions
- Exploring methodologies for promoting quality improvement

After the CC, additional workshop planning continued by e-mail; the first workshop was offered in March 2007.

This 2005 invitation to bring content on nursing research to Russian nurses began a collaborative relationship between two and then three U.S. nurse researchers (two from academia and one from clinical research with experience in inpatient and outpatient settings) and a regional RNA and national RNA leaders. This collaborative relationship continues to evolve based on mutual learning and goal setting to help Russian practicing nurses and the RNA as an organization use research to strengthen nursing practice and improve care delivery.

Over time, collaborative efforts have focused on two areas: (1) offering nursing research content in a workshop format and (2) providing consultation to the RNA as research became an organizational priority. While the nursing research workshops continued through 2011 and were offered in St. Petersburg (two), Moscow (one) (offered in collaboration with a medical academy nursing department), and Arkhangelsk (three), the focus of this case study will be on the collaborative consultation provided to the RNA as it sought to integrate nursing research into the functions and services it offers Russian nurses.

The purpose of this case study is to describe how the collaborative relationship with the RNA continues integrating nursing research into key RNA functions and services, thus establishing nursing research as an organizational priority. It also describes the process and key milestones of the collaborative relationship used to build organizational research capacity desired by the RNA and how sustainable strategies were incorporated in developing research as a priority within the RNA.

WORKSHOPS AS A VENUE FOR EDUCATION AND GOAL SETTING

Initial nursing research workshops offered in Arkhangelsk began with discussions between a regional RNA member and the RNA in St. Petersburg about nursing research and how these workshops offered opportunities for Russian nurses to gain knowledge and apply that learning to their clinical situations. Consequently, in 2010, the RNA offered a workshop for its members in St. Petersburg, home city of the RNA. As with previous workshops, participants were primarily clinical nurses including chief nurses, nurse managers, senior nurses, and staff nurses, as well as several educators. The 32 workshop participants were from regions across Russia, including Chita, in the far east of Siberia; the Mary El Republic, located in the mid–Volga River region; Omsk, in southwestern Siberia; the Leningrad region; and St. Petersburg. Participants had all completed a high nursing education program, a university-affiliated program preparing nurses for leadership positions in Russian health care. The RNA decided to invite nurses who completed the high nursing education program because they were Russian nurse leaders who could bring research knowledge to other nurses in their home organizations.

The first St. Petersburg workshop in 2010 followed the previously used 5-day format, but included a revised twofold goal for attendees to (1) examine key questions and practice issues related to their care of patients and families and (2) design projects using nursing research processes, evidence-based practice, and/or quality improvement for patient care.

Major learning activities included short presentations on nursing research, evidence-based practice and quality improvement; and small-group work facilitated by an experienced group of U.S. nurses. The small-group work allowed participants to develop project proposals they were to implement in their work settings after returning home. A related learning activity was to encourage small groups to form learning teams and networks that could help each other implement the projects as well as avail themselves of mentor opportunities with U.S. nurses using e-mail communications. Workshop evaluations were positive, suggesting that information presented was learned and would be implemented in participants' workplaces.

The RNA offered a second workshop in St. Petersburg in March 2011. Building from the first workshop, the content of this workshop was broadened to include a focus on the environment necessary to support nursing research in the clinical setting. Thus, based on the twofold objectives from the 2010 workshop, objectives for this workshop emphasized applying key nursing research, quality improvement, and evidence-based practice concepts for participants to:

1. Explore an organizational program of nursing research, quality improvement, and evidence-based practice
2. Determine strategies for creating an environment supportive of the power of nursing research in their work settings

As with the previous workshop, participants came from all over Russia. In addition, some participants who had attended prior workshops attended again because they found the first workshop helpful and wanted to have another opportunity to learn more about nursing research as well as share their projects with attendees.

On the last day of both workshops, participants presented nursing research projects they were to implement in their work settings. Participants of these workshops evaluated their learning experiences positively, confirmed they wanted to learn about the research process, and used the workshop to develop a proposal to implement in their work settings. However, long-term evaluations indicate that there was minimal implementation of study proposals, which has prompted the need to develop a plan of providing support and guidance to aid participants in implementing their research proposals in work settings after the workshops are over.

To summarize, between 2007 and 2011, U.S. nurse researchers, working collaboratively with a regional RNA president, RNA leaders, and a medical academy department of nursing in Moscow, offered six nursing research workshops. Offering these workshops demonstrated the capacity building principle of focusing on developing skills through training, then creating opportunities to apply the new skills in work settings.

NURSING RESEARCH AS AN ORGANIZATIONAL PRIORITY: RESOURCE DEVELOPMENT

After the 2010 workshop, the RNA established nursing research as an organizational priority. A first step in working on this priority was to develop resources to continue supporting Russian nurses as they learned about research. The first resource developed was an online nursing module on an introduction to nursing research. The RNA, the Arkhangelsk RNA, and the U.S. nurse researchers teaching the workshops collaborated with Sigma Theta Tau International Nursing Honor Society in developing this online module, which is an example of using and supporting networks and various skills and resources these networks bring to an endeavor. Module development identified the need to translate and interpret communication and materials from English to Russian and Russian to English, which is a consistent issue in working across languages.

The second resource was the RNA decision to create a column on nursing research in the association journal, the *RNA Tribune*, which is published quarterly. The first column appeared in the second issue of 2010, and provided a description of nursing research, how nurses' use of evidence is becoming a global expectation, and how knowledge of and involvement in research by using data and evidence improves practice and gives nurses a basis for professional communication with physicians and other health professionals. Other column topics included a definition and description of evidence-based practice, a description of an evidence hierarchy, how to frame questions to guide the conduct of a nursing research study and search for evidence to use in practice, how to critique nursing research studies, and how to search the literature.

Three U.S. nurse researchers work in collaboration with the RNA journal editor to plan column topics for 1 to 2 years. The journal editor in turn works with a committee of Russian nurses from several regions around the country to identify and confirm column topics. Members of this committee have all attended the nursing research workshops and identify column topics from the workshop and use workshop materials in their RNA regions. In addition to planning the column, the U.S. nurse researchers also author most articles. Russian nurses have been invited to serve as coauthors and, as the column continues, the goal is to identify ways for them to be more involved in authoring these articles.

As a third resource, the RNA developed a scientific committee comprised of nurses from various Russian regions who also participated in one of the RNA-sponsored nursing research workshops. The goals of the committee are to help identify clinical research topics, support nursing efforts in implementing research projects or quality improvement initiatives, communicate with colleagues in the academic setting, and advocate for support and recognition of potential funding needs for nursing research activities on the federal level. Because this committee is relatively new, it is learning and working on a plan to implement research as a priority, by helping nurses identify research topics from their daily practice. The committee also needs to learn how to work by long distance and to become comfortable with technology supporting long-distance communication. However, an important completed committee activity was planning and implementing a special session on nursing research offered as part of the All-Russian Nursing Forum held in October 2012.

Thus, in creating these three resources—an online learning module, a nursing research column, and a scientific committee—the RNA has helped encourage involvement by Russian nurses in supporting the learning of their peers. Creating resources for RNA members as well as developing a set of members with additional knowledge about nursing research are critical to initial implementation of nursing research as an organizational priority. Developing and using resources help to answer a key question posed by Ogilvie et al. (2003): how does one build capacity? The RNA has used technological innovations and captured opportunities for developing members and providing ongoing learning materials and opportunities (Ogilvie et al., 2003; Sajiwandani, 1998). The RNA selection of and development and use of these resources follows principles of research capacity building by ensuring the research is "close to practice" and investing in infrastructure and building elements for continuity and sustainability.

Nursing Research as an Organizational Priority: Development of Projects With Partners to Move the Work Forward

While developing resources is important for nursing research to be an integral part of services RNA offers members, the association also used opportunities presented by partnerships to establish research as a part of nursing practice. Therefore, during 2011, when the RNA was seeking opportunities to establish research as an organizational priority by embedding nursing research into the fabric of the organization, it became involved in grant funded projects with partners. Through continuing to have the U.S. researcher group serve as collaborative partners in capacity building and adding these projects with partners, the RNA has been able to implement two key projects. One project involves having Russian nurses conduct an evaluation study of evidence-based interventions they use with people with tuberculosis (TB). This project is being conducted in collaboration with the ICN. The ICN TB Project is supported by a United Way Worldwide grant made possible by the Lilly Foundation on behalf of the Lilly MDR–TB Partnership.

The second project involves having selected Russian oncology nurses take on a *train the trainer* role to help colleagues learn evidence-based interventions for patients undergoing chemotherapy, use quality improvement techniques to monitor practice changes, and evaluate the impact of their interventions with cancer patients undergoing chemotherapy. Currently, these projects are still being implemented and evaluated. Through these projects the RNA is striving to make nursing research an integral organizational component to ensure sustainability and further develop nursing research processes and activities (Leffers & Mitchell, 2011). A more thorough discussion of these endeavors appears below.

Project 1: Evaluate Interventions Used With TB Patients

Since 2006, the RNA has been a member of an ICN TB Project, supported by a United Way Worldwide grant made possible by the Lilly Foundation on behalf of the Lilly MDR–TB Partnership, to improve care of patients with TB. The purposes of the project are to implement a *train the trainer* model of education when caring for patients with TB and create a network of TB nurses to share and exchange learning and practice resources. The focus of the 2013 educational offering was to help attendees from the Russian nurse TB network learn about nursing research. Specifically, a nursing research workshop similar to the other RNA sponsored workshops was again held, but this one also included a session on evaluation and encouraged participants to develop study proposals that would evaluate an intervention learned in previous TB workshops that would impact TB patients, their families, or health care providers.

Project 2: Receive Grant Monies to Improve Care of Cancer Patients

In 2011, the RNA developed a proposal in response to a call from the Bristol-Myers Squibb Foundation's Bridging Cancer Care grants program. The purpose of this program is to improve care of patients with cancer in Eastern Europe and use innovative projects to strengthen nursing care to achieve this purpose. In developing this proposal, the RNA worked with Russian cancer nurses as well as one of the U.S. nurse researchers to set the focus and methodology for the project. This project was also designed to use a *train the trainer* model. However, embedded in this model was the use of oncology nursing evidence to transform nursing practice and use quality improvement processes and methodologies to monitor and evaluate the project. The project was funded in 2012 for a 2-year period and is currently in process. Therefore, the first of two oncology workshops to develop a set of trainers was held in June 2013; the second workshop is scheduled for February 2014. Two oncology nurses from each of 15 regions in Russia are selected to attend each workshop and then serve as trainers of up to 40 nurses in each of their regions. Consequently, during this 2-year project two *train the trainer* workshops will develop 60 trainers from 30 Russian regions to then train oncology nurses in their respective regions.

The RNA is working with the Oncology Nursing Society (ONS) and one of the U.S. nurse researchers to plan and implement the two workshops. A core part of implementing the new evidence-based oncology practices nurses learn is to use quality improvement processes/projects and quality-improvement methodology to contribute data for the RNA to use in monitoring and evaluating this funded project. Through this project, the RNA is using an evidence-based approach to further develop the practice of oncology nurses. Both the trainers and trainees of this program are to then form a network to share resources with each other and bring evidence-based nursing practices to oncology nurses in additional Russian regions. These projects also include ways to recognize nurses who exemplify excellence in using these research innovations in their practice.

CONCLUSION

Through these two projects the RNA is using research, by aiding nurses to both conduct studies and apply evidence, to help update clinical practice of major groups of Russian nurses: those caring for TB and oncology patients. These projects are helping the RNA bring nursing research knowledge, skills, and experience to change clinical practice and set the expectation for the way nursing is to be practiced in Russia. By engaging regional practicing nurses and leaders, the RNA is changing the nursing infrastructure and collaborating with regions to create needed resources to implement nursing research strategies in daily practice. Such engagement will advance nursing research as an integral component of the RNA, thus contributing to the sustainability of nursing research within the RNA.

With these projects, the RNA is building on strengths of using the *train the trainer* model to educate its members as well as engage the RNA regional leaders in supporting their members who become trainers to train their peers. Building on these strengths, the RNA is introducing research, both the conduct as well as use of evidence, and quality improvement initiatives in the process and activities of implementing and evaluating these projects.

Throughout the work described in this case study, facilitation, both the process and techniques, has provided the thrust to move the work along while continuing to develop the collaborative partnership that is so necessary for generating ideas and problem-solving methods to implement and evaluate these ideas. It has been challenging and rewarding to help the RNA build on its strengths while extending into new areas. Facilitation has been a prime mover in the joint learning about new ventures and how to use them in building the capacity for the RNA to commit to the development and sustainability of a major new organization priority.

In 2012, the RNA held the All-Russian Nursing Forum, which had special significance because it was a celebration of the 20th anniversary of the founding of the RNA. This forum offered two educational sessions planned collaboratively between the RNA, the Omsk Region—which took responsibility for one session—and the scientific committee, which was responsible for a presession before the actual educational forum sessions. Through these sessions, the RNA demonstrated the value of nursing research by offering educational meetings focused on research. During the forum, the RNA was awarded the Bristol-Myers Squibb grant to powerfully announce to RNA members in attendance that this multifaceted project with research as a key component is a priority of RNA emphasis for the next 2 years. As the RNA looks forward to the future, it has plans to work collaboratively with a number of groups and individuals to position its efforts to have nursing research as a core part of its function and services. Based on the work accomplished, the RNA is well positioned to meet this goal.

REFLECTIVE QUESTIONS

1. This capacity building project began with joint planning of several nursing research workshops. What factors involved in the planning and implementation of these workshops do you think helped RNA identify nursing research as an organizational priority?
2. Think about the facilitation techniques you have used and believe are useful in helping two or more individuals achieve joint work. Identify three facilitation techniques you think would be frequently used in a capacity building project and describe why each would be helpful.
3. The scientific committee described in the case study is just getting started. Which of the committee purposes would be a priority for initial focus of their work? What are two learning topics that could help the committee take on activities to successfully implement this purpose?
4. Development of resources is critical to achieving goals of a capacity building project. What criteria would you use to identify resources needed for the project?

REFERENCES

Leffers, J., & Mitchell, E. (2011). Conceptual model for partnership and sustainability in global health. *Public Health Nursing, 28*(1), 91–102.

Ogilvie, L., Allen, M., Laryea, J., & Opare, M. (2003). Building capacity through a collaborative international nursing project. *Journal of Nursing Scholarship, 35*(2), 113–118.

Sajiwandani, J. (1998). Capacity building in the new South Africa: Contribution of nursing research. *Nursing Standard, 12*(40), 34–37.

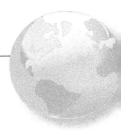

CHAPTER 7

Bridging Cultures

Luisa Barton
Jessica Larratt-Smith

Many people, including nurses, assume that living and working in an area that is considered multicultural or culturally diverse automatically makes them culturally astute or competent. However, there are far too many examples and evidence that suggest otherwise. Sadly, racism and cultural conflict continue to be pervasive, even in countries that are considered culturally diverse. In nursing, there are many models for working within cultures, yet cultural safety and cultural competence are learned skills like any other clinical competency. Working within cultures is a dynamic process, and building bridges within cultures is a skill set that should be honed.

In Canada, for instance, where culture and, specifically, multiculturalism are embraced through policy and idealism, there are still many challenges to be overcome. Nevertheless, the pivotal policy regarding multiculturalism in Canada continues to play a major role in attempts to bridge cultures within the general population. The 1987 Canadian Multiculturalism Act affirms the policy of the government to ensure that every Canadian receives equal treatment by the government, which respects and celebrates diversity. The act in general recognizes Canada's multicultural heritage and the necessity of protecting it; the rights of aboriginal peoples; that English and French remain the only official languages, but that other languages may be used; social equality within the law regardless of origins, race, or creed; and minorities' rights to enjoy their cultures (Government of Canada, n.d.). Despite policies in place, cultural tension within the nation remains a disappointing reality. Nevertheless, it behooves all citizens, particularly nurses where cultural safety and competence should be practiced, to strive for cultural harmony. This can be achieved through building bridges within cultures, in which nurses can play a pivotal role.

The approach to supporting cultures entails nurses to have a common understanding of terminology, a solid basis of transcultural theory and models, access to guidelines for cultural competence (including working with interpreters), and access to tools and resources for cultural assessment. Having adequate support and resources is crucial to working with different cultures. Moreover, other strategies such as self-reflection, mentoring/role modeling, and community engagement can be integrated into practice by nurses who are involved in the process of bridging cultures. Although they are beyond the scope of this chapter, basic community development skills are foundational to bridging cultures.

TERMINOLOGY

Culture

In 1871, anthropologist E. B. Tylor first defined culture as "that complex whole which includes knowledge, belief, art, law, morals, custom, and any other capabilities and habits acquired by man as a member of society." Tylor's perspective about culture is radically different from how it is viewed today. In his view, culture is synonymous with civilization, rather than something particular to unique societies (Charles, 2008). However, culture is perhaps most frequently used to refer to the practices and patterns that distinguish one society or group from others. In the field of sociology, culture is used to denote acquired behaviors that are shared by and transmitted among the members of the common society. In the field of nursing, Leininger (1991) refers to culture as the learned values, beliefs, norms, and way of life that influence an individual's thinking, decisions, and actions in certain ways. Some characteristics of culture specify that it is learned (rather than inherited); social (developed through social interaction); shared, transmissive, continuous, and cumulative; consistent and interconnected; and dynamic and adaptive, as well as varied from society to society. Lastly, culture is influenced by many factors, including race, religion, ethnicity, gender, sexual orientation, life experiences, economic circumstances, and political affiliation (College of Nurses of Ontario, 2009; Steckley & Letts, 2007; Wells, 2000).

Subculture

The term is used to define a group of people within a culture that differentiate themselves (having their own beliefs or interests, whether hidden or distinct) from the larger culture to which they belong. Subcultures are generally groups that are perceived to deviate from the normative standards of the dominant culture. Moreover, subcultures are live sociological phenomena that change over time. As changes occur in society and the mainstream, new subcultures emerge and old ones disappear or change. Examples of subcultures are vast and range from Goth to Hispanic, considered an ethnic subculture in the United States (Steckley & Letts, 2007).

Multiculturalism

The term is sometimes used synonymously with ethnic or cultural diversity. Multiculturalism is an ideology that embraces equality among those of different racial, religious, and cultural backgrounds, and it encourages society to learn from the contribution of those of different cultural backgrounds (Esses & Gardner, 1996). Some nations, such as Canada, have established federal policies on multiculturalism, whereas others, like the United States, do not. However, ethnic diversity in the United States is encouraged and established throughout the nation, and the metaphor of the melting pot implies that all the immigrant cultures are mixed and amalgamated without state intervention (Lee & Bean, 2004).

Cultural Awareness

Yan (2008) asserts that cultural awareness is an interactive, selective, and contingent process. Cultural awareness is observing and being conscious of similarities and contrasts between cultural groups, and understanding the way in which culture may affect different people's approach to health. In this way, cultural awareness appreciates how a person's culture may inform his or her values, behavior, beliefs, and basic assumptions (Kagawa-Singer & Kassim-Lakha, 2003; Kemp & Rasbridge, 2004).

Cultural Sensitivity

Cultural sensitivity is being aware of (and understanding) the characteristic values and perceptions of one's own culture and the way in which this may shape a nurse's approach to patients from other cultures (Yan & Wong, 2005).

Cultural Safety

As a step beyond cultural sensitivity, cultural safety is based on the understanding that inherent power imbalances exist and discrimination derives from historical relationships with people of different origins. In this way, the person has reflected on his or her own identity and the perceptions that others from different cultures may hold of him or her. Culturally safe practice implies the ability to keep these differing perspectives in mind while treating the patient as a person worthy of respect in her own right (Charles, 2008; Tucker et al., 2007; Yan & Wong, 2005).

Cultural Competence

From a general, interprofessional lens, cultural competence refers to the attitudes, knowledge, and skills of practitioners necessary to become effective health care providers for patients from diverse backgrounds (Anand, 2004; Yan & Wong, 2005). "Awareness" and "sensitivity," per previous terminology, do not necessitate action, while "competence" denotes an endpoint or mastery as opposed to a complex and dynamic process (Hixon, 2003).

Ethnocentrism

According to Hammond and Axelrod (2006), ethnocentrism consists of attitudes and behaviors, typically including in-group favoritism. The attitudes include seeing one's own group (the in group) as superior and out groups as inferior. Ethnocentrism involves using one's own standards, values, and beliefs to make judgments about someone else. Ethnocentric individuals may judge other groups relative to one's ethnicity, culture, language, behavior, or religion. Regardless of whether ethnocentricity is overt or subtle, it can lead to a myriad of negative consequences.

Stereotyping

Still a common phenomenon, stereotypes are generalizations or categorizations about a particular group based on some common feature (e.g., appearance, ethnicity, gender), usually using insufficient information and without seeking further information. Stereotyping is viewing all members of a cultural group as alike, homogeneous, leaving no room for individual variation or exception to common cultural patterns (Kemp & Rasbridge, 2004; Wells, 2000).

TRANSCULTURAL MODELS

Several transcultural models or frameworks help guide nurses toward cultural safety and competency. With the goal of improving care given to meet different health care needs of diverse cultures, Dr. Madeleine Leininger's Theory of Culture Care is seminal to nursing practice. Leininger's theory suggests that culturally competent nursing care can only occur when client beliefs and values are thoughtfully and skillfully incorporated into nursing care.

The Purnell Model for Cultural Competence is also applicable to various health care disciplines and in all practice settings. Again, cultural competence as a process embodies several assumptions, including the notion that all cultures share core similarities but that differences exist among, between, and within cultures. Moreover, as with other models, providing cultural competence enhances and improves care. In Purnell's model, 12 domains and their concepts flow from more general phenomena to more specific phenomena. The order in which the care provider uses the domains may vary. The 12 domains include overview/heritage, communication, family roles and organization, work issues, bicultural ecology, high-risk behaviors, pregnancy and childbearing practices, nutrition, death rituals, spirituality, health care practice, and health care practitioner (Purnell, 2002). The model is considered multidisciplinary and it is relevant to all aspects of health including practice, research, education, and administration.

Cultural diversity, coupled with a complex health care system, necessitates a solid understanding of transcultural theories and models. Taking action through cultural competency is integral in the provision of care to culturally diverse patients and to hopefully bridge cultures within and between nations.

CULTURAL COMPETENCY

Providing culturally competent care significantly improves patient care and outcomes, yet when culturally appropriate care is not delivered, negative patient consequences, from simple miscommunication to life-threatening incidents, may occur (Higginbottom et al., 2012). More than ever, nurses must strive for cultural competence and safety. Cultural competence can be achieved at various levels: individual, organizational, systemic. At the individual level, health care providers can hone their skills using various standards and guidelines from their professional associations. A task force of the Expert Panel for Global Nursing and Health of the American Academy of Nursing, along with members of the Transcultural Nursing Society, has developed 12 standards for cultural competence in nursing practice. These standards can be universally applied to all domains of nursing. That being said, several other jurisdictions have also developed guidelines for cultural competence that nurses and other health care providers can readily access. For example, the Nova Scotia Department of Health (2005) outlines eight steps to cultural competence:

1. Examine your values, behaviors, beliefs, and assumptions.
2. Recognize racism and the institutions or behaviors that breed racism.
3. Engage in activities that help you to reframe your thinking, allowing you to hear and understand other worldviews and perspectives.
4. Familiarize yourself with core cultural elements of the communities you serve, including physical and biological variations; concepts of time, space, and physical contact; styles and patterns of communication; physical and social expectations; social structures; and gender roles.
5. Engage clients and patients to share how their reality is similar to or different from what you have learned about their core cultural elements. Unique experiences and histories will result in differences in behaviors, values, and needs.
6. Learn how different cultures define, name, and understand disease and treatment. Engage your clients to share with you how they define, name, and understand their ailments.
7. Develop a relationship of trust with clients and co-workers by interacting with openness, understanding, and a willingness to hear different perceptions.
8. Create a welcoming environment that reflects the diverse communities you serve.

Guidelines for cultural competence include:

- Acquire cultural knowledge
- Know how to use interpreters or translators
- Establish mutual goals
- Engage in self-reflection and ongoing evaluation

- Become familiar with nonverbal cues/expressions
- Consider the patient's background rather than making assumptions; get to know the patient, asking questions
- Respect culture-specific rituals—for example, after death or during religious festivals
- Remember potential prescribing pitfalls—people from different backgrounds metabolize certain drugs differently
- Find out if a patient is using traditional or alternative treatments and remedies. Many of these remedies interact with drugs and may affect drug absorption
- Learn about cultural and religious beliefs, especially as these relate to perceptions of illness
- Explain reasons for certain questions and tests—this allays fears of discrimination or insensitivity to one's history with the health care system
- Facilitate choice; offer options for treatment
- Screen for culture-specific diseases (College of Nurses of Ontario, 2009; Nova Scotia Department of Health, 2005)

At the organizational level, Cross, Bazron, Dennis, and Isaacs (1989) list five essential elements that contribute to an institution's ability to become more culturally competent: valuing diversity; having the capacity for cultural self-assessment; being conscious of the dynamics inherent when cultures interact; having institutionalized cultural knowledge; and having developed adaptations of service delivery reflecting an understanding of cultural diversity. At the systemic level, a culturally competent primary health care system: provides health care to patients with diverse values, beliefs, and behaviors, which entails tailoring delivery to meet their needs, requires an understanding of the communities being served as well as the cultural influences on individual health beliefs and behaviors, and requires strategies for identifying and addressing cultural barriers to accessing primary health care (Nova Scotia Department of Health, 2005). Ideally, to build bridges, cultural competence should be practiced at all levels of health care.

WORKING WITH INTERPRETERS

Language barriers and cross-cultural nuances in the health care industry can lead to misdiagnosis, deferment of care, avoidance of needed services, and inconsistency in visits (Flores, 2003). Interpreters play an important role during a health care interaction. In a cross-cultural health interview, a highly skilled language professional facilitates communication between the patient and health professional. Ideally, the interpreter is capable of processing and conveying information in two languages. In health care, this becomes a complex process, because often medical terminology is used whereas personal details carry an emotional charge. In this way, interpreters are called on to balance the appropriate level of professional reserve with a compassionate and caring nature that is key in health care (Valdes & Angelelli, 2003).

Since the traditional view of interpreters as neutral conduits with no participatory role has evolved, ethical and legal principles must be balanced, including confidentiality and self-determination. The role of the interpreter does not occur in a social vacuum, because interpreters participate in the interpreted event and bring to it all the social and cultural factors that allow them to co-construct a definition of reality with the other participants in the interaction (Angelelli, 2004). It is thus important for nurses to understand the complexity of the interpretation process and to establish principles when using professional interpreters.

In some health care organizations, professional interpreters are not used; instead, family members or friends of patients take on this role. Of course, this has a very different set of ethical and legal challenges. Ideally, although not always legislated, professional interpreters should be used at all times during the health care interaction. By outsourcing an interpretation service, many legal issues such as confidentiality (using appropriate consent forms and policies) can be ameliorated.

More recently, competence standards for interpreters are now being established, including self-introduction, self-positioning, communicating all participants' content and feelings, speaking in the first person, understanding content, cultural brokering, neutrality, managing the flow of communication, and appropriate documentation (Hennepin County, n.d.). In Canada, for example, the Healthcare Interpretation Network (HIN) launched the National Standard Guide for Community Interpreting Services for the provision of quality community interpreting services to ensure reliability in the provision of such services nationwide (Healthcare Interpretation Network, 2007).

When using an interpreter, the nurse (as the provider) plays a major role in guiding the encounter as well as evaluating the quality of interpreting. Many nursing jurisdictions have developed practice guidelines to assist nurses when using interpreters during patient–nurse interactions. These general guidelines include:

- Prior to the appointment, the nurse can prepare by having translated materials and pictograms for the visit. This should also include a discussion with the interpreter about the content of the visit before the patient arrives. If this information is sensitive or includes a serious diagnosis, the more time the interpreter has to prepare for the visit, the better the communication process will be (Schapira et al., 2008). Moreover, having a discussion with the interpreter prior to the interaction may be helpful in declaring any conflicts/issues by the interpreter. For example, if the interpreter is uncomfortable with a medical situation (e.g., consent for a procedure), it is essential that the issue be resolved prior to the interaction. Again, using an interpretation service may ameliorate this type of situation. Also, prior to the interaction, the nurse should ensure confidentiality of information by using forms and ensuring that the interpreter has received appropriate training in interpreting in the health care setting.
- As the interaction progresses the nurse should be positioned in a space that is conducive to good communication; often this is in a triangle in which all parties can see and hear one another. It is imperative that the nurse always speak and look at the patient, not the interpreter, because the patient should feel that he or she is the focus of the interaction. This also helps in minimizing any power imbalance and is a basic sign of respect for the patient. That being said, in this author's experience, not all cultures are comfortable with direct eye contact with strangers, so the nurse should be cognizant of any relevant cultural nuances.
- Ensure that messages are clear and understandable. When working with an interpreter, it is important for nurses to slow down, pause often, and allow the interpreter to repeat messages whenever necessary. In this author's experience, it is essential that the health interaction be given adequate time, as interpretation itself can often double the time of contact.
- Ensuring a warm and calm tone of voice may help patients feel more comfortable during the interaction. Be mindful that body language and facial expressions are universal and should be included in the interaction. The nurse may ask the patient to repeat back, in his or her own words, the information given.
- Self-reflecting and evaluation. It is important for nurses to evaluate the quality of the interaction. Thus, asking the interpreter if there was anything about the interaction that made it difficult to interpret will help with clarification as well as the nurse's future patient interactions using interpreters (College of Nurses of Ontario, 2009; Hudelson, 2004).

CULTURAL ASSESSMENT

When clinically assessing patients, it is important to elicit relevant information. The same holds true for a cultural assessment. Asking patients open-ended questions about their culture in relation to their care is an important element of cultural competence (College of Nurses of Ontario, 2009). There are several cultural assessment tools that have an empirical basis for nursing practice. According to Higginbottom et al. (2012) these include the Sunrise model; the Culturally Competent Community Care (CCCC) model; the Family Cultural Heritage Assessment Tool (FamCHAT); Assessment, Communication, Cultural negotiation and compromise, Establishing respect and rapport, Sensitivity, and Safety (the ACCESS model); the Process of Cultural Competence in the Delivery of Healthcare Services model; the Purnell Model for Cultural Competence; the Papadopoulos, Tilki, and Taylor Model for Developing Cultural Competence; and the Giger-Davidhizar Transcultural Assessment Model (GDTAM). In light of the rise of interprofessionalism, these tools can be used by a variety of health care providers, not just in the nursing context. Choosing the appropriate assessment tool also depends on practice setting. For instance, the FamCHAT has been empirically tested for use in a primary care setting, which is very helpful for primary health care nurse practitioners and outpost registered nurses, but Higginbottom et al. (2012) noted that its succinct and user-friendly approach allows it to be transferable to the hospital setting. A comprehensive list of cultural assessment tools, prepared by Campinha-Bacote, can be readily accessed through Transcultural C.A.R.E. Associates (www.transculturalcare.net/assessment-tools.htm).

STRATEGIES FOR BUILDING BRIDGES

There is no precise recipe for bridging cultures within a nation, but nurses' ability to respond to patients' needs coupled with cultural competence serve as an important basis. Again, subsumed under cultural competence and safety, cultural knowledge is fundamental to the notion of "bridging." For example, working in Canada with aboriginal peoples, two core competencies—postcolonial understanding and indigenous knowledge—underscore the importance of cultural knowledge (Aboriginal Nurses Association of Canada, Canadian Association of Schools of Nursing & Canadian Nurses Association, 2009).

Adapted from Yoder (2001), when teaching ethnically diverse nursing students, four major strategies for bridging include (a) incorporating the student's cultural knowledge, (b) preserving cultural or ethnic identity, (c) facilitating negotiation of barriers, and (d) advocating for system change. The latter, advocating for system change, does not imply changing cultural practices within a system, but rather advocating to improve the system (such as the health care system) in order to meet the needs of diverse populations.

Similar strategies can be applied to working with different cultures within a nation. In addition to these proposed strategies, nurses and other health care providers who strive to bridge cultures should consider mentoring and support, role modeling, self-reflection, accessing resources, and participating in the communities that they serve as part of community development (College of Nurses of Ontario, 2009; Wells, 2000; Yan, 2008). For instance, nurses who work in remote or isolated communities benefit from supporting each other. Here they can learn about their cultural community through their own discussions and self-reflection. There may also be culturally competent "champions" who can serve as role models for nurses honing their culturally competence skills (Anand, 2004; Yoder, 2001). Participation in the community in which health providers serve offers a unique opportunity to learn about a culture. Cultural engagement offers many benefits, including reducing social isolation; increasing social cohesion; raising the profile of cultural organizations on the local, national, and international levels; and providing opportunities for exchange of opinions and open debates between community members to make their voice widely heard (Varbanova, 2011). Last, as previously mentioned, resources such as toolkits and guidelines are readily accessible for all health care providers who work in culturally diverse communities within a nation.

CONCLUSION

Cultural competence grows with time and experience. Fortunately, models, theories, guidelines, and other resources are readily available to those who want to enhance their cultural competence skills as means for bridging cultures. That being said, as evidenced in the following case studies, reality can often be different from theory, and there is an adjustment period that allows for this growth if given the right amount of time, patience, and self-reflection.

REFERENCES

Aboriginal Nurses Association of Canada, Canadian Association of Schools of Nursing, & Canadian Nurses Association. (2009). *Cultural competence and cultural safety in First Nations, Inuit and Metis nursing education: An integrated review of the literature.* Ottawa, ON: Aboriginal Nurses Association of Canada. www.anac.on.ca/Documents/Making%20It%20Happen%20Curriculum%20Project/FINALFRAMEWORK.pdf

Anand, R. (2004). *Cultural competence in health care: A guide for trainers* (3rd ed.). Washington, DC: NMCI Publications.

Angelelli, C. (2004). *Medical interpreting and cross-cultural communications.* Cambridge, UK: Cambridge University Press.

Charles, M. (2008). Culture and inequality: Identity, ideology, and difference in "postascriptive society." *Annals of the American Academy of Political and Social Science, 619*(1), 41–58. doi: 10.1177/0002716208319824

College of Nurses of Ontario. (2009). Culturally sensitive care. Toronto, Canada: Author. www.cno.org/Global/docs/prac/41040_CulturallySens.pdf

Cross, T., Bazron, B., Dennis, K., & Isaacs, M. (1989). *Toward a culturally competent system of care,* Vol. 1. Washington, DC: Georgetown University.

Esses, V. M., & Gardner, R. C. (1996). Multiculturalism in Canada: Context and current status. *Canadian Journal of Behavioural Science, 28,* 145–152.

Flores, G. (2006). Language barriers to health care in the United States. *New England Journal of Medicine, 355*(3), 229–231.

Government of Canada. Canadian Multiculturalism Act (R.S.C., 1985, c. 24 (4th Suppl.). http://laws-lois.justice.gc.ca/eng/acts/c-18.7/page-1.html#h-3

Hammond, R. A., & Axelrod, R. (2006). The evolution of ethnocentrism. *Journal of Conflict Resolution, 50*(6), 926–936. doi: 10.1177/0022002706293470

Healthcare Interpretation Network. (2007). National standard guide for community interpreting services. http://healthcareinterpretationnetwork.ca

Hennepin County. (n.d.). *Ethics and competency standards for interpretation.* Training documents for interpreters.

Higginbottom, G., Richter, M. S., Young, S., Ortiz, L. M., Callender, S. D., Forgeron, J. I., & Boyce, M. L. (2012). Evaluating the utility of the FamCHAT ethnocultural nursing assessment tool at a Canadian tertiary care hospital: A pilot study with recommendations for hospital management. *Journal of Nursing Education and Practice, 2*(2), 24–40.

Hixon, A. L. (2003). Beyond cultural competence. *Academic Medicine, 78*(6), 634.

Hudelson, P. (2004). Improving patient-provider communication: Insights from interpreters. *Family Practice, 22*(3), 311–316.

Kagawa-Singer, M., & Kassim-Lakha, S. (2003). A strategy to reduce cross-cultural miscommunication and increase the likelihood of improving health outcomes. *Academic Medicine, 78*(6), 577–587.

Kemp, C., & Rasbridge, L. (2004). *Refugee and immigrant health: A handbook for health professionals.* Cambridge, UK: Cambridge University Press.

Lee, J., & Bean, F. D. (2004). America's changing color lines: Race/ethnicity, immigration, and multiracial identification. *Annual Review of Sociology, 30,* 221–242.

Leininger, M. (1991). Becoming aware of types of health practitioners and cultural imposition. *Journal of Transcultural Nursing, 4*(2), 39–40.

Nova Scotia Department of Health. (2005). A cultural competence guide for primary health care professionals in Nova Scotia. www.healthteamnovascotia.ca/cultural_competence/Cultural_Competence_guide_for_Primary_Health_Care_Professionals.pdf

Purnell, L. (2002). The Purnell Model for Cultural Competence. *Journal of Transcultural Nursing, 13*(3), 193–196. doi: 10.1177/10459602013003006

Schapira, L., Vargas, E., Hidalgo, R., Brier, M., Sanchez, L., Hobrecker, K. I., et al. (2008). Lost in translation: Integrating medical interpreters into the multidisciplinary team. *Oncologist, 13,* 586–592.

Steckley, J., & Letts, G. K. (2007). *Elements of sociology: A critical Canadian introduction.* Oxford University Press.

Tucker, C. M., Mirsu-Paun, A., Van den Berg, J. J., Ferdinand, L., Jones, J. D., Curry, R. W., . . . Beato, C. (2007). Assessments for measuring patient-centered cultural sensitivity in community-based primary care clinics. *Journal of National Medical Association, 99*(6), 609–619.

Valdes, G., & Angelelli, C. V. (2003). Interpreters, interpreting, and the study of bilingualism. *Annual Review of Applied Linguistics, 23,* 58–78.

Varbanova, L. (2011). Cultural participation in education and lifelong learning: A catalyst for personal advancement, community development, social change and economic growth. Access to Culture Platform.

Wells, M. I. (2000). Beyond cultural competence: A model for individual and institutional cultural development. *Journal of Community Health Nursing, 17,* 189–199.

Yan, M. C. (2008). Exploring the meaning of crossing and culture: An empirical understanding from practitioners' everyday experience. *Families in Society, 89*(2), 282–292.

Yan, M. C., & Wong, Y. L. R. (2005). Rethinking self-awareness in cultural competence: Towards a dialogic self in cross-cultural social work. *Families in Society, 86*(2), 181–188.

Yoder, M. (2001). The bridging approach: Effective strategies for teaching ethnically diverse nursing students. *Journal of Transcultural Nursing, 12*(4), 319–325.

Bridging Cultures Within Nations

Jessica Larratt-Smith
Luisa Barton

CONTEXT: ABORIGINAL HEALTH CARE IN CANADA

Aboriginal peoples are the descendents of the original inhabitants of North America. The Canadian constitution recognizes three groups of aboriginal peoples: Indians (commonly referred to as First Nations people), Métis, and Inuit, yet the constitution does not define any of these groups. According to the 2006 Canadian Census, 3.8% of the Canadian population was comprised of aboriginal peoples. Canada's aboriginal population is growing faster than the general population, increasing by 20.1% from 2001 to 2006. This is due to a higher fertility rate among aboriginal women than among other Canadian women. Aboriginal communities are located in urban, rural, and remote locations across Canada, including First Nations or Indian bands (generally located on lands called reserves); Inuit communities located in Nunavut, NWT, Northern Quebec (Nunavik), and Labrador; Métis communities; and communities of aboriginal people (including Métis, nonstatus Indians, Inuit, and First Nations individuals) in cities or towns that are not part of reserves or traditional territories, such as the aboriginal community in Winnipeg.

Health Canada works with First Nations, Inuit, other federal departments, and provincial and territorial partners to support healthy First Nations and Inuit (FNI) individuals, families, and communities. The responsibilities for aboriginal health are shared through federal and provincial/territorial governments and First Nations self-government arrangements. While Health Canada's First Nations and Inuit Health Branch (FNIHB) oversees health programming for FNI peoples, Aboriginal Affairs and Northern Development works with First Nations, Inuit, and Métis individuals, families, and communities to improve their health and social well-being. In doing so, Health Canada strives to improve health outcomes by providing access to quality health services and support. Although FNI health has improved, gaps remain in the overall health status of FNI individuals when compared to other Canadians. Health Canada's First Nations and Inuit Health Branch (FNIHB) works with numerous partners to carry out many activities aimed at improving health outcomes (Health Canada, 2010).

FNIHB, now known as First Nations and Inuit Health (FNIH), aims for "health self-determination." Almost three-quarters of the 680 FNI communities in Canada are now served predominantly by First Nations organizations (Health Canada, 2010). Regions with higher levels of self-determination tend to be those with developed capacity and greater access to other sources of health care services, such as FNI communities within British Columbia, Alberta, Saskatchewan, Quebec, the Atlantic Provinces, and the Territories (Health Canada, 2010). Manitoba and Ontario FNI communities remain particularly reliant on Health Canada for health care provision in remote and isolated areas due to infrastructure and geographical barriers (i.e., no road access) (Health Canada, 2010). Of the 57 nursing stations across Canada under direct control of Health Canada, the majority are in remote and isolated First Nations communities in northern Ontario and Manitoba, with 24 and 22 nursing stations, respectively (Health Canada, 2011). In Manitoba, more than 60% of First Nations people, approximately 40,000 people, live on reserves north of the 53rd parallel (Health Canada, 2011).

Comprising three divisions, the Community Programs Directorate (CPD) aims to improve the health of FNI people on reserves by promoting health and preventing disease among children and youth and persons at risk of chronic disease, mental illness, and addictions. According to Health Canada, CPD does this through funding of community-based programs focused on providing the following:

- A healthy start in life for children
- Community mental wellness
- Youth suicide prevention programming
- Addictions prevention and treatment programming
- Healthy nutrition and activity promotion programming
- Disease/injury risk-factor prevention programming

In some provinces, such as Saskatchewan, improving health outcomes for aboriginal peoples appear to be a priority. According to the Saskatoon Health Region (2010), the aboriginal health strategy aims to honor the spirit and intent of the original treaties. Some of the guiding principles of aboriginal services include being cognizant of the holistic approach regarding all developmental stages of life; meaningful engagement of community elders to provide guidance and input into the design, delivery, implementation, and evaluation of programs and services; meaningful and inclusive collaboration between the aboriginal community, the Saskatoon Health Region, and various government stakeholders; increased access and effectiveness of programs and services delivered to aboriginal people; patient-centered care as regards alternative healing methods; and respect for the interrelatedness of all things in life (environment). The Saskatoon Health Region (2010) asserts that in order to have a positive impact on health outcomes, aboriginal and nonaboriginal people need to jointly commit to actions ensuring that aboriginal health programs meet the needs of aboriginal communities.

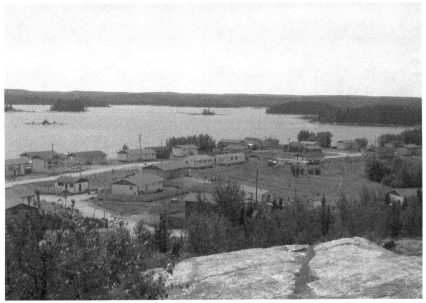

Overlooking the landscape at Pukatawagan reserve, Manitoba, Canada.   *Credit*: J. Larratt-Smith

POPULATION HEALTH

There are significant health disparities between the First Nations, Inuit, and Métis peoples and the general Canadian population. First Nations populations tend to have a higher burden of chronic disease within reserve communities as opposed to the general Canadian population. Among the aboriginal population, there are high rates of mental illness, substance abuse, fetal alcohol syndrome, domestic violence, diabetes, tuberculosis and other infectious diseases, obesity, and hypertension. Diabetes is almost 3.8 times more prevalent among registered First Nations (RFN) adults on reserves than among the general Canadian population (Health Canada, 2009). Incidence of tuberculosis is also significantly higher among RFN populations than the general Canadian population (Health Canada, 2009). The overall human immunodeficiency virus (HIV) infection rate among RFN persons is approximately 2.8 times higher, and the rate of new hepatitis C virus infections is 5.8 times higher than in the general Canadian population (Health Canada, 2009). The most frequent long-term health-related conditions among First Nation children living in reserves include asthma, allergies, chronic ear infections, chronic bronchitis, and learning disabilities (NCCAH, 2009). Relative to the general Canadian population, the life expectancy of aboriginal peoples is 7.4 and 5.2 years shorter for males and females, respectively. Infant mortality in Manitoba among RFN populations is twice that of the general regional population (Health Canada, 2010). Suicide rates are five to seven times higher for aboriginal youth than the national average, and suicide is also one of the greatest causes of injury-related deaths (Health Canada, 2009). Death rates are higher among RFN populations in western Canada than in the corresponding general Canadian population, with one-third of all deaths caused by accidental poisoning, transport accidents, and intentional self-harm (Health Canada, 2010).

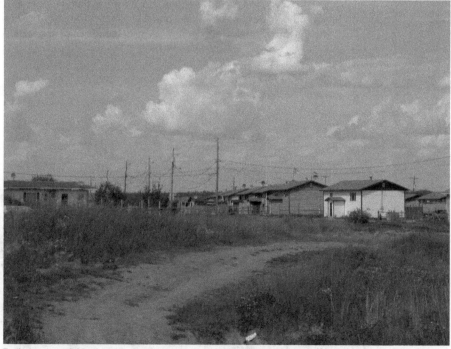

Exploring the neighborhood on Pukatawagan reserve, Manitoba, Canada.   *Credit*: J. Larratt-Smith

NURSING'S ROLE

Remote nursing stations are staffed predominantly by registered nurses (RNs) working within a broadened scope of practice supported by the FNIH clinical guidelines (Health Canada, 2010). As the first point of contact in the health care system for FNI people, RNs triage a client's health needs and, in partnership with the client, decide to initiate services independently within FNIH clinical guidelines or in consultation with another health care provider or refer to the provincial health system (Health Canada, 2010). During regular clinic hours (Monday through Friday, 8 a.m.–5 p.m.) RNs provide communities with primary care nursing services, including preventative health care; episodic health assessments; population health services; family care, chronic care, and follow-up; and the provision of consultation and referral services with other health care providers and institutions (Health Canada, 2010). In addition, RNs provide critical, emergent, and urgent care 24 hours a day, 7 days a week (Health Canada, 2010). RNs work in consultation with a physician (often off site) to address any immediate threat to life or function, acute trauma, or illness and frequently secure and coordinate medical transportation if care requires a more advanced treatment team (Health Canada, 2010).

During a client encounter an RN could, within FNIH guidelines, be responsible for as much as obtaining a complete health history; performing a focused or complete physical assessment; performing and interpreting in-house diagnostic tests, such as x-rays, ECGs, and point of care tests such as urine dip, blood glucose or hemoglobin testing, a urine pregnancy test, or a quick strep test; ordering and obtaining samples for referred-out diagnostic tests such as swabs or for blood samples spun and separated on location; determining and communicating a diagnosis within FNIH clinical guidelines; determining a treatment plan in partnership with the client; prescribing and dispensing medications; and educating the client on expected outcomes and follow-up care.

According to Health Canada, the 3-year departure rate for RNs working in remote and isolated FNI communities was 55% in 2010 (Health Canada, 2010). Among younger RNs, these rates are even higher, with 83% loss of RNs younger than 30 and 69% loss of RNs aged 30 to 40 (Health Canada, 2010). Due to difficulties in recruitment and retention of regular full-time RNs, the government has become more reliant on contracted agency staff to fill the staffing gaps (Health Canada, 2010). In 2009, at least 41% of Manitoba's RNs working remotely were agency staff (Health Canada, 2010).

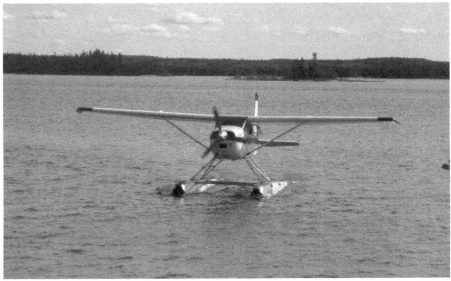

Transportation home from Pukatawagan reserve.   *Credit:* J. Larratt-Smith

One of the complications of agency RNs is the continued turnover and variation in nursing station staff, which has the potential to negatively impact continuity of care for First Nations clients (Health Canada, 2010). The alternative to filling the gaps with contract staff is not for nursing stations to close but rather to continue understaffed, resulting in a heavy work burden for the remaining nurse(s) who continue to provide services around the clock (Health Canada, 2010). In fact, even with contract RN staff in place, some nursing stations have annual vacancies in excess of 20% (Health Canada, 2010).

CULTURAL SAFETY AND COMPETENCY

Most jurisdictions in Canada require that nurses be culturally competent. Cultural competence is defined by Canadian Nurses Association (CNA) as "the application of knowledge, skills, attitudes and personal attributes required by nurses to provide appropriate care and services in relation to cultural characteristics of their clients" (CNA, 2010, p. 1). According to the National Aboriginal Health Organization (NAHO), cultural safety within a First Nations, Inuit, and Métis context means that the practitioner, whether aboriginal or not, can communicate competently within the patient's social, political, linguistic, economic, and spiritual realm.

In 2009, the Aboriginal Nurses Association of Canada, the Canadian Association of Schools of Nursing, and the Canadian Nurses Association outlined core competencies: postcolonial understanding, communication, respect, inclusivity, indigenous knowledge, and mentoring and supporting students for success. Understanding postcolonial theory helps nurses examine the relationship between residential schools and historic trauma transmission and its impact on the lives of aboriginal peoples. Of course, communication, the cornerstone of all nursing competencies, is particularly important when interacting with First Nations, Inuits, and Métis peoples.

Inclusivity is part of the engagement process and relationship building with the aboriginal community and, with it, respect for First Nations, Inuit, and Métis cultural integrity. Also, nurses should have substantial indigenous knowledge, which includes traditional knowledge, oral knowledge, and literate knowledge. It also includes understanding First Nations, Inuit, and Métis ontology, epistemology, and explanatory models related to health and healing, as well as First Nations, Inuit, and Métis cosmologies. Nurses must mentor their nursing students in fostering their success in these competencies.

PERSONAL PERSPECTIVE

I've worked as a contract RN for multiple northern nursing agencies for more than 3 years on remote Manitoba reserves. To access these remote communities, I've flown low across the marshy Canadian shield in a wide assortment of small aircraft (between 4 and 20 seats); the most memorable was a four-seat twin otter seaplane. I've worked in a variety of nursing stations, from small stations with just one other RN to bigger stations with 8 to 10 RNs. The size depends on both how large the community is and how great the health care need. RNs staff the station 24/7 with an administration assistant and a housekeeper during the daytime hours but only a security guard during the nights. Often a patient driver provides transportation to the station for community members without access to a vehicle. Many large communities have a physician on site as often as 3½ days a week, but most are small and only have a physician in the community for a total of 1 to 3 days a month. There is always a physician available to the RNs by phone.

Personal Attributes and Expectations

I completed a bachelor of nursing science degree in conjunction with a bachelor of arts minor in global development studies at Queen's University in Kingston, Ontario, Canada. I had a strong interest in nursing with developing communities, so I did my final 10-week

RN consolidation on a fly-in reserve in northern Ontario. I enjoyed my experience, but I quickly realized that I needed to acquire some significant nursing experience before pursuing remote nursing any further.

There are some major challenges to this role. One of these challenges is the isolation, both professional and personal. As the only health care professional in the facility, I need to be able to competently provide both primary and emergency care to adult and pediatric patients. I have delivered a baby, run a pediatric code, cardioverted an adult using adenosine, managed overdoses, stabilized patients with sepsis or gastrointestinal bleeds, been in a pertussis (whooping cough) outbreak, and worked with actively suicidal patients. In addition, the more voluminous primary care I provide on a routine basis includes well-child exams, immunizations, prenatal visits, hypertension and diabetes disease promotion and prevention, insulin initiation education, suturing lacerations, contraception discussions, Pap testing, and treating episodic complaints like pneumonia, otitis media, and febrile children.

Every patient encounter makes me thankful for my accumulated years of emergency and acute care experience that solidified my wealth of clinical knowledge and skills. I am also extremely fortunate that I completed my primary care nurse practitioner degree during my northern experiences. This gave me much-needed assessment and diagnostic resources for the expanded scope of an RN working remotely. Without both of these I would have felt lost and unsafe in the broadened scope and minimal training of an agency RN working remotely.

Most of the nurses younger than age 50 who I meet in the north are either divorced or single. It is incredibly hard to have normal relationships while living remotely for weeks at a time. Even part-time work means you are remote for 2 out of every 4 weeks; when travel time is factored in, you are away 17 out of every 28 days. I've always enjoyed alone time, so I bring books and movies north with me to bury myself in. I explore the communities by walking or running along the main roads despite the dust in the summer, the mud in the spring and fall, and the cold in the winter. Due to the daytime clinic shifts plus nighttime on-call hours, I often work 14- to 18-hour days for the whole 2-week stint, so much of my spare time is spent trying to catch up on sleep.

Cultural Differences

Both the culture of the First Nations people and the remoteness of the location affect the health care experience on reserves.

Postcolonial Understanding

I have witnessed multigenerational substance misuse, abuse, and family dysfunction on the reserves as a result of traumatic residential school experiences. During most of the 20th century, these federally run boarding schools were imposed on aboriginal children with the intention of assimilating them into mainstream modern Canadian society by teaching them Christianity and replacing their native languages with either English or French (CBC News, 2010). Unfortunately, many students lived in substandard conditions, endured physical, emotional, and sometimes sexual abuse, and had little opportunity to learn parenting skills through a significant deficit in normal family life experiences (CBC News, 2010).

As the only health care provider in the community I often treat both victims and abusers, which can be emotionally and ethically difficult. Understanding the roots of the problem and lingering postcolonial effects in communities helps me understand my experiences. It has also allowed me to see that as both an outsider and a short-term contract worker, I am not an instigator for major change and growth in First Nations communities. This needs to happen at the community roots level. When I'm working in a community, I see a connection between the physical and mental health of that community and the strength and innovation of the community leaders. The most difficult clinical situations I've seen included rape, scalping, and pediatric death by drowning and by accidental strangulation—all in the same few communities. But I've also seen many positive things: people taking charge of their health by doing blood glucose checks or seeking contraception education proactively, breastfeeding instead of bottle-feeding Carnation condensed milk, and running water in most homes.

Date of Confinement

Women have to leave the remote community at 36 weeks gestation, or 34 weeks if they are high risk, to go to a major city with a tertiary care hospital. Nursing stations are just not equipped to handle deliveries on a routine basis. Flights to and accommodations in the city are paid for the mother, but if she is older than 18, then any accompanying escort has to pay his or her own way. Most people cannot afford to pay for an escort, or their closest relative is taking care of the other young children at home on the reserve. I can only imagine how isolating and frustrating this period of "confinement" is for First Nations women. Some women actually return to the community before the baby is born or hide to avoid leaving due to the stress of this imposed isolation. At that time I, as the remote RN, am responsible for informing the Royal Canadian Mounted Police (RCMP) so they can search for the woman and force her to leave the community to ensure safe birthing for the neonate. It is a challenging situation to be in ethically: I enforce a system that I did not create and cannot control.

Infectious Diseases

Skin infections are rampant in the Northern reserves. I have seen 3-month-old infants with a "boil" that cultures positive for methicillin-resistant *Staphylococcus aureus* (MRSA). There are usually cramped living conditions and often no running water in many of the community homes. Attracting plumbing experts into a remote reserve requires much money and training them requires sending the community member away, potentially never to return. No running water means difficulty treating scabies and lice—also a complication of overcrowding. I once diagnosed a young girl and her brother with scabies, explained to the mother how to treat with the Nix rinse and to wash all bedding and towels, and sent them home with a note to excuse them from school for 2 days while this was done. But 2 days later they were back for another note to excuse them from school again. When I delved into the situation further, it turned out that they did not have running water—I had not individualized my treatment to meet their situation. Fortunately, it was winter, so we had alternate ways of treating the linen, bagging and leaving it out in the cold for 2 days.

Attitudes Toward Disease

There are very high rates of diabetes in First Nations communities. I have learned to tailor my patient care to include a random peripheral blood glucose as part of my basic assessment for most patient care scenarios. This has often led to new diagnoses of diabetes or awareness of poorly controlled diabetes. I have found that looming diabetes does not motivate effectively for lifestyle changes and prevention techniques on remote reserves. Often the attitude is not "*if* I get diabetes" but "*when* I get diabetes." Diabetes is such a common health condition that it has been accepted as inevitable by many members of these communities. I am still frustrated when I encounter an apathetic attitude to looming diabetes, but I know that the necessary change in attitude needs to come from influential community members. I can offer support, education, and an open door, but I cannot make people change unless they want to.

Communication

Language and cultural expressions can be very different among First Nations communities. Some groups have retained their native language quite intact despite colonialism, and I find I need interpreters just as often in those remote reserves as I have in a busy downtown

Toronto emergency department. Nonverbal communication can also be quite common. A unique grunt or vocal sound to indicate yes or no can leave a newcomer confused. Pointing with the lips is another subtle cue that is often missed by outsiders.

Government Organization and Expectations

Working indirectly for an organization can be challenging. My employer is the agency that is contracted by FNIH to fill staffing holes created by illness, vacation, or vacancies. As a temporary relief worker, I am never sure what situation I will find. I might arrive to an overworked nursing station with burned-out staff members due to an epidemic of influenza, pertussis, or suicide. I have arrived to the overwhelming setup of a brand new nursing station and the middle of a forest fire evacuation. I have also arrived to find a nurse in charge (NIC) who was not aware that I was coming for a 4-week stint.

As a contract worker, I need to make sure I am effective in the role I am filling. Otherwise, I just create more work for the permanent staff to clean up after I leave. Each nursing station has particular ways of doing things: covering on-call shifts, filling out laboratory requisitions, filing patient charts, consulting physician services, and processing medical evacuations. I orient myself on day 1 in a new station using a list of these basic nursing rituals and then focus on complying with the routine.

As I've said, I understand that I am not making profound changes or rescuing communities when I work in a nursing station for 2 weeks. This would not be my role as a guest in the community in any circumstance. However, I do focus on making small but meaningful impacts to a handful of people each contract I work. This attitude started with my first contract when I had a patient in supraventricular tachycardia who I successfully cardioverted with adenosine one night. When I reviewed his chart, I realized that he was going into this non-life-sustaining rhythm every 2 weeks and had been referred to a cardiologist 6 months before but had not yet been seen. It took me 2 weeks of follow-up to get everything set up because of staff vacations and busy physicians at the cardiology clinic, but the day I left the community, he had a date for his treatment procedure. Now I frequently have sticky notes on my desk regarding various patients who I am following in that community throughout my contract. Sometimes it is to follow a child who is not up to date on his or her immunizations, to motivate the parent to bring him or her in, or it might be to monitor a patient's recovery from Bell's palsy so that he or she can be referred to a specialist if he or she misses a milestone in his or her recovery; sometimes it is to receive a specialist's response to a patient's inquiry about the next steps for his or her condition.

Politics

Being a guest on Northern reserves involves politics. The reserve's governing body can vote to withdraw a visitor's welcome status at any time. This is called a BCR (Band and Council Resolution), and the person implicated must leave reserve land within a specified time period of notification (often a few hours). I know many nurses who have had a difference of opinion on the ethics of a clinical situation with the leaders of a community and received a BCR. I have never personally encountered an overt threat of a BCR, but it is something that lingers above my head as I work, and I am mindful to be diplomatic while also trying to work within my professional scope of practice. For example, I am frequently pressured to approve a medical escort for patients who do not qualify for one. It is a difficult position to be in, because I could push beyond my authority and override the system for a few cases, but I ultimately risk my job or license when I go too far beyond my authority. However, I often feel that I risk a BCR if I do not comply with local band authority pressures.

On the other hand, local authorities have been an asset when I used the local radio station to call patient names for overdue pediatric immunizations. Many families have six to seven children, so immunizations always seem to be late.

One time I had a suicidal patient run out of the clinic when I explained that I needed to evacuate him out of the community to the closest city for psychiatric assessment. I asked the security guard to call the band constables to search for the patient, and the chief himself assisted in the search and recovery of the patient. I do not think the response would have been quite so efficient if the chief had not become involved.

When you are an isolated practitioner, you are often the key medical decision maker and you need to take control and be decisive lest you risk losing control of medical situations or passively allowing errors to occur. However, swing too far on the confidence scale and you risk developing a god complex. I have found that it is important to continue to actively use my resources and double check my logic and decisions with other practitioners to prevent this. Access to a physician by phone and working with other experienced remote RNs have been invaluable resources in the remote north.

CONCLUSION

My experience working on remote reserves in northern Canada has been fantastic. I love the job. But I have realized during my time in the north that it is similar to any other nursing position: You need to leave before you burn out. I have always been realistic about there being an end to my remote nursing time due to the personal isolation attendant on the role. I have made sure to enjoy the experience while in the job and then to translate my favorite part of the experience—the expanded scope—into my future nursing practice, wherever it is.

REFLECTIVE QUESTIONS

1. What knowledge, skills, or experiences do you have from your background to work in an expanded nursing scope?
2. How would you manage working in a remote or isolated community? What character strengths or home supports would be available to you?
3. How will you ensure that you work within your professional scope of practice even when there is pressure from authority figures to push the boundaries? What checks can you put in place for yourself to ensure that you work safely and competently? How will you handle a situation where someone is pushing you beyond your knowledge or skill level?
4. As a short-term nurse in a foreign community how will you ensure that you work effectively in the role you are filling? What orientation will you seek when you arrive in the community to feel confident that you are competent in your temporary role?

REFERENCES

Canadian Nurses Association. (2010). Promoting culturally competent care. Ottawa, ON: Author. http://www.cna-aiic.ca/~/media/cna/page%20content/pdf%20en/2013/09/04/16/27/6%20-%20ps114_cultural_competence_2010_e.pdf

CBC News. (2010). Residential schools: A history of residential schools in Canada. www.cbc.ca/news/canada/story/2008/05/16/f-faqs-residential-schools.html

Health Canada. (n.d.). First Nations and Inuit Health. www.hc-sc.gc.ca/fniah-spnia/index-eng.php

Health Canada. (2009, December). A statistical profile on the health of First Nations in Canada: Self-rated health and selected conditions, 2002 to 2005. www.hc-sc.gc.ca/fniah-spnia/pubs/aborig-autoch/2009-stats-profil-vol3/index-eng.php#a2

Health Canada. (2010, October). Health Canada's northern nursing community. www.hc-sc.gc.ca/ahc-asc/pubs/_audit-verif/2010-06/index-eng.php#rec

Health Canada. (2011). Manitoba Region. www.hc-sc.gc.ca/ahc-asc/branch-dirgen/rapb-dgrp/reg/mb-eng.php

National Collaborating Centre for Aboriginal Health. (2009). Health inequalities and social determinants of aboriginal peoples' health. www.nccah-ccnsa.ca/docs/social%20determinates/nccah-loppie-wien_report.pdf

Saskatoon Health Region. (2010). Strengthening the circle: Partnering for improved health for aboriginal people. www.saskatoonhealthregion.ca/about_us/documents/STC-Aboriginal-Health-Stragety-summary.pdf

From Global Support to Local Change: The Impact of the Aga Khan University School of Nursing Throughout Pakistan

Jacqueline Maria Dias

CONTEXT: PAKISTAN

The history of nursing education in Pakistan parallels the country's independence. Nursing education in Pakistan began before partition with India in 1947. In 1952, the Pakistan Nursing Council (PNC) was formed, and a standard curriculum was developed. It reflected the medical model and nurses were primarily taught by physicians using traditional teaching methodologies—namely, lectures.

The Image of Nursing in Pakistan and the Role of Women

In Pakistan women have a uniquely defined identity as a Muslim, a Pakistani, and a woman (Carbonu & Soares, 1997). This identity dictates the way the women live and are influenced by custom, religion, norms, mores, laws, rules, and regulations (Carbonu & Soares, 1997). Despite the social orientation of the Islamic faith, nursing is seen in Pakistan as a menial occupation and consequently unsuitable as a field of study for daughters of the middle- and upper-class Muslim families. Nursing is not seen as a professional career with a future and is terminated by marriage, pregnancy, family demands, or emigration. The concept of "nurse" is inseparable from the concept of women as obedient and subject to the authority of fathers, husbands, and brothers (Harner, Amarsi, Herberg, & Miller, 1992).

My journey in nursing began over 25 years ago. Nursing today is undergoing an unprecedented change in the country. I have seen nursing evolve over the years; I have witnessed a movement where nursing in Pakistan has moved out of the hospitals with the apprenticeship model into universities and found its rightful place in higher education (Dias, 2013).

CURRENT SCENARIO

Currently in Pakistan, for every 2,500 people there is only one nurse, while in developed countries approximately 150 to 200 people are served by one nurse. Furthermore, the doctor–nurse ratio is 3:1 (Settle, 2010). According to international standards, the ratio should be reversed: three nurses to one doctor. Greater and better quality health workers mean that the general population has better access to a good health care system, which automatically improves the general health of the country. The need to increase the quality of education for nurses has been recognized for many years by the provincial and federal governments. Aga Khan University School of Nursing (AKUSON) has sought to improve nursing education

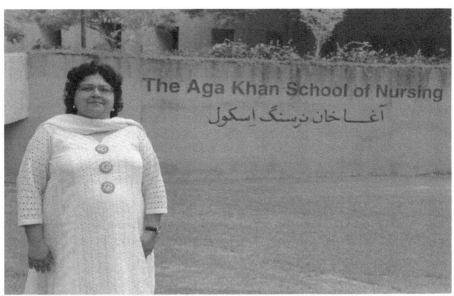

Author in front of Aga Khan School of Nursing building.   *Credit*: J. Dias

and professional standards in the country by working with the PNC, the regulatory body for nursing; the Pakistan Nursing Federation (PNF), a professional body; nursing authorities within the country's provinces; examination boards; other schools of nursing; and various health service institutions throughout Pakistan. The efforts of AKUSON in facilitating change across schools of nursing is acknowledged on all fronts with the nursing leaders at the PNC and the PNF. Thus, AKUSON is seen as a trendsetter for nursing education across the country (Dias, Ayaz, & Barolia, 2013). The significant contribution of this university effect has been felt across the country and the surrounding regions in the areas of curriculum, policy and higher education, testing, and assessments. Through the efforts of AKUSON, women have been empowered.

As the university's first academic institution, AKUSON began operating in 1980, with a view to educate nurses to provide exemplary patient care and demonstrate leadership in nursing education, practice, administration and research. In addition, AKUSON was the first to offer professional qualifications and degree programs in the field of nursing up to the master of science in nursing (MSN) level. Today, work is under way to begin a doctoral program in nursing.

Since its inception, AKUSON has played a leading role in establishing an internationally acceptable model for nursing education and practice in Pakistan. The community-oriented high-quality education at AKUSON has been pivotal in raising the status of nursing in Pakistan and in changing public perceptions toward the profession and its role in health care. Over the past 3 decades, AKUSON has not only established itself as the premier nursing school in the country, but has also become a strong regional center for nursing education. Finally, AKUSON aspires to encourage young women throughout Pakistan to choose a nursing career in order to strengthen the health services in the country. In the process, women are encouraged to play a more meaningful role in the nation's development (Karamliani, 2011).

FACILITATING CHANGE IN NURSING SCHOOLS ACROSS PAKISTAN

AKUSON, in keeping with its mission, has contributed toward enhancing the status of the nursing profession by offering continuing education activities and organizing academic events for national nursing leaders and educators. Its faculty have conducted and facilitated several local, national, and international workshops over the past 30 years. The first seminar, "The Role of Nurses in the '80s," was hosted in February 1981. The objective of the seminar was to share ideas with nurses from Pakistan and abroad on the role of nursing with reference to primary health care. The late Dr. Virginia Henderson, professor emeritus, School of Nursing, Yale University, was the distinguished keynote speaker at the seminar.

Another cardinal event that took place was the first National Workshop on the Nursing Process, in August 1984. AKUSON organized its first national workshop, "The Nursing Process: A Means to Improving Nursing Care." The 27 participants, representing eight hospitals and maternity homes in Karachi, discussed the methodology of planning, implementing, and evaluating care. This was the first time that national faculty were introduced to the concept of the nursing process (Cassum & Eijaz, 2000).

CURRICULUM REFORM

The Aga Khan University has been instrumental in the revision of nursing curricula at all levels. In 1992, with the assistance of the WHO (World Health Organization) and CIDA (Canadian International Development Agency), community health nursing was introduced into the nursing curriculum with emphasis on primary health care and an understanding of the various health issues that confront the Pakistani people. Concerns such as population growth, antenatal programs, treatment of diarrheal diseases, and immunization were included (Harner, Amarsi, Herberg, & Miller, 1992). In addition, AKUSON facilitated the inclusion and development of mental health nursing as part of the PNC general nursing diploma. The highlight of this curriculum revision was that AKUSON undertook the responsibility of training nurse educators across the country. Thus, for the first time, nursing faculty began to take over teaching nurses, rather than physicians. This significant achievement occurred through several faculty development workshops in which nursing faculty were taught concepts in community health nursing, mental health nursing, and how to use the nursing process.

As the only institution offering baccalaureate programs in the country, AKUSON is seen as a national resource. In 2006, the Higher Education Commission and the PNC called on AKUSON to lead the development of a standardized national curriculum for baccalaureate nursing in the country (Higher Education Commission Islamabad & Pakistan Nursing Council, 2006). Five years later, in 2011, the baccalaureate curriculum was again revised and, once again, AKUSON was called on to lead the review (Higher Education Commission Islamabad & Pakistan Nursing Council, 2011). I was honored to be the convener for the revision.

Curriculum reform also includes testing and examinations at the national level. Over the years, AKUSON has strengthened the national licensure examination through the introduction of a table of specifications, multiple choice questions, item analysis, viva examination (oral examination to assess student knowledge), and training for examiners on an ongoing basis.

LINKAGES WITH OTHER NATIONAL INSTITUTIONS

National universities are at our doorsteps. Our faculty are working closely with several institutions in the country to help them set up their baccalaureate programs across Pakistan. A recent undertaking of the Aga Khan University has been with the provincial government of Khyber Pakhtunkhwa for capacity building of nurses through higher education in the post–RN bachelor of science in nursing (BSN) and MSN programs.

AKUSON'S WORK WITH POLICYMAKERS

AKUSON has lobbied for change through the introduction of degree programs in nursing. In order to upgrade nursing qualifications to an undergraduate degree, AKUSON embarked on a post–RN degree program in 1988—the first program of its kind in the country—to prepare nurses for higher education and leadership roles in Pakistan. Until this point, the highest academic qualification was the registered nurse (RN) diploma, for which matriculation was the basic application requirement. By graduating over 3,000 nurses to date, this has led to a role model effect in enhancing the quality of nursing care overall in the country as the graduates of these programs have gone on to become principals and heads of nursing in their respective schools.

Another significant change occurred in the PNC regulations for the diploma program so that married women became eligible to apply and age limits were relaxed from 16 to 35 years and up to 40 years in some cases. Moreover, day students were permitted to enroll, and hostel (dormitory) accommodation was no longer a requirement. Furthermore, AKU-SON introduced the direct entry route into the BSN program in 1997. Subsequently, for the first time, both female and male candidates could apply to nursing after completing grade 12. For the first time, males and females took classes together, a radical change from the previous PNC diploma policy which had students segregated by gender, taught separately, and unable to share the same premises.

Another milestone that followed the baccalaureate program was the introduction of the MSN program in 2001. All these programs, post–RN BSN and prelicensure BSN and MSN, are the first programs of their kind in Pakistan, thereby upgrading nursing education to the university level.

SCHOLARSHIP

The Aga Khan University School of Nursing Honor Society (AKUSON-HS) became a chapter of Sigma Theta Tau International (STTI) at the 35th biennial convention, held on November 10, 1999, in San Diego, California. Pakistan is the first Muslim country to achieve chapter status, another milestone in the history of nursing in Pakistan. This has become an avenue for faculty across the country to participate in online certification, receive grants, and showcase their research work at national and international conferences. It is also an opportunity for nursing faculty to network and share ideas with colleagues from around the world.

FACILITATING CHANGE REGIONALLY

As the university has grown internationally, AKUSON has used various approaches to respond to the human resource challenges of different countries. Since 2001, for instance, AKUSON has offered an advanced nursing studies program in Kenya, Uganda, and Tanzania. Developed at the request of nursing leaders and the respective governments, the program offers continuing and higher education up to a BSN level to working nurses, allowing them to remain at their workplaces while pursuing professional development. In Syria and Afghanistan, AKUSON is providing technical assistance for baccalaureate education and for strengthening the national examination systems.

All these regional events would not have been possible were it not for a simultaneous investment of resources and a reliance on partnerships and collaborations with other universities. The Aga Khan University has invested heavily in faculty development. Universities have excellent instructors when there is an investment in faculty development (Whitcombe, 2003). Wilkerson and Irby (1998) state that faculty development plays a pivotal role to ensure academic excellence and innovation (Wilkerson & Irby, 1998). Faculty development is usually a planned program designed to prepare institutions and faculty members for their various roles in teaching, administration, and research (Steinhert, 2010). By providing the appropriate faculty development activities, the nursing faculty at the Aga Khan University have grown both professionally and personally in their multiple roles. Faculties have been granted support to upgrade their educational profile and complete undergraduate studies (post–RN BSN) and graduate studies (master's and PhD).

PARTNERSHIPS AND COLLABORATIONS

AKUSON has supported the ongoing development of nursing faculty from sources outside of Pakistan since its inception in 1980. This was achieved through partnerships and collaborations with other universities, including McMaster University in Canada, Sheffield University in the United Kingdom, and Karolinska Institute in Sweden. AKUSON has been fortunate to have had assistance in faculty capacity building from McMaster University, funded by CIDA, to develop educational programs, especially the post–RN BSN. Diploma-educated faculty were sent for baccalaureate education outside the country to McMaster University in Canada from 1983 until 1998, when AKUSON began its own BSN program. Today, 95% of AKUSON faculty members have the MSN, and seven faculty have a doctorate. These programs prepared the faculty as well as nursing leaders at AKU in the areas of service and education. This is evident from the nursing leadership at the school. The former dean and the author of this case study are both graduates of McMaster University.

Another significant milestone was the Development of Women Health Professionals (DWHP) program. This venture aimed at sustainable human resource development in Pakistan as it opened up avenues with the Ministry of Health, which prepared women professionals, both nurses and female health visitors, in leadership positions to participate effectively in health policy and planning activities. The outcome of the DWHP program was institutional development for nursing across Pakistan and capacity building related to the nursing profession with a view to empowering women.

Collaboration with the University of Sheffield through a link with the British Council facilitated the development and marketing of MSN programs with nursing leaders (Upvall, Karmaliani, Pirani, Gul, & Khalid, 2004) while with Karolinska Institute faculty and student exchanges were initiated and led to faculty enrollment in PhD programs. Another, more recent partnership with the University of Alberta has opened up avenues for faculty to pursue their doctoral studies in Canada.

EMPOWERMENT OF WOMEN

Nurses directly improve the health status of their families and the communities in which they live. Women from disadvantaged backgrounds who become well-qualified nurses often become the primary breadwinners of families who otherwise have no income source. AKUSON has seen that its alumnae, especially those from marginalized areas, such as the poor localities of Karachi, rural Sindh, the northern areas of Pakistan, and the like, often return to become leaders in their communities and have a greater voice in health issues and policymaking at the local and national levels. Furthermore, AKUSON motivates young women from all over Pakistan to choose nursing as a career in order to strengthen the delivery of health care services. In the process, women are encouraged to play a more meaningful role in the nation's development and in advancement for women that is in harmony with the traditions of an Islamic society. Through AKUSON's efforts, nursing has evolved into an academic profession that women choose to enter, rather than simply being a service profession. This has changed the image of the profession and has resulted in the empowerment of women, who are now able to independently make decisions affecting them and their families. Furthermore, nurses have become role models for other women in this profession, resulting in a larger number of women entering this profession by choice (AKUSON Student Handbook, 2012; Higher Education Commission & Pakistan Nursing Council, 2011).

CHALLENGES

One of the biggest challenges is how to formalize the partnerships. Once formalized, how we sustain these partnerships remains an ongoing challenge. Over half our faculty have less than 5 years of experience. The current geopolitical situation has affected us in many ways.

Attracting expatriate faculty has been unsuccessful, yet is essential for the start of new programs. The pool of experienced faculty is therefore very limited. Retention of national faculty is another big challenge as many leave for better opportunities in North America and the United Kingdom. Our students hail from places ranging from the shores of Africa to the hilly regions of Afghanistan and Tajikistan, as well as Syria. This diversified student population is both a success and a challenge for us at the school of nursing. Families have been reluctant to send their daughters to Pakistan because of the current geopolitical situation. Nevertheless, the institutions with which we partner stand to benefit as well. By learning about the health issues and academic needs of the developing world, these universities have gained stature as international universities.

CONCLUSION

Faculty development is the lifeline of a university. This case study illustrates how one university has transformed the face of nursing education and empowered women in the developing world by heavily investing in faculty development. Bridges have been built between AKSUON and universities throughout the world, including those in both high- and low-income countries. Challenges continue to exist, but this case study demonstrates that positive change can occur at all levels: international, national, local. Lessons learned from AKUSON can be a source of inspiration for helping other countries build capacity of their nurses and other health care professionals.

REFLECTIVE QUESTIONS

1. What challenges may exist when collaborating with local nursing institutions? How could you address these challenges?
2. Think about the concepts of time and change within the nursing profession. What would your expectations be in promoting change to the profession within the context of another country such as Pakistan?
3. How can you adapt your current nursing practice to meet the needs and expectations of nurses in other countries? What factors would you need to consider? How would you begin to make this connection?
4. Changes to a profession may have implications for society. Discuss the potential implications, comparing high-income and low-resource countries.

REFERENCES

AKUSON Student Handbook. (2012). http://portal.aku.edu/son

Carbonu, D. M., & Soares, J. M. (1997). Forensic nursing in Pakistan bridging the gap between victimized women and health care delivery systems. *Journal of Psychosocial Nursing, 35*(6), 19–27.

Cassum, S., & Eijaz, A. (2000). *The Aga Khan University School of Nursing: Two decades of accomplishments 1980–2000.* Unpublished manuscript.

Dias, J. (2013). The future of nursing education. *Canadian Medical Education Journal, 4*(1), 113–114.

Dias, J. M., Ayaz,. B., & Barolia, R. (2013). Accelerated programmes: The way forward in curriculum development and innovation. In *ELT in a changing World: Innovative approaches to new challenges.* New Castle: Cambridge Scholars Publishing.

Harner, R., Amarsi, Y., Herberg, P., & Miller., G. (1992). Health and nursing services in Pakistan: Problems and challenges for the nurse leader. *Journal of Nursing Administration Quarterly, 16*(2), 52–59.

Higher Education Commission Islamabad & Pakistan Nursing Council. (2006). *Curriculum of nursing education BScN.* Islamabad, Pakistan: Higher Education Commission.

Higher Education Commission & Pakistan Nursing Council. (2011). *Revised curriculum of nursing BS (4-year degree program)*. Islamabad, Pakistan: Higher Education Commission.

Karamliani, R. (2011). *Proposal for financial support to the scholarship program of Aga Khan University School of Nursing and Midwifery*. Unpublished manuscript.

Settle, A. (2010). *Federal budget: Briefing paper*. www.sanianishtar.info/pdfs/CP-PB.pdf

Steinhert, Y. (2010). Becoming a better teacher. In J. Ende (Ed.), *Theory and practice of teaching medicine*. Philadelphia: American College of Physicians.

Upvall, M. J., Karamliani, R., Pirani, F., Gul, R., & Khalid, F. (2004). Developing nurse leaders through graduate education in Pakistan. *International Journal of Nursing Scholarship*, www.bepress.com/ijnes/vol1/iss1/art27

Whitcombe, M. (2003).The medical school's faculty is its most important asset. *Academic Medicine*, *78*(2), 117–118.

Wilkerson, L., & Irby, D. M. (1998). Strategies for improving teaching practices: A comprehensive approach to faculty development. *Academic Medicine*, *73*, 387–396.

CHAPTER 8

Collaboration With International Organizations

Jeanne M. Leffers

Globally there are more than 32 million nurses in practice. While nurses deliver almost 90% of care to patients globally, in most countries nurses are not well represented at the decision-making level in international agencies or in government offices (Davis, 2012). In low- and middle-income countries (LMICs) nurses often serve as the sole health care provider to millions of people living in poverty worldwide. There is a profound need for nurses, nurse faculty, and support for professional development in lower-income countries that can be addressed through collaborative nurse partnerships (George & Meadows-Oliver, 2013; Frenk et al., 2010). While approximately 90% of the global burden of disease occurs in low-income countries, only 10% of the world's health research funding addresses that burden (Doyal, 2004). Additionally, great inequities exist between countries in relation to availability of educational institutions for health care professional development and ability to address the shortage of skilled professionals to address the global burden of disease (Frenk et al., 2010). Consistent with the Leffers and Mitchell (2011) model, DeSantis (1995) offers a model for partnership that emphasizes a counterpart concept to explain how partnerships must address the needs, resources, and development potential of the LMIC partners; address social, political, cultural, and economic factors for partnership; negate the need for donations from the high-income country partners; and develop the potential of nurses from both low-income and higher income countries. George and Meadows-Oliver (2013) emphasize that nurses from high-income countries who work in global settings must include nurses from the respective LMICs to form partnerships based on the expressed needs by the low-income country partners. Working with organizations globally provides an opportunity for nurses to form such important partnerships, as well as to collaborate to effect change at the health system level (Frenk et al., 2010).

Amieva and Ferguson (2012) suggest that nurses can impact the achievement of the UN Millennium Development Goals (MDG) by collaborative partnerships, research, and policy development. Several examples in the case studies in this book shared by nurse partners in the United States and nurse colleagues in Haiti and Rwanda illustrate the variety of partnerships that involve nursing organizations. In collaboration with Partners in Health (PIH) partnerships between nurses from higher income settings with more resources can have a positive impact on health. The Dana Farber Cancer Institute, based in Boston, Massachusetts, has an oncology nursing partnership with Inshuti Mu Buzima (IMB), the Rwandan oncology nursing organization, to promote the development of specialized skills to advance oncology care. Another example is the partnership, highlighted in a case study in this chapter, of Regis College in Weston, Massachusetts; the Haitian Ministry of Health; and PIH to develop and administer a collaborative master's in nursing program for Haitian nursing faculty. Through this initiative to strengthen nursing education in Haiti, the master's-prepared faculty will become the educational leaders for future generations of nurses in Haiti (Davis, 2012).

Professional nurses who work in global settings almost always participate as part of an organization, whether in their home country or in another country or region. Previous chapters and case studies provided examples of a variety of both academic and professional partnerships. In these examples, visiting nurse partners frequently represent one organization but are likely to interact with several organizations.

The purpose of this chapter is to highlight the critical importance of nurse collaboration in international settings, particularly with nursing organizations across borders. Such collaboration is essential in partnership formation and builds on the concept of bridging cultures and mutual respect of both nurses and host partners (Leffers & Mitchell, 2011; George & Meadows-Oliver, 2013). In many cases, such collaboration builds capacity for nurse partner organizations. In this chapter, types of organizations relevant to global health are defined, examples are shared, the importance of nursing organizations to the advancement of the profession is addressed, and the mandate to collaborate globally with nurses and nursing organizations is articulated. The examples do not represent all international organizations but do offer a sample of the global organizations in operation. Examples of organizations in the United States are included to offer a comparison for emerging organizations in distant global settings.

TYPES OF INTERNATIONAL ORGANIZATIONS

A great number of organizations focus their efforts on international and/or global health. These include large organizations such as the World Health Organization (WHO) and smaller nonprofit aid organizations. They can be defined as multilateral, bilateral, and nongovernmental (International Medical Volunteers Association, 2013). The largest organizations are referred to as multilateral because their funding comes from the governments of many countries and the organizations support a variety of programs across a wide range of countries. The United Nations (UN) and the WHO are two such multilateral health organizations. The United Nations has several programs that focus on health, primarily the United Nations Children's Fund (UNICEF), as well as other development-, nutrition-, and health-related programs. Formed after World War II, the main functions of the UN are to keep peace and foster friendly relations among nations as well as to work to improve lives worldwide by addressing hunger, illiteracy, disease, and human rights (United Nations, 2013b). With its focus on worldwide development, the UN established the Millennium Development Goals (MDG) in 2000 to address the health and well-being of people worldwide by 2015 (www.un.org/millenniumgoals/bkgd.shtml). The health of the world's population would greatly improve if these goals were met (UN, 2013b) (see Table 8.1 for the MDG).

The WHO is the coordinating health authority of the United Nations, formed in 1948 to meet the UN mission to address health worldwide. According to the WHO website, the organization is "responsible for providing leadership on global health matters, shaping the health research agenda, setting norms and standards, articulating evidence-based policy options, providing technical support to countries and monitoring and assessing health trends" (2011, 2013a). To accomplish its goals, the WHO has a six-point agenda to promote development; foster health security; strengthen health systems; harness research, information, and evidence; enhance partnerships; and improve performance. Just as noted in the UN MDG, poverty and underdevelopment contribute to poor health outcomes. Using a health equity approach the WHO gives priority to health outcomes for poor, disadvantaged, or vulnerable groups (World Health Organization, 2013b).

Other governmental organizations are generally bilateral in nature. That is, one government funds projects that are developed in a second country. In Denmark, the bilateral development organization DANIDA strategically focuses on human rights and democracy,

TABLE 8.1 United Nations Millennium Development Goals

Eradicating extreme poverty and hunger

Achieving universal primary education

Promoting gender equality and empowering women

Reducing child mortality rates

Improving maternal health

Combating HIV/AIDS, malaria, and other diseases

Ensuring environmental sustainability

Developing a global partnership for development

TABLE 8.2 Focus of USAID Projects

Agriculture and food security

Democracy, human rights, and governance

Economic growth and trade

Education

Environment and global climate change

Gender equality and women's empowerment

Global health

Science, technology, and innovation

Water and sanitation

Working in conflict and crisis

Source: www.usaid.gov/what-we-do

green growth, social progress and stability, and protection. Most important to stability and protection are basic human needs such as water, food, shelter, education, health, and employment. Through health sector programs in Ghana, Uganda, Kenya, and Mozambique, the Danish government agency DANIDA provides millions of dollars, aid, and expertise (DANIDA, 2013). The Canadian International Development Agency (CIDA) is a bilateral organization that focuses on meeting the MDG by addressing five key areas: food security, children and youth, sustainable economic growth, democratic governance, and security and stability (Canadian International Development Agency, 2013). An example of a bilateral organization is the United States Agency for International Development (USAID, 2013). This organization addresses a variety of issues to improve well-being in international settings (see Tables 8.2 and 8.3). Later in this chapter there is an example of a USAID project with the Uganda National Association for Nurses and Midwives.

Governmental Health Structures: The Ministry of Health

While nurses in the United States are familiar with a governmental structure that includes a cabinet-level leader as the secretary of health and human services, a surgeon-general, and chief nurse of the U.S. Public Health Service, most other countries have a different form of administration for their health system. In most other countries a minister of health oversees the Ministry of Health for the country. The health ministry is usually responsible for setting

TABLE 8.3 Specific Health Focus of USAID Projects

Family planning
HIV and AIDS
Health systems
Malaria
Maternal child health
Neglected tropical diseases
Nutrition
Pandemic and other emerging diseases
Tuberculosis

Source: www.usaid.gov/what-we-do

and enforcing standards for health management in the country, regulating health professions, monitoring health system and programs, and regulating pharmaceuticals and medical devices and their quality for the overall health of the population. The minister of health is ultimately responsible for the administration of the country's health care system. While health systems and administrative structure might vary across countries, each country will have some form of leadership for health. Within the Ministry of Health organizational structure is a chief nurse officer (CNO). The CNO oversees the nursing role for public health, registration and disciplinary functions for nursing practice, and nursing administration in government hospitals and health care facilities. CNO roles can vary across international settings. Our case studies illustrate how nurses or the organizations for which nurses might work partner with both the Ministry of Health and the nursing associations and councils in the host country. In particular, Case Study 8.2, "Rwanda Human Resources for Health Program," details the collaboration between various partners while led by the Ministry of Health.

The U.S. governmental system partners with ministries of health (MOHs) through systems such as the partnership with the Centers for Disease Control and Prevention (CDC). Based on "mutual respect, joint mission, and a shared long-term vision of sustainable institutional capacity" (CDC, 2013), the CDC provides direct technical assistance, trains health practitioners and leaders, and helps the MOH strengthen its capacity for prevention and treatment programs.

Nongovernmental Organizations

The organizations referred to as nongovernmental organizations (NGOs) are generally smaller in scope and funding and frequently are associated with religious sponsors. Thousands of nurses participate in global health programs with nongovernmental organizations each year. The role of nongovernmental organizations varies by size, scope, origin, sponsorship, funding and partnership with host country organizations. Health NGOs most often provide basic health services, donate medical supplies, and provide a variety of medical services. Most NGOs define themselves as nonprofit, autonomous, and private. In many LMICs where the infrastructure for health services is not as well developed as in higher income countries, NGOs can serve a vital role in helping to build capacity for health, to educate health care providers, and to provide essential health services. Precise numbers are difficult to obtain, because not all NGOs register with the national health system or government in the country in which they operate. For example, in Haiti, often referred to as the "Republic of NGOs," it is estimated that anywhere between 300 and 20,000 NGOs provide as much as 70% of health care (Center for Global Development, 2013). This is the case in many other countries. In Uganda, estimates cite approximately 200 NGOs in 1986, 5,500 by the end of 2005, and as many as 8,000 at present (Ssewakiryanga, 2009).

One of the largest of these NGOs, Project HOPE (Health Opportunities for People Everywhere), was founded in 1958 in the United States. Beginning with a donated former U.S. naval ship, the program began as *S.S. Hope*, a ship that traveled the world to bring medical care to those in need. Today Project HOPE serves more than 35 countries and in 2012 provided $1.7 million in donated services (Project HOPE, 2013). Project HOPE's headquarters are in the United States, with offices in the United Kingdom and Germany. Their stated mission is "to achieve sustainable advances in health care around the world by implementing health education programs and providing humanitarian assistance in areas of need" (Project HOPE, 2013).

Another large nongovernmental organization based in the United States is Oxfam America. While the focus of this organization is poverty and hunger, Oxfam programs address many of the MDG such as gender equality, global development, climate change, and poverty and hunger. Programs that focus specifically on health include access to medications and disaster relief (Project HOPE, 2013).

PIH began in 1987 to provide health care to the Haitian people living in the Artibonite region of the country. Their mission to provide a preferential option for the poor in health care is operationalized by the establishment of long-term partnerships with local organizations in settings where the poor and most vulnerable live. Currently they serve in Haiti, Russia, Peru, Rwanda, Leshsoto, Malawi, Mexico, Kazakhstan, the United States, and the Dominican Republic, offering programs in partnership with local health care systems. From their beginning 26 years ago, they have come to now work in 12 countries and number more than 15,000 health care workers. Through their partnerships they provide medical care for millions of patients, build their community-based model of care, train health care workers, conduct research, and advocate for health policy change to promote global health for the most vulnerable (PIH, 2013).

Disaster Response and Relief Organizations

There are many organizations that focus primarily on disaster response and relief both nationally and internationally. While the focus of this book is neither disaster response nor the nursing role in disaster, the examples here are provided to identify the variety of NGOs that deliver relief in times of crisis and disaster. Many books speak to nursing roles in disaster (Leffers & Plotnick, 2011; Veenema, 2012). Those organizations whose work is reported frequently include the International Red Cross, Médecins Sans Frontières (MSF)—known in the United States as Doctors Without Borders—and Catholic Relief Services. Each of these NGOs address health as central to its mission. The International Committee of the Red Cross is a humanitarian organization that coordinates international activities in regions where there is crisis due to violence, conflict, or disaster. Health activities include direct emergency care, provision of surgical and medical treatments, provision of medications, reconstruction of medical facilities, and other preventive and restorative care (International Committee of the Red Cross, 2013).

Médecins Sans Frontières (MSF), known as Doctors Without Borders in the United States, is an international medical humanitarian organization that provides emergency relief to people affected by natural disasters, epidemics, and armed conflict. Founded in France in 1971, it is based in Switzerland and delivers services in 70 countries globally (Médecins Sans Frontières, 2013). Nurses frequently serve with this organization for long-term assignments in priority settings.

Catholic Relief Services is the official humanitarian organization of the Catholic Church in the United States. Formed in 1943, its mission is to "promote human development by responding to major emergencies, fighting disease and poverty, and nurturing peaceful and just societies" (Catholic Relief Services, 2013b) and to engage U.S. Catholics in international work to serve the needs of those most in need across the globe (Catholic Relief Services, 2013a). While Catholic Relief Services with its $700 million in donations in 2011 to 2012 provides a broad array of services beyond health, they emphasize community capacity for local governments to manage their own health programs (Catholic Relief Services, 2013a).

Preparation and registration with an organization that provides relief and response in disasters and emergencies is essential for health care providers to serve effectively and not burden local resources during relief efforts. Working with those organizations described above, rather than undertake well-intended but harmful assistance on an individual basis, promotes partnerships worldwide in times of emergency.

Despite the services that NGOs provide, their role is not without critics. Some note that the exponential growth of NGOs in many countries undermines the efforts of the local health system and fragment health services (Pfeiffer, 2003). Other critiques suggest that many NGOs lack accountability, fail to adequately evaluate their impact, and are negatively influenced by their major donors (Johnson, 2009). To counter the possibility of negative effects of NGO actions, the "NGO Code of Conduct for Health System Strengthening" was developed. Included in this code are articles that emphasize long-term health system sustainability by hiring practices, human resources training, and employee compensation; supporting and collaborating with ministries of health in ways that minimize burdens on the ministry; and advocating for policies to promote the public sector. By working with the government sector in a given country, the NGO will build successful partnerships and foster sustainability within the host country. NGOs must be flexible in order to adapt to the needs of the local health system and must not duplicate programs that the national health system offers, but should support the health system to build capacity (Pfeiffer, 2011).

Private Foundations

Other types of NGOs are private foundations that focus on global health initiatives. Examples of these include the Rockefeller Foundation, the Clinton Foundation, and the Bill & Melinda Gates Foundation. The oldest of these is the Rockefeller Foundation, and among their initiatives addressing many of the MDG such as gender equity, climate change, cities, and food security, they focus on health systems and provide financial support and guidance through their grant funding (Rockefeller Foundation, 2013). The Bill & Melinda Gates Foundation focuses primarily on infectious diseases such as malaria, tuberculosis, and HIV/AIDS, as well as leading causes of morbidity and mortality in low-income countries, such as diarrhea and pneumonia. With more than 1,000 employees, the foundation provides billions of dollars in grant-funded projects (Bill & Melinda Gates Foundation, 2013).

The Clinton Foundation, begun by former U.S. president Bill Clinton, was formed after he left government office in 2001. Working with governmental partners globally, the foundation focuses on global health in addition to health and welfare, childhood obesity, climate change, and economic inequalities (Clinton Foundation, 2013). A significant part of the Clinton Foundation, which became a separately incorporated entity in 2010, is the Clinton Health Access Initiative (CHAI). Initially focused on HIV/AIDS when it was formed in 2002, CHAI now focuses not only on programs for HIV/AIDS and access to medications, but also on malaria, maternal child health, and health systems. Since its formation, millions of people in the developing world are receiving antiretroviral medications. One of the newer projects is the Human Resources for Health program, which seeks to improve the health care systems in lower resource countries by increasing the capacity of the health care providers (Clinton Health Access Initiative, 2013).

PROFESSIONAL NURSING ORGANIZATIONS

Professional nursing organizations promote the profession and improve nursing practice. Professional organizations have been found to assist in the development of the profession, raise standards for the profession's education and practice, foster professional identity, sustain a professional culture, regulate professional practice, and establish an authority recognized by the wider society (Japanese Nursing Association, 2013; Matthews, 2012; National Council of Nurses and Midwives, 2013). Such associations can serve as a voice for health policy locally and globally (Benton, 2012). Furthermore, the participation in a professional social network where nurses receive support and professional advice can promote solidarity among nurses, reduce stress, and create opportunities to learn best practices for nursing care (Zuyderduin, Obuni, & McQuide, 2010).

The International Council of Nurses (ICN), founded in 1899, represents more than 13 million nurses worldwide through the representation of more than 130 national nurses associations (Bush et al., 2001; International Council of Nurses, 2007; Matthews, 2012). The ICN works to advance the nursing profession globally by advancing nursing knowledge, ensuring quality nursing care by a competent nursing workforce, and advocating for and influencing health policy. By working with national nursing associations around the world, the ICN supports policies that advance the health of populations, promote the security of nursing and health care professionals, and foster sustainable development (ICN, 2013a, 2013b). The ICN leadership believes that nurses can best serve patients worldwide by coordinating nursing actions, fostering solidarity in the profession, and shaping health policy through strong nursing leadership (Benton, 2012; ICN, 2013c, 2013d). Nurses who work in global health settings should first identify the role of ICN in relationship to the nursing profession where the global health work occurs.

An example offered by the ICN is the advancement of the nursing profession in Rwanda. Following this chapter are case studies highlighting the development of the nursing profession in Rwanda. The chief nursing officer and the president of the national nursing association in Rwanda recognized the need to introduce professional regulation and licensure in the country but knew that such legislation might be time-consuming and challenging. Seeking support from the ICN to lobby the government on their behalf, working to gather local support for their proposal, and persuading local nurses to operate as if the legislation was passed, the Rwandan nurses were successful in their efforts. Presently the National Council of Nurses and Midwives in Rwanda has completed the educational and practice standards to improve nursing practice (Benton, 2012).

Nursing Organizations in the United States as an Example

The development of the nursing profession in the United States is similar to what has occurred or is currently occurring in other countries. By using this U.S. example, the intention is not to presume that nurses in other global settings did not demonstrate their leadership to advance nursing education and practice in their own countries. The Royal College of Nursing was founded in 1916 in the United Kingdom, the Danish Nursing Association formed in 1899 in Denmark, and modern nursing began in Japan in 1895, with professional standards formalized in 1899. When ICN was formed in 1899, the United Kingdom, United States, and Germany were the charter members. In addition, advancements in nursing education were not limited to only higher income countries such as the United States and United Kingdom, but also occurred in other regions of the world such as the Middle East (Frenk et al., 2010). With this important fact in mind, the U.S. example is used simply because there is so much literature available about the history of the nursing profession in the United States to offer as a comparison for professional advancement globally.

Nursing in the United States began as a vocation wherein nurses were trained in hospitals to provide care to the sick. Through the work of nursing organizations, the education and practice of nursing evolved into the profession as it exists today. The nursing associations and councils that have been developed in most countries worldwide parallel examples of the

American Nurses Association (ANA) and the National Council of State Boards of Nursing (NCSBN). The ANA formed as the Nurses Associated Alumnae of the United States and Canada in 1896 and was renamed the ANA in 1911; it has served to advance education and practice for more than a century. As the only U.S. nursing full service organization representing the more than 3 million registered nurses in the United States, the ANA works in collaboration with its constituent state associations to "advances the nursing profession by fostering high standards of nursing practice, promoting the rights of nurses in the workplace, projecting a positive and realistic view of nursing, and lobbying the Congress and regulatory agencies on health care issues affecting nurses and the public" (American Nurses Association, 2013). By first organizing as a voice for nurses, the ANA spurred on the development of nursing to become a profession and advocated for licensure to ensure quality and safety. As shown in Table 8.4, the timeline for nursing professional development in the United States during the past 150 years offers an example of the types of advances that are comparable to those currently occurring in many countries.

In the United States there are more than 100 nursing specialty organizations dedicated to improving education and practice for the respective specialty. Many sponsor journals dedicated to the specialty offer continuing education and promote certification, practice, and patient advocacy. In other countries a growing number of nursing journals advances their professional practice, education, and research as well.

The examples of nursing organizations and boards of nursing in the United States provide a comparison with nursing organizations in other countries. Most LMICs today have some form of nursing association and a nursing council within the Ministry of Health structure. Some of our case studies include examples of partnerships or consultation with the country's nursing organization.

Boards of Nursing

Across the United States, the state boards of nursing are agencies of the state governments that protect the public by ensuring nursing competence and enforcement of standards of nursing practice. They are responsible for the regulation of nursing, administration of licensure examinations, oversight of nurse competency by handling complaints and disciplinary actions, enforcement of the relevant nurse practice act, and accreditation or approval of nursing educational programs (ANA, 2012).

In the United States, the NCSBN was formed in 1978 to oversee the licensure of nurses across all 50 states. Prior to that time, individual state boards of nursing administered their own licensing examinations and set their own passing standards. Founded in 1978 as an independent, 501(c)(3) not-for-profit organization, NCSBN can trace its roots to the ANA Council on State Boards of Nursing. The impetus for its creation arose out of recognition that in order to guard the safety of the public, the regulation of nurses needed to be a separate entity from the organization representing professional nurses. The member boards that comprise NCSBN protect the public by ensuring that safe and competent nursing care is provided by licensed nurses. NCSBN is the vehicle through which boards of nursing act and counsel together on matters of common interest. These member boards are charged with providing regulatory excellence for public health, safety, and welfare (National Council of State Boards of Nursing, 2013).

While the U.S. structure has boards of nursing in each of its 50 states and the District of Columbia, the structure differs in other countries, and global health nurses must consider how to locate the comparable regulatory agency. In most countries it is a nursing council functioning as part of the Ministry of Health. In Canada, for example, the Canadian Council of Registered Nurse Regulators represents Canada's 12 provincial/territorial bodies and regulates the practice of registered nurses. An example of a capacity project for the Uganda National Association for Nurses and Midwives (UNANM) is the Capacity Project in partnership with USAID. Established in 1964 as an NGO, the UNANM association became a member of the ICN in 1969, as well as a member of the Commonwealth Nurses Federation

TABLE 8.4 Timeline for Nursing Professional Development in the United States

Year	Example
1873	First training school for nurses, Linda Richards becomes first nurse to graduate from U.S. nursing school
1893	Lillian Wald begins public health nursing
1896	American Society of Superintendents of Training Schools of Nursing support licensure for nurses
1897	First meeting of American Nurses Association
1901	U.S. Army Nurse Corps begun
1903	North Carolina institutes permissive licensure for nurses
1915	ANA drafts for nurse practice act model
1923	All 48 states have permissive licensure laws
1923	Yale School of Nursing begins
1923	Mary Breckinridge begins Frontier Nursing Service
1935	New York passes first mandatory licensure law
1944	State Board Test Pool Examination created
1956	Columbia University awards first master's degree in nursing
1950s–1960s	Revision of nurse practice acts
1970s	Regulation begun for advanced practice nurses
1978	National Council of State Boards of Nursing created

Source: http://doh.sd.gov/boards/nursing/Documents/WhitePaperHistory2000.pdf

and Eastern, Central, and Southern African College of Nurses. The purpose of the collaborative project is to strengthen the association in order to retain nurses and improve the nursing workforce in Uganda (Zuyderduin et al., 2010).

Nursing Collaboration Imperative

To meet the mandates put forth by organizations such as the ICN and meet the recommendations of the Conceptual Model for Partnership and Sustainability in Global Health (Leffers & Mitchell, 2011), nurses who work in global health settings must collaborate with international and local nursing organizations and the host country's Ministry of Health (Frenk et al., 2010). Nurse partners who work with a large organization or with most NGOs will most likely learn that the leadership of their sponsoring organization has some type of partnership with the national health system in the host country. Many visiting partner nurses must obtain a nursing license in order to practice nursing in the host country. For many smaller NGOs and for shorter terms of service, the sponsoring NGO organization will have a formal agreement or memorandum of understanding with the Ministry of Health whereby the visiting nurse or other health professional will provide a copy of his or her license and any relevant certification to the NGO. These are then kept on file in country with the NGO. Nurses who work or volunteer across international borders must be licensed in the host country or have some cooperative agreement through the governing body such as the Ministry of Health. Ensuring

that patients in all countries receive the same quality of care is an ethical and moral imperative for nursing (Levi, 2009). The author of this chapter was recently working with an NGO
in Haiti that has such an agreement with the Haitian Ministry of Health (see Case Study 2.2,
"Building and Sustaining an Academic Partnership in Haiti"). During her stay, the Haitian
Ministère de la Santé Publique et de la Population (MSPP) made a site visit to the clinic to
evaluate services much the way that U.S. nurses are familiar with during a Joint Commission
visit at home. One criterion for evaluation was that all American visitors be licensed and registered appropriately for their role in Haiti.

To ensure that nurse partners who travel to another country for global health work
show respect to the host country nurses, do not duplicate services, and do not undermine
the host country nursing profession or take away from the essential services provided by
the local health system, we suggest taking the following steps:

1. Contact the ICN to identify any current partnerships or nursing associations in the
   country where the nurse partner will work.
2. Seek information about the host country nursing association and nursing council.
   While many countries are working toward professional standards, regulation, and
   licensure, most have some form of nursing association. It is imperative to know about
   the status of nursing in the host country.
3. Ensure that regulations for license or formal agreements with the host country are followed. Learn about the chief nurse officer in the host country.
4. Once in country, make every effort to make connections with the host country nursing
   association. Nurse partner guests can offer their expertise to build capacity for host
   country nurse partners, and vice versa.

When a guest nurse partner works collaboratively with nurses in the host country,
partnerships are built that can improve nursing education and practice, build capacity for
the nursing profession, and ensure sustainability to improve the health of populations. In
order to foster partnerships, working with government organizations such as a Ministry of
Health, the nursing council, and nursing associations in the host country is imperative. The
ICN can be a significant resource for nurses working across international borders.

REFERENCES

American Nurses Association. (2012). Roles of state boards of nursing: Licensure, regulation
and complaint investigation. http://nursingworld.org/MainMenuCategories/Tools/State-
Boards-of-Nursing- FAQ.pdf

American Nurses Association. (2013). About ANA. www.nursingworld.org/FunctionalMenu
Categories/AboutANA

Amieva S., & Ferguson, S. (2012). Moving forward: Nurses are key to achieving the United
Nations Development Program's Millennium Development Goals. *International Nursing
Review, 59,* 55–58.

Benton, D. (2012). Advocating globally to shape policy and strengthen nursing's influence.
OJIN: The Online Journal of Issues in Nursing, 17(1), Manuscript 5. doi: 10.3912/OJIN.
Vol17No01Man05

Bill & Melinda Gates Foundation. (2013). The Bill & Melinda Gates Foundation. www.gatesfoun-
dation.org

Bush, B. L., Lynaugh, J. E., Boschma, G., Rafferty, A. M., Stuart, M., & Tomes, N. J. (2001). Nurses
of all nations: A history of the International Council of Nurses 1899–1999. Philadelphia, PA:
Lippincott Publishing, Ltd.

Canadian International Development Agency. (2013). Foreign affairs, trade and development:
Canada. www.acdi-cida.gc.ca/home

Catholic Relief Services (CRS). (2013a). Mission statement: Health. www.catholicrelief.org/health

Catholic Relief Services (CRS). (2013b). www.catholicrelief.org/about/mission-statement

CDC. (2013). Ministry of Health partnerships. www.cdc.gov/globalaids/leverage-partnerships/ministry-of-health- partnerships.html

Center for Global Development (2013). Is Haiti doomed to be the Republic of NGOs? www.cgdev.org/blog/haiti-doomed-be-republic-ngos

Clinton Foundation. (2013). The Clinton Foundation. www.clintonfoundation.org.

Clinton Health Access Initiative. (2013). The Clinton Health Access Initiative. www.clinton-healthaccess.org

DANIDA. (2013). Udenrigsministeriet. Ministry of Foreign Affairs of Denmark. About DANIDA. http://um.dk/en/danida-en/about-danida

Davis, S. (2012). Why nurses are the unsung heroes of global health. www.huffingtonpost.com/sheila-davis-dnp-anpbc-faan/international-nurses- week_b_1499802.html?view=print&comm_ref=false

DeSantis, L. (1995). A model for counterparts in international nursing. *International Journal of Nursing Studies, 12*(2), 198–209.

Doyal, L. (2004). Gender and the 10/90 gap in health research. *Bulletin of the World Health Organization. 82*(3), 162.

Frenk, J., Chen, L, Bhutta, Z, Cohen, J., Crisp, N., Evans, T., . . . Zurayk, H. (2010). Health professionals for a new century: transforming education to strengthen health systems in an independent world. *The Lancet, 376*, 1923–1958.

George, E. K., & Meadows-Oliver, M. (2013). Searching for collaboration in international nursing partnerships: A literature review. *International Nursing Review, 60*(1), 31–36.

International Committee of the Red Cross. (2013). Health overview 29-10-2010. www.icrc.org/eng/what-we-do/health/health-overview.htm

International Council of Nurses. (2007). Vision for the future of nursing. Geneva, International Council of Nurses. www.icn.ch/about-icn/icns-vision-for-the-future-of-nursing

International Council of Nurses. (2013a). Position statements. Geneva, International Council of Nurses. http://www.icn.ch/images/stories/documents/publications/position_statements/B04_Nsg_Regulation.pdf

International Council of Nurses. (2013b). Leadership in negotiation. Geneva, International Council of Nurses. www.icn.ch/pillarsprograms/leadership-in-negotiation

International Council of Nurses. (2013c). Global nursing leadership institute. Geneva, International Council of Nurses. www.icn.ch/pillarsprograms/global-nursing-leadership-institute

International Council of Nurses. (2013d). Leadership for change. Geneva, International Council of Nurses. www.icn.ch/pillarsprograms/leadership-for-change

International Medical Volunteers Association. (2013). The major international health organizations. www.imva.org/Pages/orgfrm.htm.

Japanese Nursing Association. (2013). Nursing in Japan: History and system. https://www.nurse.or.jp/jna/english/nursing/system.html#history

Johnson, L. (2009). *The contributions of NGOs to health in the developing world.* Dissertation at University of Texas–Arlington.

Leffers, J., & Mitchell, E. (2011). Conceptual model for partnership and sustainability in global health. *Public Health Nursing, 28*(1), 91–102. doi: 10.1111/j.1525-1446.2010.00892.x

Levi, A. (2009). The ethics of nursing student international clinical experiences. *Journal of Obstetric, Gynecologic & Neonatal Nursing, 38*(1), 94–99. doi: 10.1111/j.1552-6909.2008.00314.x

Matthews, J. H. (2012). Role of professional organizations in advocating for the nursing profession. *Online Journal of Issues in Nursing, 17*(1).

Médecins Sans Frontières. (2013). www.msf.org/about-msf

National Council of Nurses and Midwives. (2013). http://ncnm.gov.rw/aboutus

National Council of State Boards of Nursing. (2013). https://www.ncsbn.org/181.htm

Partners in Health (PIH). (2013). Health is a human right. www.pih.org

Pfeiffer, J. (2003). International NGOs and primary health care in Mozambique: The need for a new model of collaboration. *Social Science Medicine, 56*(4), 725–738.

Pfeiffer, J. (2011). Strengthening the health system: The role of NGOs. GHD Online. www .ghdonline.org/strengthening-health- systems/discussion/panel-discussion

Project HOPE. (2013). Assets. www.projecthope.org/assets/documents/2012PHope-AR.pdf

Rockefeller Foundation. (2013). The Rockefeller Foundation. www.rockefellerfoundation.org

Ssewakiryanga, R. (2009). NGOs working to reduce poverty. *The Independent.* www.independent .co.ug/supplement/105-role-of-ngos-in-poverty-eradication-/1581-ngos-working-to-reduce-poverty

United Nations. (2013a). Millennium Development Goals: Background. www.un.org/ millenniumgoals/bkgd.shtml

United Nations. (2013b). UN at a glance. www.un.org/en/aboutun/index.shtml

United States Agency for International Development (USAID). (2013). What we do. www.usaid .gov/what-we-do

Veenema, T. G. (2012). *Disaster nursing and emergency preparedness: For chemical, biological, and radiological terrorism and other hazards* (3rd ed.). New York, NY: Springer Publishing.

World Bank. (2011). Healthy partnerships: How governments can engage the private sector to improve health in Africa. Washington, DC: World Bank. https://www .wbginvestmentclimate.org/advisory-services/health/upload/Healthy-Partnerships_Full-Rpt-bkmarks-2.pdf

World Health Organization. (2011). Strategic directions for strengthening nursing and midwifery services 2011–2015. Geneva, World Health Organization. www.who.int/hrh/resources/ nmsd/en/index.html

World Health Organization. (2013a). About WHO. www.who.int/about/en

World Health Organization. (2013b). The WHO agenda. www.who.int/about/agenda/en/index .html

Zuyderduin, A., Obuni, J. D., & McQuide, P. A. (2010). Strengthening the Uganda nurses' and midwives' association for a motivated workforce. *International Nursing Review, 57*(4), 419–425. doi: 10.1111/j.1466-7657.2010.00826.x. Epub 2010 September 14.

Collaboration With Rwanda After the 1994 Civil War

Julia Plotnick

CONTEXT: RWANDA

Rwanda, also known as the land of a thousand hills, is a landlocked country situated in central Africa The country lies 75 miles south of the equator in the Tropic of Capricorn, almost midway between the Indian Ocean and the Atlantic Ocean. Rwanda is bordered on the north by Uganda, on the east by Tanzania, on the south by Burundi, and on the west by the Democratic Republic of Congo. It is a land of volcanoes, lakes, and rivers, and home to an estimated 12 million people (Rwanda, 2013).

Rwanda was ruled by a series of Tutsi kings until becoming a colony of Belgium in 1899. During the independence movement that swept sub-Saharan Africa in the late 1950s, Rwanda's colonial government came under attack. Upheaval continued, leading to the 1994 civil war.

After the death of the presidents of Rwanda and Burundi in a suspicious plane crash on April 6, 1994, intense rioting erupted in Rwanda between the Hutu militia and Tutsi rebel forces. It is estimated that between April and July 1994, between 600,000 and 1 million unarmed men, women, and children were systematically massacred. When the new government was formed in July 1994, the country's infrastructure and public service system had been severely damaged and the fighting had brought the economy to a virtual standstill.

Many UN agencies, such as the World Health Organization (WHO), the United Nations Children's Fund (UNICEF), and the United Nations High Commission for Refugees (UNHCR), with support from the World Bank, helped the government reestablish the Ministry of Health. Priorities were to restore the water supply, control the spread of disease, and provide essential medications and medical services.

Thousands of Rwandans fled their country during the genocide. Almost 50,000 children who had been separated from their parents or orphaned were in camps in the neighboring country of Zaire, now the Democratic Republic of the Congo. UNICEF was staffing the children's camps with local women from Zaire.

MOBILIZATION OF NURSES FOR DISASTER RESPONSE

The U.S. Department of Health and Human Services received a request from UNICEF to detail pediatric nurse practitioners to Zaire to teach the new hires to care for the physical and emotional needs of the children. At this time I was chief nurse of the U.S. Public Health Service (USPHS). Dr. Donna Shalala, then secretary of Health and Human Services, requested my office to select 11 other pediatric nurse practitioners, a nutritionist, and a psychiatric nurse, all officers in the USPHS, and travel to Zaire for 6 weeks to provide this service under the auspices of UNICEF. Departing in late September 1994, our assignment was to train the local health workers to help with the care of the children who had been separated from their families and moved to Zaire. This team of nurse practitioners worked tirelessly to teach the care workers to provide physical and psychological care for severely traumatized children. Some of these camps had as many as 2,000 unaccompanied children. Simple protocols to address pediatric care were developed by these outstanding nurses that the caregivers could use to assist the most traumatized children.

While on assignment with this team, I was asked to travel to Kigali, the capital of Rwanda, to meet with the new director of the Ministry of Health to discuss with him how the United States could assist in re-establishing the health system after the civil war. According to the Rwanda Ministry of Health, at that time there were only 8 physicians and 32 nurses serving more than 6 million people.

BUILDING A PROGRAM FOR NURSING EDUCATION IN RWANDA

In February 1995, Dr. Joseph Karemera, minister of health in Rwanda, met with Dr. Shalala during his visit to Washington. Dr. Karamera requested that I return to Kigali to work with two nurses that he had hired at the ministry to assist them in developing a plan to re-establish community health services throughout the country. Dr. Shalala directed me, as chief nurse officer of the public health service, to assist the ministry in developing a training program for auxiliary health workers.

My assistant, Commander Mary Pat Couig, and I traveled to Kigali in February 1995. Our assignment was to assist the Rwandan Ministry of Health in developing a program to educate community health workers who would be assigned throughout the country. Priorities for health were to restore the water supply, provide essential medications, control the spread of communicable diseases, and provide some level of health care to the population. According to data presented by the U.S. Department of State fact sheet for 1994, health indicators at the time showed that three diseases/conditions caused 90% morbidity in the country—respiratory illness, diarrhea, and malaria. We had two wonderful Rwandan nurses to work with, one of whom is currently the chief nurse officer in Rwanda. They had been educated in Uganda and had been hired by the ministry. The four of us developed a proposal for a 12-week standardized curriculum for health auxiliaries. The program included teaching modules and educational materials for a 5-week training curriculum to specifically address the three priority problems of malaria, respiratory diseases, and diarrhea. In addition, the program was designed to meet the specific needs in Rwanda at that time. In addition to the standard content of anatomy, physiology, and pathophysiology, the Rwandan nurses sought to learn about ethics and other topics relevant to their practice. To be eligible, prospective trainees must have completed the primary level of education and have successfully completed an entry examination in their native language. Following the 5-week training, the health workers pass an examination. On successful completion of the course, the graduate would receive a certificate as a primary health care health auxiliary.

It was proposed that the course would be presented in five areas of the country, with 25 students in each class; the course would be presented four times so that in 1 year there would be 500 health auxiliary personnel working in all parts of the country. I proposed that the USPHS detail two nurses for assignment to the U.S. Agency for International Development (USAID). These nurses would then be assigned to the Rwandan Ministry of Health for 3 months. The USPHS nurses had expertise in education and training, community health, and public health nursing management. There were many nongovernmental agencies working in Rwanda, and many of their nurses collaborated on this program and taught at many of the programs throughout the country.

During the time I was assigned to Rwanda, I witnessed the leadership and commitment of the Rwandan nurses. Barely 1 year after the end of the Rwandan Civil War, in spring 1995, a proud group of nurses held a parade to celebrate Nurses' Day. The leadership for the nursing profession was remarkable and positioned them to rebuild the nursing workforce for Rwanda.

About 6 months later, I was invited to again travel to Rwanda for the graduation of the first class of health auxiliaries. With concerted effort from the Ministry of Health, many nongovernment agencies, the international organizations, and the USAID, the program was a rousing success.

MOVING FORWARD AFTER THE PARTNERSHIP ENDS

Although my formal partnership with the Rwandan nurses ended in 1996 with my third trip to Rwanda, I have maintained contact with nursing colleagues to the present day. In 1997, the International Council of Nurses met in Vancouver, Canada. I was invited to be the Florence Nightingale speaker. With funding from USAID and 3M Corporation, my two Rwandan nurse colleagues attended the meeting. In my presentation I was able to highlight the amazing accomplishments that they had achieved in their country in 3 short years. They received a well-deserved standing ovation.

I remained involved with my Rwandan colleagues and supported them with consultants and funding throughout the 1-year program. Over the past 19 years I have continued to support my Rwandan colleagues by e-mail and letters as they continue to develop the nursing and midwifery education programs in their country. Partnerships with professional nurse colleagues offers opportunities to assist them in their professional development and also bring the benefits of lifelong friendships once the formal partnership ends.

REFLECTIVE QUESTIONS

1. Why must nurses who serve during times of international disasters collaborate with sponsoring organizations?
2. Consider how you personally might respond to deployment to an assignment such as the one described here. What are the particular housing, food, water, sanitation, health, psychological, cultural, and language needs considered in settings such as Rwanda after a disaster?

REFERENCE

Rwanda. (2013). *Brief history of Rwanda.* Republic of Rwanda. www.gov.rw/History

Rwanda Human Resources for Health Program

Anne Sliney
Catherine Uwimana

"The Human Resources for Health Program will address the acute human resources shortage in Rwanda and allow the country to meet these challenges while advancing the Government of Rwanda's drive for sustainable and equitable economic development."

Agnes Binagwaho, Honorable Minister of Health, Rwanda, July 19, 2012, at the launch of the Human Resources for Health Program, Rwamagana School of Nursing and Midwifery

CONTEXT: RWANDA

Rwanda is a country located in central and east Africa that has contiguous borders with Tanzania, Uganda, Burundi, and the Democratic Republic of Congo. About the size of Maryland, it has a population of nearly 11 million people. It is the most densely populated country in sub-Saharan Africa.

In the past 30 years, Rwanda has suffered a civil war and a genocide in which up to 1 million lives were claimed. Many Rwandans were forced to flee the country to escape the violence and death surrounding them in the early 1990s. After the genocide, nearly 2 million people were left homeless and only 5% of the nation's people had access to clean water. The post-genocide years were marked by a severe shortage of professionals in all essential sectors, including education and health care.

Although the economy has made slow but steady progress, it is still highly dependent on subsistence agriculture. According to the World Bank, the GDP per capita in 2012 was $644.

In the early 1990s, Rwanda had the lowest life expectancy of any country in the world— 28 years. It currently stands at 56 years. Demonstrating a serious commitment to improved health care, Rwanda is one of the first countries in Africa to exceed the Abuja Declaration target of dedicating at least 15% of government spending to health, and is currently on track to achieve the health-related Millennium Development Goals (MDG) before 2015. Rwanda has significant accomplishments in major public health areas, including immunization rates of 93% coverage for nine vaccines, including 93.2% coverage of all three doses of HPV vaccine for eligible girls, over 80% of eligible patients receiving antiretroviral therapy, and 69% of women delivering in a health facility (National Institute of Statistics Rwanda, 2010). Figure 8.1 highlights other major public health accomplishments.

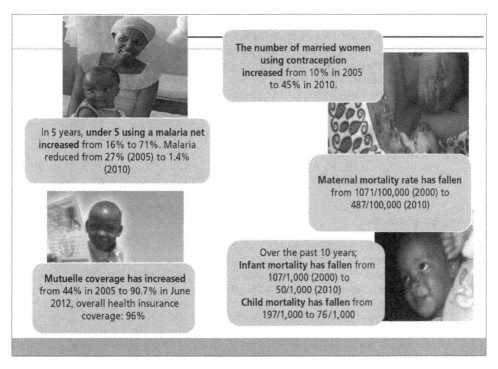

The number of married women using contraception increased from 10% in 2005 to 45% in 2010.

In 5 years, under 5 using a malaria net increased from 16% to 71%. Malaria reduced from 27% (2005) to 1.4% (2010)

Maternal mortality rate has fallen from 1071/100,000 (2000) to 487/100,000 (2010)

Mutuelle coverage has increased from 44% in 2005 to 90.7% in June 2012, overall health insurance coverage: 96%

Over the past 10 years; Infant mortality has fallen from 107/1,000 (2000) to 50/1,000 (2010) Child mortality has fallen from 197/1,000 to 76/1,000

FIGURE 8.1 Key Achivements in the Public Health Sector

Rwandan Health Care System

Rwanda has a decentralized model of health care delivery. There are 438 health centers, 44 district hospitals, and five referral hospitals, including one psychiatric hospital. Primary health care is delivered at the health center level, including prenatal care, vaginal deliveries, childhood immunizations, diagnosis and treatment of HIV and other infectious diseases, immediate management of acute illness and trauma, and referral to district hospitals for more complex care and/or surgery. These health centers are managed by nurses, most of whom are educated to an A2 or secondary school level. Rwanda has additionally mobilized a cadre of 45,000 community health workers who work within local sectors and in close conjunction with the health centers to monitor the health care of members of their community. Community health care workers provide the most fundamental primary care services, including malaria tests, malnutrition screening and support, and drug treatment adherence.

Rwanda has a national health insurance program called *Mutuelle de Sante*, which significantly increases access to health services for most Rwandans. Current coverage is at more than 90% of the population (Ministry of Health Rwanda, 2010).

In 2011, the Ministry of Health (MOH) developed a strategic plan for Human Resources for Health (HRH), 2011–2016. According to the executive summary,

> There is still much more work to be done to increase the quantity, quality, and overall management/coordination of HRH. There is a general shortage of health professionals, particularly amongst more highly skilled groups. As geographic distribution favors urban areas, there are still health facilities that are understaffed. There is a major shortage of midwives, exacerbating the high rate of maternal mortality. (Ministry of Health Rwanda, 2011, p. 5)

The total number of nurses at the time of this report was estimated to be 6,629. Prior to 2011, registration of nurses was not well organized, so numbers of nurses may not be entirely accurate. Of the 6,629 nurses, only 20 held a bachelor's degree or above. In fact, the overwhelming majority of nurses had a high school–level education or less (6,152). In 2011, there were only 240 professional midwives in the country. The ratio of nurses and midwives to population was determined to be 0.70 nurses or midwives per 1,000 people. The goal of the government of Rwanda, as articulated in the Vision 2020 document, which outlines an ambitious plan for establishing health and well-being in the country, sets a goal of two nurses/midwives per 1,000 people. The WHO has established guidelines for the ratio of health professionals (physicians, nurses, midwives) to population as 2.28. The plans for scaling up health profession education will position Rwanda well above this suggested minimum ratio (Ministry of Health Rwanda, 2011).

Nursing Education

Traditionally, nurses in Rwanda were educated while in secondary school in a vocational training–type program. These curricula were generally affiliated with either faith-based or government-supported programs. The graduates were designated as A2 or certificate-prepared nurses. In the late 1990s, Kigali Health Institute (KHI) developed a 3-year diploma in nursing (A1) and produced the first cadre of professional nurses, most of whom served as educators in the regional schools of nursing.

In 2005, the MOH made the decision to close all A2 nursing programs and set the 3-year diploma as the entry level for nursing practice. Over the next 2 years, all A2 programs were phased out, and five government-affiliated schools of nursing and midwifery (SNMW) were approved to educate nurses and midwives to the A1 level. These five schools share a common curriculum and issue what is called an "advanced diploma." Around this same time frame, KHI began the bachelor of science in general nursing (A0) program while continuing to educate midwives and mental health nurses at the diploma level.

The 3-year advanced diploma programs for generic students begin with general nursing for all students in year 1. In year 2, students choose between general nursing and midwifery. A2 nurses are given the opportunity to upgrade to A1 by enrolling in one of the schools of nursing and midwifery. They are given credit for year 1 and enter at year 2 in either nursing or midwifery.

Clinical education is a particular weakness of the Rwandan nursing education system, as is true for most programs in low-income countries that are transitioning from hospital-based nursing and midwifery programs to college-based programs. Although students have extensive clinical rotation hours (26 weeks in year 3), most of that experience is accomplished with the student acquiring any on-site teaching from mentors (staff nurses) within the clinical setting. Clinical instructors are responsible for up to 30 students at several sites, often geographically distant from each other, during a clinical rotation timeframe. Technically, the hospital nurses and midwives are supposed to teach the students, but this is often suboptimal due to staffing shortages, the hospital nurse being at a lower level than the student, or lack of confidence on the part of the hospital nurse or midwife in his or her ability to teach.

In 2012, the MOH instituted an e-learning program for A2 nurses to upgrade to A1 level while continuing to work in their health facilities. Nurses enrolled in the program access classroom training via the Internet and participate in 2-week face-to-face interactions with faculty at the schools three times each year while conventional students are at their clinical placements. The program takes 3 years to complete. The first class, which entered in January 2012, was made up of 300 students (mostly heads of health centers). The second class entered in January 2013, completing the enrollment of health center heads who want to upgrade. The next priority for enrollment was A2 nurses who are working in referral hospitals. In January 2015, the first class of e-learning graduates will graduate, and each subsequent year will be a big step toward professionalizing the nursing workforce.

The move to the advanced diploma as entry level for nursing and midwifery required educators who did not previously exist in Rwanda. In the early years, foreign faculty from Nigeria provided the teaching. KHI developed a 1-year program called bachelor's in nursing education to prepare advanced diploma nurses to become the faculty of the five schools. Ongoing efforts to strengthen the academic preparation of faculty members and to increase the number of qualified educators continue both through study abroad masters programs and in-country mentoring by U.S. institution faculty as part of the HRH program.

Throughout this evolution of nursing education there has been somewhat of a disconnect between the five public schools of nursing and midwifery (SNMWs) and KHI. The SNMWs have been governed by the Ministry of Health, and KHI has fallen under the authority of the ministry of education by design. In September 2013, all nursing and midwifery education will be organized within the new school of nursing (SON) within the college of medicine and health sciences at the newly established University of Rwanda. Along with this major reorganization of medical and nursing education will be a redesign of the role of teaching hospitals. Plans call for nursing and midwifery clinical faculty to be permanently assigned to the hospitals, thereby ensuring on-site teaching and supervision for all students.

DEVELOPMENT OF THE RWANDA HUMAN RESOURCES FOR HEALTH PROGRAM

As the HRH strategic plan was taking shape, the then permanent secretary of the MOH, Dr. Agnes Binagwaho, reached out to trusted development partners and advisors to explore the possibility of designing a radical and comprehensive approach to producing Rwandan health care professionals. She had a vision of how to get to the targets being set by the strategic plan. Her vision was to engage with U.S. universities to provide highly qualified and experienced medical, nursing, midwifery, health management, and dentistry educators to Rwandan teaching institutions.

Dr. Binagwaho, now Rwanda's minister of health, had many years of experience with how foreign aid was provided in the health sector, having previously been the director of the National AIDS Control Program. Her request to the U.S. government; the Global Fund for AIDS, Tuberculosis, and Malaria; and the U.S. universities was for a sustainable model of aid that would allow Rwanda to educate its own doctors, nurses, midwives, and health managers, who would then improve the quality of health services provided to all Rwandan citizens.

In March 2011, Dr. Binagwaho visited Boston, Massachusetts, to describe her vision to representatives of major U.S. schools of nursing, medicine, dentistry, and health management. This proposed program would require U.S. institutions to join a consortium in which all partners agreed to some unique and unconventional terms. The minister proposed that funding be provided directly to Rwanda's MOH and that institutions agree to work with no overhead and only a 7% administrative fee. She requested that each institution respond on its willingness and ability to join the consortium within 3 weeks.

In April of 2011, representatives of six U.S. schools of nursing joined their medical school colleagues at a meeting in Kigali to begin the process of collaboratively building the Rwanda HRH program for nurses and midwives. Those schools were the New York University College of Nursing, the University of Maryland School of Nursing, the Duke University School of Nursing, the Howard University School of Nursing, the University of Illinois at Chicago College of Nursing, and the University of Texas–Houston School of Nursing. Over 5 days of meetings with Rwandan nurse educators and leaders, the framework of a program was developed. Rwandan nurses and midwives described what their needs were and what their vision of nursing/midwifery education was. The two groups talked through the kind of faculty that should be recruited, the specific skills required, and where those faculty members should be assigned. In June 2011, a $152 million, 7-year proposal was developed and submitted to the U.S. government and the Global Fund for approval. Funding for the program's first 2 years was confirmed in February 2012. Figure 8.2 depicts the traditional model of foreign aid for health-related projects and the new model on which the HRH program is built.

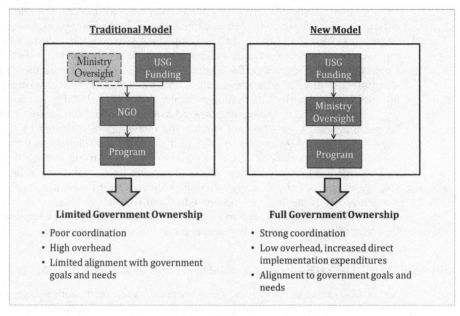

FIGURE 8.2 The HRH Program: A New Model for Foreign Aid

Design and Implementation of the Rwanda HRH Program

U.S. institutions have signed memoranda of understanding with the government of Rwanda. Funding goes directly from the U.S. government and Global Fund to the government of Rwanda. Governance of the HRH program lies with Rwandan health educators and officials. The nursing and midwifery subcommittee meets monthly to set policy, review candidates for faculty positions, and address challenges that arise. Only four U.S. institution representatives sit on the subcommittee as voting members, ensuring that the program is governed and implemented by Rwandan nurses and midwives. Figure 8.3 indicates the makeup of the Nursing and Midwifery Subcommittee.

In year 1, 32 U.S. nursing and midwifery faculty members were recruited and relocated to Rwanda. Faculty members are required to commit to a minimum of 1 year, except in rare instances when a nursing specialty is especially difficult to recruit. These are salaried positions with full benefits. Salaries are consistent across universities. Each faculty member also receives a housing allowance. Nursing and midwifery faculty have two levels of responsibility: educators, who serve as advisors at the highest levels, and clinical nurse mentors, who are primarily engaged in teaching students and staff in the clinical settings.

In year 1, funding was available for 42 nursing/midwifery faculty members, but due to delays in contracting, some of those positions were not filled. Thirty-two educators and mentors were deployed. Year 2, which began on August 1, 2013, includes 46 faculty members. During years 1, 2, and 3, faculty numbers will be approximately 40, gradually decreasing during years 4 to 7 as Rwandan faculty members' numbers and capacity increase (see Figure 8.4).

Recruitment

Rwandan nursing and midwifery educators indicated the need for experienced nurse educators to partner with the dean of the faculty of nursing sciences and the directors of the five SNMWs. They also requested an e-learning advisor, a simulation advisor, a

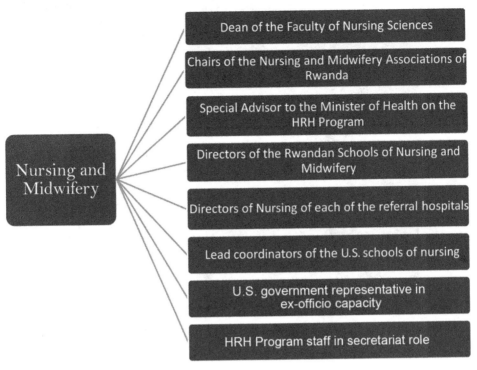

FIGURE 8.3 Nursing and Midwifery Subcommittee

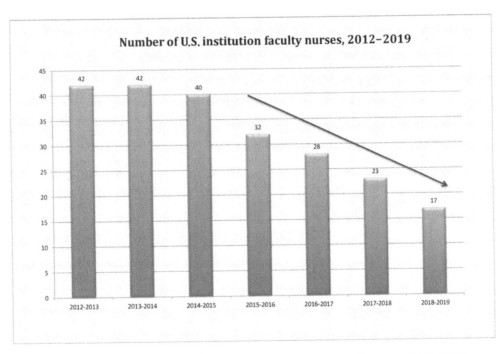

FIGURE 8.4 Scale-Up and Scale-Down Plan for U.S. Institution Program, 2012–2019: Nurses

Position Title	Year 1 2012–2013	Year 2 2013–2014
Mentors Adult Med Surg Mentor	X	X
Critical Care Mentor	X	X
Emergency / Trauma Mentor	X	X
Mental Health Mentor	X	
Midwifery Mentor	X	X
Neonatal Mentor	X	X
Neurosurgery Mentor		X
Pediatric Mentor	X	X
Perioperative Mentors	X	X
PICU Mentors	X	
Educators Advisor to the Director of the SNMW	X	X
Advisor to the Director of Nurses – Referral Hospital		X
Curriculum Advisor		X
E-Learning Advisor	X	
Infection Control Advisor	X	X
Partner to the Dean	X	X
Professional Standards Advisor	X	X

FIGURE 8.5 U.S. Institution Faculty Specialties (Nursing & Midwifery)
Source: Human resources for health program, Republic of Rwanda.

curriculum advisor, an infection control nurse educator, and a professional standards advisor. The U.S. SON were able to recruit highly qualified faculty members for these positions. They Rwandan nursing leadership also made specific requests for nurses/midwives with at least 3 years' clinical experience in a nursing specialty area. Some experience in teaching or mentoring is also required for these clinical nurse mentors (see Figure 8.5).

Each U.S. SON estimated the number of faculty members it could recruit and hire. Each school began by recruiting within its own faculty, alumni, and networks. They then reached out to professional organizations and listservs reaching nurses and midwives interested in global nursing. Many applicants came to the program through the HRH website and were referred to one of the U.S. SONs according to a set rotation. These six schools held a conference call every 2 weeks for more than a year to ensure that they were on track to recruit faculty with the appropriate qualifications. They exhibited a tremendous willingness to be collaborative. If one school found a highly qualified candidate for a position, the other schools were quick to agree to allow the first school to fill the position.

Once a candidate was thoroughly vetted by the specific U.S. SON and a decision made that he or she was a candidate that would be recommended, the candidate's CV and letter of recommendation were sent to the nursing and midwifery subcommittee in Rwanda. Each candidate was thoroughly reviewed at the monthly meeting, and decisions were made on whether the candidate would be sent on to the minister of health for final approval. On several occasions, candidates that were recommended by the U.S. school failed to gain approval by the subcommittee—the policy put the control over the program squarely in the hands of the Rwandan nursing leadership. Carefully developed relationships and constant communication, plus mutually agreed-on principles of Rwandan ownership of the program, led to a trusting relationship between the U.S. university coordinators and the subcommittee members.

All U.S. faculty members are required to be licensed to practice nursing or midwifery in Rwanda. They submit their applications and supporting documents to the National Council of Nurses and Midwives before beginning work. Although they are licensed, direct patient care is only provided in the context of teaching.

Midway through year 1, it became apparent that there were many issues in the teaching hospitals that were impacting the ability of the clinical nurse mentors to teach students or staff nurses. The honorable minister requested that nurses with management experience be recruited to partner with the directors of nursing of the four referral hospitals. A request was made from the surgical faculty to recruit experienced OR nurse educators, and the neurosurgeons requested a neurosurgery nurse mentor. The U.S. SONs were able to recruit highly qualified nurses for each of these positions for year 2.

Role of U.S. Institution Faculty

Each U.S. faculty member is "twinned" to one or more Rwandan nurses or midwives. For the educators, their twin is an obvious individual who is in a unique leadership position at one of the SNMWs. The professional standards advisor is partnered with the registrar of the National Council of Nurses and Midwives. The simulation advisor is partnered with the skills lab coordinators at each SNMW. The e-learning advisor is partnered with the e-learning coordinator in the Ministry of Health.

The position of advisor to the director of the SNMW (six individuals) had the following job description:

- Working with the director and faculty members to improve teaching techniques, integrate simulation into the curriculum, and address all other aspects of the functioning of the school
- Working with faculty at an SNMW, as well as the clinical mentors at the partner institutions where students have clinical placements, to ensure integration of theory into clinical instruction
- Working collaboratively to develop management and leadership courses
- Mentoring nursing faculty in the development and implementation of research projects
- Providing lectures in faculty area of expertise
- Participating in national meetings related to nursing and midwifery education and curriculum development as requested

In year 1, the clinical nurse mentors were assigned to teaching hospitals—both referral hospitals and district hospitals attached to SNMWs. They provided bedside teaching, continuing professional development courses, and education and supervision of students. Their job description included:

- Modeling the knowledge, skills, and attitudes relevant to the clinical nurse mentor role within the area of nursing/midwifery practice
- Serving as part of the professional development team at the clinical teaching sites
- Providing continuing education collaboratively with Rwandan colleagues to the current nursing and midwifery staff
- Working with physician mentors, as applicable, to foster integrated education of medical, nursing, and midwifery students and medical residents
- Serving as a resource for SNMW by providing lectures, faculty development programs, and advice on curriculum development in specialty areas
- Performing needs assessment of current nursing and midwifery staff practices and collaborating with unit leaders to implement changes in practice to reflect evidence-based care

- Providing teaching and supervision of students in the mentor's nursing specialty as well as in one of the following areas: general nursing, general pediatrics, or midwifery
- Collaborating with and mentoring clinical instructors from KHI and the schools of nursing and midwifery in order to ensure a positive clinical experience for students

Twinning Model

Rwandan nurses and midwives were chosen by their director of nurses to "twin" with U.S. institution faculty. These were staff nurses working in the specialty area of the U.S. faculty member. Many of these twinning relationships were mutually satisfying and resulted in improved nursing practice on the wards. Each U.S. faculty member tried to assess the needs of his or her twin and the unit and teach according to the priority needs. This resulted in some exceptional projects being implemented in referral hospitals and district hospitals alike. There certainly were challenges—language barriers, mismatch of interests, and nurses with little time to engage in the twinning relationship. It became apparent that the twinning model, while having a significant impact on individual nurses, was not accomplishing the primary goals of the program to do the following:

- Develop the clinical, teaching, and research skills of current and future nursing and midwifery faculty
- Improve the quality of nursing and midwifery education at clinical sites

These concerns were shared by both the Rwandan nursing leadership and the U.S. faculty. The subcommittee discussed these concerns and made significant adjustments to the model for year 2. In year 2, twins were selected using new criteria. A twin should be a nurse or midwife who

- Is A1 or above
- Speaks English
- Volunteers to participate
- Is in a position to effect change in the clinical setting

Clear expectations were established that U.S. clinical nurse mentors should spend 70% of their time focusing on students or faculty and 30% of their time on hospital nurses. This readjustment of the role of the clinical nurse mentors was a wonderful example of collaboration and compromise among all the nursing and midwifery stakeholders.

SUCCESSFUL PARTNERSHIPS FOR NURSING EDUCATION AND PRACTICE IN RWANDA

In order to make a complex program like this work and stay true to the principles of country ownership, the partnerships must be strong and mutually beneficial. The success of one partner depends on the success of the other. Each must deliver on what it has promised. This program has several layers of partnerships.

Ministry of Health and U.S. Institutions

The memorandum of understanding between the MOH and each U.S. institution laid out the legal obligations for each of the parties. This is standard practice. The difference in this program is that the MOH is the party contracting with the U.S. institutions, not the the U.S. government or Global Fund. The U.S. institutions are acknowledging that they work for the government of Rwanda. The government of Rwanda is taking full responsibility for the success or failure of the program, since it is reporting to the donors directly. The U.S.

institutions agree to 7% administrative costs, to the Rwandans having the final say in hiring faculty, and to taking direction from the professional subcommittees. These are unique and bold steps by both parties.

U.S. Schools of Nursing With Each Other

The six SONs in the consortium worked collaboratively every step of the way. They were honored to be included in the first year of the program and understand that the success of this program may determine what other funding becomes available for nursing and midwifery education. They appreciated the value of finding the very best nurse educators regardless of which school hired them.

U.S. Schools of Nursing With Rwandan Nursing Leadership

The honorable minister of health pushed for nursing and midwifery to have equal importance to medical education in this program. Indeed, half the U.S. faculty members are nurses or midwives. The Rwandan nursing leadership was clear in its assessment of its strengths and weaknesses. They communicated clearly to the U.S. SONs what they needed and wanted from them. U.S. SONs respected these requests and recruited accordingly. University coordinators offered insights and suggestions to their Rwandan colleagues, which were carefully considered in-country.

U.S. Institution Faculty With Their Rwandan Twins

The U.S. nursing and midwifery faculty formed extraordinary partnerships with their Rwandan counterparts. The assignments lasted for 12 months, giving them time to develop trust and an appreciation of each other's strengths. The clear message that the HRH faculty members were advisors—that they were not in country to develop their own program but rather to carry out a mandate from the MOH—helped enormously to keep everyone focused on the goals of the program. Each U.S. faculty member reported to the director of nurses within her or his hospital or school. Rwandan nurses, who were used to groups coming in and out to do brief visits, teaching whatever the group thought was appropriate, came to realize that these HRH faculty were actually there to stay, and that they worked for the MOH just as the Rwandan nurses did.

CONCLUSION

These multiple layers of partnership have worked extremely well. The common thread is that there is respect for the country ownership. There is acknowledgment that all faculty members are working for the MOH, there is genuine respect for the knowledge, skills, and experience of Rwandan colleagues, and there is a sense of control that the Rwandans have over a global health program that they have never had in the past.

REFLECTIVE QUESTIONS

1. How has the Rwanda HRH program developed a model for sustainable partnerships? Are there strategies that they have used that you can employ in your own global health work?
2. Collaboration with global health organizations and with professional nursing organizations is evident in all phases of the program. Identify ways in which this collaboration has contributed to the success of the program thus far.

REFERENCES

Ministry of Health Rwanda. (2010). Rwanda community-based health insurance policy. http://moh.gov.rw/english/wp-content/uploads/2012/05/Mutual_policy_document_final1.pdf

Ministry of Health Rwanda. (2011). Human Resources for Health Strategic Plan 2011–2016.

National Institute of Statistics Rwanda. (2005). Macro international. Rwanda demographic and health survey. http://measuredhs.com/what-we-do-survey/survey-display-252cfm

National Institute of Statistics Rwanda. (2010). Macro international. Rwanda demographic and health survey. http://measuredhs.com/what-we-do-survey/survey-display-364cfm

Promoting the Profession of Nursing Through Collaboration With Nursing Organizations in Romania

Julia Plotnick

Consultation is frequently time-limited, with specific objectives or terms of reference. In contrast, my involvement with Romania, through my work with orphans, the health care system, nursing education, professional development, and organizational development, lasted for more than 12 years and involved many individuals and organizations. This case study highlights the importance of working with organizations, particularly nursing organizations, to advance nursing education and practice. The best example of nursing collaboration is that of nurse partnerships with host country nursing associations. However, in many low- and middle-income countries (LMICs), nursing associations are not well established or are still becoming fully operational.

CONTEXT: ROMANIA

Romania is located between central and southeastern Europe on the Black Sea, sharing borders with Hungary, Serbia, Ukraine, Moldova, and Bulgaria. Coming under military dictatorship during World War II, Romania became a people's republic from 1947 to 1965 (Gulie, 2011). At that time, Nicolae Ceausescu took leadership and created the Socialist Republic of Romania in 1965.

Romania remained under communism until the Romanian Revolution of 1989. After the revolution, the world became aware of the disastrous crisis in Romania of an estimated 200,000 children who were living in orphanages where the care was inadequate and conditions deplorable. This situation was the direct result of the dictator Ceausescu's decree that all women bear at least five children in order to increase the future workforce. Due to the health care issues of the mothers themselves and the financial burden resulting from this policy, large numbers of sick, small, and disabled children were placed in orphanages (Paton & Purvis, 1995).

Prior to the suppression of nursing in 1978 by Ceausescu, Romanian nurses had been members of the International Council of Nurses (ICN) beginning in 1937 and were organized professionally. Three-year diploma schools were opened in Romania as early as 1919. Ceausescu closed all the nursing schools and eliminated the position of nursing across Romania. The former nurses were no longer part of the health care system and were placed as medical assistants to the physicians. Former nurses were required to serve in orphanages or go to jail.

INITIAL CONSULTATION TO ROMANIA

In 1990, my initial assignment from the secretary of Health and Human Services was to go to Romania for several months and assess the situation of the orphaned children. There had been very disturbing exposés on television, some taken with hidden cameras, of the situation in the orphanages throughout Romania.

Hundreds of governmental, nongovernmental, and volunteer organizations, as well as well-intended individuals, flooded into the country, some to adopt orphans, some to provide care to them, and others to deliver supplies and medicines. This was allowed by the Romanian government without an organized structure in place.

I was selected for this assignment for several reasons. During my career in the USPHS, I developed a strong background in public health and maternal and child health, as well as working as a pediatric nurse practitioner. I had worked with disabled children in various assignments in the United States. Also dealing with a previous foreign assignment during the famine crisis in Sudan and health issues on the U.S.–Mexican border prepared me for this consultation.

I was seconded to the World Health Organization, European Office, in Copenhagen under directions from the U.S. Department of Health and Human Services (USDHHS) with directions to assess the situation and report how the United States could be of help. During my 5-month stay it became evident that the situation in the orphanages was just one of many issues that related to health in Romania (Vladescu, Scintee, & Olsavszky, 2008). Of particular importance to me as a nurse was the state of nursing practice in Romania. The government had cancelled nursing education in 1976, and "medical assistants," as nurses were called at that time, had 2 years of health education in high school. They were then assigned to hospitals and were considered helpers to the doctors. Their education consisted of learning by observation.

I worked at the Romanian Ministry of Health, Department of Maternal and Child Health. Initially my colleagues at the ministry were very suspicious of me, because most of them had never had dealings with a foreigner. Winning their trust and trying to identify a process for assessment and planning took considerable time. I did identify a strong nurse leader, Gabriela Bocec. She had been educated in the traditional post-basic program before 1976, had experience with the Rockefeller Foundation, and understood and firmly believed in nursing education that built upon the theoretical perspective of American nurse leader Virginia Henderson. It was clear to me, almost from the very beginning of my assignment, that to improve the orphanage situation, the provision of health care for the entire population needed to be addressed.

COLLABORATING ORGANIZATIONS

During this initial assignment, a team from the World Bank visited Romania several times. Its purpose was to negotiate a loan to the government of Romania for the improvement of health care to the population. As a consultant who had been in country for about 2 months, I saw this as an opportunity to influence the government to include basic nursing education in its proposal to the World Bank. Gabriela and I met with the parliament to create a proposal for the development of basic nursing education programs in each judet (county). The World Bank approved a multimillion-dollar loan to build the health workforce in Romania, with a significant portion directed to nursing education.

The next task was the development of a curriculum for these new schools of nursing. WHO–Copenhagen suggested that the Danish nursing education system would be the most accepted model by Romania and identified two Danish nurse consultants who were funded by the World Bank loan for an 18-month assignment to Bucharest to develop a 30-month curriculum that would be used throughout Romania. Gabriela, through her network, was able to identify some Romanian nurses educated before 1976 to assist in the curriculum development and begin the first programs of post–high school nursing education.

Another issue that needed immediate attention was to provide some continuing education for the current nurses working in hospitals and clinics throughout Romania. The individuals currently working as medical assistants had only minimal training at the high school level. It was imperative that education programs for these caregivers, which we called "bridging courses," be developed at the same time as the new nursing schools were being created. President George H.W. Bush had instituted his "Points of Light" program in the United States during his presidency. Humana Health Care System and Baylor University chose Romania's health care system as their contribution to this Points of Light program. The Romanian Assistance Project was created to serve as a humanitarian effort to help the people of Romania in meeting the country's health care needs. The project offered training programs for Romanian medical professionals and donated equipment, supplies, and technical literature.

During the initial assessment to determine how contributions could be made, one of the Baylor representatives was a nurse administrator, William Denton. The Romanian Ministry of Health referred him to me. Together we devised a program for a group of Romanian nurses to travel to the United States for several months to prepare them to teach in the continuing education programs. Gabriela was responsible for the selection of this initial group of eight nurses. The group of eight Romanian nurses traveled to Baylor University in Dallas, Texas, for a 7-month course in community health nursing, psychiatric/mental health nursing, nursing management, how to develop programs, teaching/learning techniques, and nursing leadership. When the Romanian nurses had returned home, a team from Baylor traveled to Romania to continue the collaborative educational program (Garner & Bufton, 2001).

WHO and UNICEF were two organizations that worked with me to strengthen nursing education throughout the country. Because of their vast experience, they were able to build on existing structures within the country and to encompass the new strategies of nursing programs.

By this time I had completed my initial on-site assignment and had returned to my USPHS position with the USDHHS as deputy director of the children with special needs department. The Romanian Ministry of Health continued to refer individuals and organizations to me for consultation on their programs in Romania. A sense of trust and overall confidence had been built during my initial assignment so that they felt that my advice would be beneficial to their programs and the health needs of the population.

ONGOING CONSULTATION WITH ROMANIA

Many times during the following 6 years, while I was still on active duty with the USPHS, I was requested by international organizations to travel to Romania to assist with issues affecting nurses and nursing programs.

On my retirement from the USPHS in 1996, the Baylor program invited me to be a consultant to their team to continue the project of both basic nursing education as well as continuing nursing education in Romania. It was decided that if the Romanian government was to take responsibility for its nursing programs, a "stakeholders forum" should be held. The purpose of this forum, jointly sponsored by Humana and Baylor, was to provide focus for a recent upsurge of interest in nursing education, regulation, and practice by government and nongovernmental groups in Romania. A basic premise of consultation is to involve the client as much as possible. Approximately 50 people were invited from universities, ministries, the WHO and UNICEF, and Baylor and Humana, as well as politicians.

The meeting objectives were as follows:

- Discuss the current status of nursing and allied health professionals in Romania
- Identify global nursing standards governing nursing education, regulation, and practice
- Explore pathways for nursing in education, practice, and regulation
- Develop a strategic plan
- Create an implementation plan

One tangible outcome of this collaborative forum was action to support the proposal to develop a university program for the education of nurses at Cluj in Transylvania. This was a challenge for all of us who had been involved with nursing, due to the severe shortage of potential well-educated nursing faculty. There were very few nurses who had any university degrees, so no nurses were identified who could teach in a university system. Several U.S. nurse educators were invited to consult with the university. This was also funded by Baylor.

While this potential university educational program was investigated, Baylor and Humana agreed to provide continuing education for practicing nurses. Nurses were sent to Romania several times a year for about 5 years to provide continuing education in operating room techniques, neonatal care, and general nursing care. These programs were very well received and well attended. A continuing education center was established in Bucharest. This entire project was funded by the Health Care Leadership Council, a collaboration between Humana and Baylor. It included a computer laboratory and employed a computer technician to introduce the students to computer technology.

It became obvious that some regulation of the practice of nursing was essential for the safety of the population. The ICN was identified as the appropriate group to provide this information and guidance. Again, funding from the Baylor project paid for the consultant from ICN to provide this information on licensure and credentialing. There was resistance to licensure mainly from the trade unions. Every employed individual had to pay dues to the union. There was considerable concern that licensure would allow nurses to opt out of union membership. Again, I was asked to assist in mediating this issue. This required several visits and discussions at the government level.

As nursing grew as a profession, Gabriela, Bill Denton, and I realized that one more thing was needed to improve the image of nursing as well as to bolster the confidence of the practicing nurses: a professional association. Many national associations offered to assist in this project, including the Danish Nurses Association; the Royal College of Nursing, UK; the American Nurses Association; and the ICN. Gabriela was invited to attend a 2-week program on professional association development held in the United States in New Jersey. Although it was a short, intensive course, Gabriela felt empowered to begin the process in Romania. I invited the executive director of the New Jersey Nurses Association to act as a consultant to Gabriela and the association board. We traveled to Bucharest several times as the association took small steps to become the premier nurses association in Romania. The first national conference for nurses was held in 1996 and was a great success. I was able to attend with Bill Denton and several nurses who had consulted over the years. Its success proved a psychological boost for the Romanian attendees. This was the first time many of them had ever had an opportunity to present to their colleagues.

The Baylor project assisted Gabriela to publish a quarterly journal. Contributions to the journal were provided by consultants that had served in Romania as well as by Romanian nurses who had been educated before 1976. As the schools of nursing began to graduate its first classes, the faculty and new nurses were anxious to be published. The journal also provided valuable information about the health care system as it was evolving in Romania.

In 1997, the Romanian Nurses Association—Asociatia de Nursing din Romania—was formally accepted into the ICN. This was a crowning achievement for the nurses who had struggled so hard to be recognized professionally in their own country.

CONCLUSION

From 1998 to 2002, I continued to provide assistance to the nurses, sometimes visiting the country and through letters and more and more through e-mail correspondence. These were not formal consultations, but rather informal advice on nursing education and practice issues. To this day, I correspond with the current executive director of the association.

It has been a long and rewarding relationship over the past 12 years, starting with a consultation assignment of 5 months in 1990, which led to a lasting professional and personal relationship, as well as an example of partnership across organizations worldwide.

REFLECTIVE QUESTIONS

1. Think about the professional nursing organizations that you belong to. How are you involved, actively or sporadically?
2. Do organizations to which you belong have a role in global health? Do they have a special-interest group or international collaboration?
3. Identify specific ways that your organization can collaborate with nursing organizations in other countries as the New Jersey Nurses Association did.

REFERENCES

Garner, L. F., & Bufton, K. A. (2001). History of nursing at the Baylor University Medical Center. Proceedings of the Baylor University Medical Center, *14*(4), 385–405. www.ncbi.nlm.nih.gov/pmc/articles/PMC1305904

Gulie, E. (2011). The history of nursing in Romania. *Nursing History Review, 19*, 175–178.

Paton, D., & Purvis, C. (1995). Nursing in the aftermath of disaster: Orphanage relief work in Romania. *Disaster Prevention and Management, 4*(1), 45–54.

Vladescu, C., Scintee, G., & Olsavszky, V. (2008). Health systems in transition. *Romania Health System Review, 10*(3). http://www.euro.who.int/__data/assets/pdf_file/0008/95165/E91689.pdf

CHAPTER 9

Making Collaborative Research Work

Linda Ciofu Baumann

The health challenges and disparities faced by developing nations of the world have increased attention to the need for more global nursing research. Contemporary global health is guided by the ethical principles of respect for persons, beneficence, and social justice. These principles are vital to the conduct of nursing research for it to contribute to an evidence-based model needed to guide practice, research, and policy development. This chapter reviews contextual factors that influence global nursing research, models used to guide the development of sustainable partnerships, ethical issues of global nursing research, and research methods appropriate for global settings. Finally, community-based participatory research (CBPR) is reviewed as an approach to engage communities and address global health challenges.

Historically much of the international research conducted by U.S. researchers has involved collection of data and conduct of clinical trials in another setting. In many low- and middle-income countries there is a long history of the west or north exploiting entire populations with colonization, racism, and extreme economic inequities. In this context, the research administrative structure often inhibited the development of partnerships that were truly collaborative. However, to achieve dissemination and application of research evidence to address real issues, global nursing research must be based on equitable partnerships. These partnerships can be among academic institutions, government agencies and ministries, and civil society organizations (CSOs) that aim to further the interests of the communities they serve and include community-based, faith-based, and nongovernmental organizations (Bhan, Singh, Upshur, Singer, & Daar, 2007; Oldenberg, 2012).

The process of engagement and partnerships must precede planning and intervention to create sustainable partnerships (Leffers & Mitchell, 2010), since community participation is a requisite for conducting health research. Time spent assessing setting-specific health priorities, beliefs, and health systems will help to divert precious resources and time if not addressed (Baumann, 2011).

CULTURAL AND ENVIRONMENTAL CONTEXT

A prominent cultural difference between the United States and other societies is the high value placed on individualism. In contrast, most other countries have more collective societies characterized by shared responsibility for community and family members (Epping-Jordan, 2004; Landrine & Klonoff, 2001). Although some level of cultural awareness or competence is requisite for conducting global research, a spirit of cultural humility may help to bridge the power and resource disparities that may exist between partnerships whose members are from developed and developing countries. Cultural humility incorporates a lifelong commitment to self-evaluation and self-critique, to redressing the power imbalances in cross-cultural relationships, and to developing mutually beneficial and non-paternalistic partnerships with communities on behalf of individuals and defined populations (Tervalon & Murray-Garcia, 1998).

Environmental assessment of the local physical, health care system, and political context assessment is a practical approach to conducting international nursing research and involves visiting a site before beginning a project (Ketefian, 2000; Leffers & Mitchell, 2010; NLN, 2012). This approach may be seem obvious, but international travel is costly and scouting or meet-and-greet visits are often not covered in research grants. To make the most of this initial visit, visitors need to be prepared. Many websites provide profiles of a country that include descriptions of the physical, socioeconomic, political, and health indicators. The Internet can be used to exchange written documents that briefly identify who is involved and the purpose of a visit.

Skilled research personnel, available technology, library, and institutional resources can present challenges in global nursing research. The Health InterNetwork Access to Research Initiative (HINARI) is a significant resource for public institutions from low-income countries that provides access to health and social science journals free or at very low cost. It is used extensively in Bhutan and by other members of the World Health Organization (WHO) South-East Asian Regional Office (SEARO) (Glover et al., 2004). Research projects that require skilled full-time workers might need to recruit them from public or governmental sectors, contributing to an internal brain drain and weakening public service sectors (Parry, 2000). This issue is especially acute in countries with severe shortages of health care workers, where up to half of available positions in the public sector remained unfilled.

In many developing regions nurses are not recognized as researchers. There is often a social stigma to nursing as a vocation, and although the work that nurses do is respected, it is not viewed as a profession. In addition, women as leaders in a research project may not fit the traditional gender roles in some settings. Finally, the role of nurses in global health research is often not recognized or acknowledged, yet they have had a major role globally in establishing new models for delivering health care. The President's Emergency Plan for AIDS Relief (PEPFAR), for example, has adopted a strategy of task shifting, or giving nurses more advanced roles in patient management (McCarthy et al., 2013).

Level of Poverty

Large economic disparities between researchers from a high-income country doing work in a low- or middle-income country often raise the issue of coercive incentives. However, poor participants need money for transport and food. In our study in Uganda (Fisher et al., 2010), the average distance to the diabetes clinic from home was 11 kilometers, a distance many probably walked. Incentives can drive participation. We paid each participant about US$5 to attend a community meeting, even though some participants were closer and would not use the entire amount for transport. Ugandans on our research team thought this might appear that some profited more from participation. We provided everyone a meal because we knew that in this setting many adults with type 2 diabetes do not eat regularly throughout the day and the risk of hypoglycemia on the journey home could be life-threatening. In our first community meeting we recruited fewer participants than we had hoped because of a road rally that disrupted transportation that day. However, at our second community meeting, once the word was out that transport money, food, and a cell phone would be provided, we had 46 potential partners arrive when we only wanted to recruit 30. We did not over-enroll into the study because of resources, but allowed those who showed up to sit in on the program.

Language

Language can be a complex issue in countries where multiple tribal or local languages are used despite English being the official language. In south-central Uganda, the predominant languages are Luganda and Acholi, so even bilingual written materials in English and Luganda did not reach everyone. The multiple regional languages used in many African countries present challenges for ministries of health in developing any written public health materials. Even written materials that match the language of most participants do not address the low literacy level of many rural residents or account for poor eyesight and lack of corrective lenses that may prevent someone from reading any printed document. Language and literacy differences in the meanings and understandings of words pose challenges for developing written instruments and ensuring that the same meaning is translated. These issues can be partially addressed by using local workers; explaining the study in written, pictorial, and verbal modes, since some cultures rely on oral communication; and piloting instruments and procedures.

MODELS TO GUIDE PARTNERSHIPS

Global nurse leaders have developed models for developing transformative and sustainable partnership for global nursing practice, education, and research. Leffers and Mitchell (2010) used a grounded theory methodology in interviews with global health nursing experts and captured the following themes that guide global health nursing: engagement, cultural bridging, collaboration, capacity building, and mutual goal setting.

Powell and colleagues (Powell, Gilliss, Hewitt, & Flint, 2010) use a consensus community engagement model as a framework for conducting nursing research in low-resource settings globally: inform, consult, involve, collaborate, and empower.

Differences in the state of nursing education and delivery systems in a country can affect the availability of nurses prepared to conduct research (Uys & Klopper, 2013). Research is required in most undergraduate nursing curricula, but students may have minimal research training and work with faculty who are often overburdened to be able to produce well-designed research and disseminate results through publications. Increasing requirements for nursing faculty in baccalaureate programs to have doctorates require that faculty find support from international partners to receive doctoral training abroad. This may involve leaving the faculty temporarily, creating further shortages in country, and obtaining this education abroad for 2 or 3 years.

ETHICAL ISSUES

A fundamental principle of conducting global health research in low-resource countries is that the health issue being studied must be relevant to the needs and issues in that country. Historically, research has been conducted in low-resource settings because of easy access to subjects and fewer restrictions in research conduct and administration. Several organizations have proposed ethical guidelines for conducting international research.

The Working Group for the Study of Ethical Issues (2003) specified three criteria for ethical conduct of international nursing research: (1) there must be a mechanism for input from local communities about the research methods, purpose, and goals; (2) the design must generate knowledge that can potentially benefit the community from which participants are recruited; and (3) it must provide ethical justification for selecting the population from which participants are recruited.

Ethical guidelines for conducting international biomedical research involving human subjects have been published by the Council for International Organizations of Medical Sciences (CIOMS) (www.cioms.sch/frame_guidelines). The council presents 21 guidelines with commentary that are designed to be of use to countries in defining national policies on the ethics of biomedical research, applying ethical standards in local circumstances, and establishing or improving the ethical review mechanisms. A particular aim is to reflect the conditions and the needs of low-resources countries, as well as the implication for multinational or transnational research in which they may be partners.

Recognizing the growth of international research, the Office for Human Research Protections (OHRP) has developed an International Compilation of Human Subject Research Protections for research sponsored by the U.S. Department of Health and Human Services (USDHHS). The compilation lists the laws, regulations, and guidelines of over 50 countries where USDHHS-funded or USDHHS-supported research has been conducted (www.hhs.gov/ohrp/international/index.html#NatlPol).

Federal regulation *Title 45, Code of Federal Regulations, Part 46* requires that all institutions receiving federal funds that conduct research using living humans as subjects establish and operate an institutional review board (IRB). The purpose of the IRB is to ensure the protection of these human subjects. To comply with this federal regulation, all key research personnel must participate in the collaborative institutional training initiative (CITI) in the ethical conduct of research. Since academic health science centers in the United States are guided by these policies, all research that is reviewed must satisfy this requirement. CITI training can be completed online or in a printed form and provides a standardized education in the ethical conduct of research.

The approaches described above prominently reflect the traditional ethical standard of research to populations in developing countries. It assumes ethical principles are universal and not culturally bound. However, even the concept of informed consent may have different meanings and applicability in cultures and contexts where females have fewer rights, paternalistic health care systems are not patient-centered, or access to therapy that meets standards of care is only available through participation in a clinical trial (Kent, Mwamburi, Bennish, Kupelnick, & Ioannidis, 2004). Ethical multiculturalism is a perspective that protects the peculiarities of different cultures and can be promoted in the conduct of global nursing research (Crigger, Holcomb, & Weiss, 2001).

ISSUES IN THE CONDUCT OF RESEARCH

A useful model for establishing and sustaining global research partnerships was developed by Maselli and colleagues (Maselli, Lys, & Schmid, 2006) and is based on 11 key principles that are particularly relevant to the African context (see Table 9.1). Using these principles, de-Graft and colleagues (de-Graft Aikins et al., 2012) monitored both barriers and enabling factors in a case study of a UK–Africa research partnership on chronic disease. They identified five critical ingredients needed to sustain a research partnership: (1) social capital, or shared understandings, values, and links that engender trust and collaboration, (2) measurable goals that can be used to track progress and maintain transparency to all partners, (3) administrative support, (4) creative and innovative strategies, and (5) funding, especially in moving from small-scale to large-scale research projects. Other aspects of conducting research in global settings include the following.

Institutional Review Board Approval

IRB approval for international studies is required from all members of a partnership. A list of the appropriate review boards that grant approval for biomedical research from a country or institution within the country can be obtained online. However, sometimes this information is outdated, and consulting with local researchers is critical. Most IRBs require a small fee to review any potential project.

Recruitment/Informed Consent

Research conducted in developing countries often recruit poor people. There is debate over incentives for engaging poor subjects in research, arguing that the compensation is so great

TABLE 9.1 Criteria for Developing Successful Communities of Research Excellence

 1. Set agenda together
 2. Interact with stakeholders
 3. Clarify responsibilities
 4. Account to beneficiaries
 5. Promote mutual learning
 6. Enhance capacities
 7. Share data & networks
 8. Disseminate results
 9. Pool profits & merits
10. Apply results
11. Secure outcomes

Source: Stockli, Weismann, and Lys (2012).

that it is a form of coercion. However, the level of poverty is so great that few potential participants can participate in a study without being reimbursed for a phone call, travel, or a meal. The need for this compensation can also apply to research personnel.

Gaining access to the participants in some communities may require permission from local authorities such as a village chief and/or village elders. These individuals act as gatekeepers between the researcher and community members, and although some researchers may feel this is a limitation to the research, in reality it may promote stronger communication between the researcher and the community participants (Tindana et al., 2011).

Data Management

Continued data monitoring for adherence to informed consent procedures and mortality or serious morbidity and safety is required. This should be done at regular intervals throughout the research project. Data that are collected using paper and pencil instruments need to be converted to an electronic database that conforms with the conditions required for handling data on IRB approval. Secure space can be at a premium in some settings. Managing data in an equitable partnership requires that all parties have access to files during the study as well as after a study is completed.

Research Methods

Randomized clinical trials are designed to provide the gold standard of evidence, but in resource-poor settings, randomized trials may be neither possible nor appropriate and more general evidence needs to be examined, such as descriptive studies, pre- and post-analyses, and qualitative methods. And an issue arises when a new intervention is tested that might treat or manage a disease condition, such as HIV/AIDS: When the study ends, what plans are made for the participant to continue to receive appropriate health care services, and are the standards of care offered according to what is locally available or what is available in the country funding the study (Parry, 2000)?

Epidemiologic studies and descriptive surveys can provide important baseline information on which to build further projects. For example, a recent survey of nurse and midwifery regulations for practice provides baseline data for country-level comparisons for 11 African countries (McCarthy et al., 2013). Qualitative methods are suited to global nursing research to discover the meaning of processes and contexts (Harrowing, Mill, Spiers, Kulig, & Kipp, 2010).

A participatory approach to research diverges from the traditional research approach. In a traditional research approach, issues are identified by funding priorities, and the researcher controls the research design, recruitment of participants, implementation of the study or intervention, and dissemination of results. However, the traditional research

TABLE 9.2 Principles of Community-Based Participatory Research (CBPR)

1. Acknowledges community as the unit of identity
2. Builds on strengths and resources within the community
3. Facilitates a collaborative, equitable partnership in all phases of research, involving an empowering and power-sharing process that attends to social inequalities
4. Fosters colearning and capacity building among all partners
5. Integrates and achieves a balance between knowledge generation and intervention for the mutual benefit of all partners
6. Focuses on local relevance of public health problems and on ecological perspectives that attend to the multiple determinants of health
7. Involves systems development using a cyclical and iterative process
8. Disseminates results to all partners and involves them in the wider dissemination of results
9. Involves a long-term process and commitment to sustainability

Source: Israel, Eng, Schulz, and Parker (2012). This material is reproduced with permission of John Wiley & Sons, Inc.

approach fails to incorporate the social, cultural, and economic contexts where health issues occur to be able to provide research that can be implemented effectively in diverse populations. CBPR emerged from public health as a research approach that examines health issues affecting populations associated with racial, ethnic, and socioeconomic disparities in health (Israel, Eng, Schulz, & Parker, 2012). The methods used aim to identify and build on existing resources and relationships to improve health. CBPR depends on partnerships devoted to meaningful change and progress. The nine guiding principles of CBPR are listed in Table 9.2.

The key dimensions to a successful CBPR approach are (1) sustaining relationships with partners, (2) sustaining knowledge and values generated by the partnership, and (3) funding, staffing, and the partnership itself (Israel et al., 2006). Although CBPR has proven value in leading to positive changes in communities, it requires ongoing commitment to the communities being studied.

Participatory action research (PAR) emerged from the social sciences and is focused less on democratic processes and egalitarian decision making and more on understanding organizational problems through the eyes of the participants (Glassman, Erdem, & Bartholomew, 2013). PAR integrates participation (life in society and democracy), action (engagement with experience and history), and research (soundness in thought and the growth of knowledge) (Chevalier & Buckles, 2013). It shares with CBPR the commitment to conducting research that shares power with and engages community partners and benefits the communities involved using research evidence that can be translated into programs and policies within diverse settings.

CONCLUSION

Making nursing research work in global settings requires attention to the health needs and priorities of a population and an investment of time in finding and working with partners committed to mutual goals and equitable relationships. Table 9.1 summarizes the elements of building a research community of excellence from initiation to ongoing project development.

Because global nursing research often involves researchers from high-income countries working with people from low- and middle-income countries, ethical principles of respect for persons, beneficence, and social justice must be foremost in engaging with partners to build trust, respect, and hope for sustainability. Useful models have been proposed to help guide the process of research as well as global standards and policies for the ethical conduct of human subject research. Although a variety of research methods can be used, action research approaches may be best suited for global research that acknowledges the socioeconomic and cultural contexts that contribute to global health inequities.

REFERENCES

Bahn, A., Singh, J. A., Upshur, R. E. G., Singer, P. A., & Daar, A. S. (2007). Grand challenges in global health: Engaging civil society organizations in biomedical research in developing countries. *PLos Medicine, 4*,1456–1459.

Baumann, L. C. (2011). Insights on conducting research in low-resource settings: Examples from Vietnam and Uganda. *Translational Behavioral Medicine, 1*(2), 299–302. doi: 10.1007/s13142-011-0040-4

Chevalier, J. M., & Buckles, D. J. (2013). *Participatory action research: Theory and methods for engaged inquiry.* London, UK: Routledge.

Crigger, N. J., Holcomb, L., & Weiss, J. (2001). Fundamentalism, multiculturalism and problems of conducting research with populations in developing nations. *Nursing Ethics, 8,* 459–468.

de-Graft Aikins, A., Arhinful, D. K., Pitchforth, E. M., Ogedegbe, G., Allotey, P., & Agyeman, C. (2012). Establishing and sustaining research partnerships in Africa: A case study of the UK–Africa academic partnership on chronic disease. *Globalization and Health, 8,* 29. doi: 10.1186/1744-8603-8-29

Epping-Jordan, J. E. (2004). Research to practice: International dissemination of evidence-based behavioral medicine. *Annals of Behavioral Medicine, 28,* 81–87.

Fisher, E. B., Boothroyd, R. I., Coufal, M. M., Baumann, L. C., Mbanya, J. C., Rotheram-Borus, M. J., . . . Tanasugarn, C. (2012). Peer support for self-management of diabetes improved outcomes in international settings. *Health Affairs, 30,* 130–139. doi: 10.1377/hlthaff.2011.0914

Glassman, M., Erdem, G., & Bartholomew, M. (2013). Action research and its history as an adult education movement for social change. *Adult Education Quarterly, 63,* 272–288.

Glover, S. W., Joshi, R., Thapa, G., Sonam, K., Cheata, T., & Gleghorn, C. (2004). International training course on Health InterNetwork Access to Research Initiative (HINARI). *Health Information and Libraries Journal, 21,* 193–196.

Harrowing, J. N., Mill, J., Spiers, J., Kulig, J., & Kipp, W. (2010). Critical ethnography, cultural safety, and international nursing research. *International Journal of Qualitative Methods, 9,* 240–251.

Israel, B. A., Eng, E., Schulz, A. J., & Parker, E. A. (2012). Introduction to methods for CBPR for health. In B. A. Israel, E. Eng, A. J. Schulz, & E. A. Parker (Eds.), *Methods for community-based participatory research for health* (2nd ed., pp. 4–37). San Francisco, CA: Jossey-Bass.

Israel, B. A., Krieger, J., Vlahov, D., Ciske, S., Foley, M., Fortin, P., . . . Tang, G. (2006). Challenges and facilitating factors in sustaining community-based participatory research partnerships: Lessons learned from the Detroit, New York City and Seattle urban research centers. *Journal of Urban Health: Bulletin of the New York Academy of Medicine, 83,* 1022–1040.

Kent, D. M., Mwamburi, D. M., Bennish, M. L., Kupelnick, B., & Ioannidis, J. P. A. (2004). Clinical trials in sub-Saharan Africa and established standards of care. *JAMA, 292,* 237–242.

Ketefian, S. (2000). Ethical considerations in international nursing. *Journal of Professional Nursing, 16,* 257.

Landrine, H., & Klonoff, E. A. (2001). Cultural diversity and health psychology. In A. Baum, T. A. Revensen, & J. E. Singer (Eds.), *Handbook of health psychology* (pp. 851–891). Mahwah, NJ: Lawrence Erlbaum Associates.

Leffers, J., & Mitchell, E. (2010). Conceptual model for partnerships and sustainability in global health. *Public Health Nursing, 28,* 91–102.

Maselli, D., Lys, J. A., & Schmid, J. (2006). *Improving impacts of research partnerships.* Berne Swiss Commission for Research Partnerships with Developing Countries, Geographicia Berensia, Berne, Switzerland.

McCarthy, C. F., Voss, J., Verani, A. R. Vidot, P., Salmon, M. E., & Riley, P. L. (2013). Nursing and midwifery regulation and HIV scale-up: Establishing a baseline in east, central, and southern Africa. *Journal of International AIDS Society, 16,* 18051. http://dx.doi.org/10.7448/IAS.16.1.18051

National League for Nursing. (2012). *Faculty preparation for global experiences toolkit.* New York: National League for Nursing. www.ghdonline.org/nursing/discussion/nln-faculty-preparation-for-global-experiences-t-2

Parry, E. (2000). The ethics of clinical research in developing countries. *Journal of the Royal College of Physicians of London, 34,* 328–329.

Powell, D. L., Gilliss, C. L., Hewitt, H. H., & Flint, E. P. (2010). Application of a partnership model for transformative and sustainable international development. *Public Health Nursing, 27,* 54–70.

Stöckli, B., Wiesmann, U., & Lys, J.-A. (2012). *A guide for transboundary research partnerships: 11 principles.* Bern, Switzerland: Swiss Commission for Research Partnerships with Developing Countries (KFPE).

Tervalon, M., & Murray-Garcia, J. (1998). Cultural humility versus cultural competence: A critical distinction in defining physician training outcomes in multicultural education. *Journal of Health Care for the Poor and Underserved, 9,* 117–125. doi: 10.1353/hpu.2010.0233

Tindana, P. O., Rozmovits, L., Boulanger, R. F., Bandewar, S. V. S., Aborigo, R. A., Hodgson, A. V. O., & Lavery, J. V. (2011). Aligning community engagement with traditional authority structures in global health research: A case study from northern Ghana. *American Journal of Public Health, 101,* 1857–1867.

Uys, L. R., & Klopper, H. C. (2013). *The state of nursing and nursing education in Africa: A country-by-country review.* Sigma Theta Tau International.

Working Group for the Study of Ethical Issues in International Nursing Research. (2003). Ethical consideration in international nursing research: A report from the International Centre for Nursing Ethics. *Nursing Ethics, 10,* 123–137.

Conducting Nursing Research in Uganda

Linda Ciofu Baumann

I first traveled to Uganda in 2000 to explore the development of an academic exchange program with a U.S. university for the purpose of providing global health learning experiences for graduate, undergraduate, and health profession students. During this initial visit, accompanied by two physician faculty members from Wisconsin, we met with faculty at Makerere University in the schools of medicine, nursing, and public health to explore what each of us would offer in an academic partnership. A timely development was the implementation of an interprofessional problem-based learning curriculum in the health science schools at Makerere. This learning model emphasizes interprofessional teams and a focus on learning about the health problems that occur most often in community settings. It also emphasizes more learning experiences outside of hospitals and in communities. Our Makerere partners agreed that U.S. students could participate in these rotations alongside Ugandan students.

During this visit I also met with health care providers at Mulago Hospital and others who worked in the Kampala area to learn more about their health care delivery system. The people I met were most interested in the work I did in diabetes care in Vietnam, conducting research and helping build the health workforce capacity (Baumann, Blobner, Binh, & Lan, 2006). Diabetes is a global epidemic, worldwide and in many low- and middle-income countries (International Diabetes Federation, 2012), and has created concerns about the ability to address the growing noncommunicable disease burden within existing health care systems and with the current health care workforce, especially in low-resources countries. In approaching my work in Uganda I was guided by a few basic principles: (1) ensure that research fits local needs and priorities; (2) know the environment; (3) adapt to language, literacy, and culture; (4) ensure sustainability.

ENSURE THAT RESEARCH FITS LOCAL NEEDS AND PRIORITIES

From 2001 to 2009, I supervised U.S. students in a 3-week study abroad immersion program to learn about Ugandan health care, public health, and culture. We planned the curriculum with Makerere faculty and staff, and they accompanied us on many of the site visits. Through this exposure I met many nurses, physicians, and community leaders who were interested in working with us to develop more training opportunities in diabetes care and research.

Our first diabetes study, begun in 2006, was a descriptive study on beliefs and knowledge of adults with type 2 diabetes about their disease and self-management. We first conducted a small pilot to assess the feasibility of carrying out such a study in this setting. I worked with a community physician, Dr. Marcel Otim; a hospital-based physician, Dr. Kenneth Opio; and Sister Josephine Ejang, one of the few diabetes specialist nurses in Uganda. In the next study, I was able to hire three Ugandan baccalaureate nursing students to conduct interviews and assist with data management, giving them direct experience with nursing research (Baumann, Opio, Otim, Olson, & Ellison, 2010).

In 2008, I returned to Uganda for a sabbatical semester as a Health Volunteers Overseas (HVO) volunteer to learn more about how diabetes was managed and about how I could contribute to improving diabetes care through research. By working as a nurse volunteer in the diabetes clinics at Mulago, I was able to learn first-hand the needs, resources, and acceptable approaches for diabetes care in this setting. This visit also allowed me the opportunity to conduct the final data analysis and study debriefing and write up the results of our diabetes study. While working as a nurse in this setting, I appreciated the scarcity of resources in the health care system for managing and treating diabetes and became more aware of the significant role nurses were assuming in managing diabetes as well as many other conditions, such as HIV/AIDS.

During this visit I was invited to attend a diabetes education program funded by the World Diabetes Federation (WDF) with the purpose of training teams of nurses, medical technicians, and medical officers to establish diabetes care clinics at 20 district hospitals throughout Uganda. This health system change was needed because the Mulago hospital weekly endocrine clinic was becoming overwhelmed with the increased number of patients wanting to be seen. To meet this growing demand, diabetes care needed to be provided locally. In a country with severe shortages in the health care workforce, innovative models were needed. The 20 diabetes teams attended a 2-week workshop based on the International Diabetes Federation curriculum to learn about diabetes diagnosis, management, and treatment and were given basic materials needed to operate a clinic, such as sphygmomanometers, stethoscopes, weight scales, record books, and blood testing supplies.

I approached the physician in charge of the project, Dr. Agatha, and shared with her my interest in diabetes, especially diabetes education and self-management, and that I would be interested in working with her on the project. She was a bit surprised that I didn't have an idea already in mind, but viewed this as an opportunity to work with a U.S. researcher, who had some resources to work with, to develop a project that would enhance the ongoing effort to improve diabetes care by training local diabetes care teams.

My initial contribution to the project was to obtain a small faculty grant to develop a pictorial diabetes foot care poster that reflected the Ugandan setting and distribute these to each of the diabetes teams' district hospitals. In our first diabetes study, we gave all participants a pictorial foot care poster, but the research assistants observed that many patients didn't recognize a nail clipper, since most cut their toenails with razor blades; that foot cream was unfamiliar, since petroleum jelly is the more common skin softener; and that the people in the posters were not black enough to identify with. These revisions were briefly field tested and a new poster was created by a graphic artist from a vocational school that was part of a faith-based community organization to help support jobs and education for residents of one of the worst slums in Kampala. I knew of this site through our student visits and had developed a great respect for their community development work.

KNOW THE ENVIRONMENT

After 2008, most of my efforts in Uganda were directed toward research. When I told people back in the United States that I was doing research in Uganda, they were often surprised to hear that I was studying diabetes, not thinking that it was in Africa. However, Uganda was the epicenter of the HIV/AIDS epidemic and is recognized for reducing HIV/AIDS prevalence as well as the research partnerships with major U.S. universities to study HIV/AIDS. Later that year a funding opportunity arose to examine the feasibility of diabetes self-management support provided by peers in developing countries. I asked my Ugandan colleagues to serve as co-investigators for a study to examine this question. We aimed

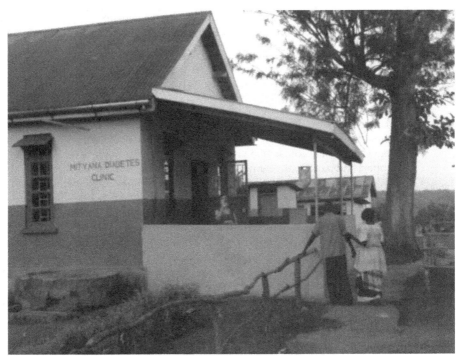

Mityana Diabetes Clinic, Mityana District Hospital, Uganda.   *Credit*: L. Baumann.

to conduct this initial study in one site drawing from the 20 teams that were trained. We applied two criteria to select a site: the site had to be within a 2-hour drive from Kampala, and the diabetes care team selected should be a best example of the diabetes teams trained to operate a district hospital diabetes clinic. A rural district hospital 50 kilometers west of Kampala was chosen as the study site.

Our first contact at this potential study site was a meeting between Mulago physicians, a diabetes specialist nurse, me (introduced as the "donor from the United States"), and, from the district hospital, the chief administrator, medical director, and chief nurse. The purpose of the meeting was to explain the study, address any concerns or questions, and obtain permission to conduct it in their setting. My role as "donor" is one that Ugandans are familiar with, since often it is the *muzungu* (White person) who has the money. It also conveyed that the Ugandans would have a major role in the project, and I suspect that culturally it was not common that a nurse would be the leader of a research project. The project was described as one that was testing how to best care for adults with type 2 diabetes, and that involving patient peers to provide support to each other could improve the experience of living with diabetes. The spokesperson for the hospital acknowledged their appreciation for us asking permission, since some researchers, both domestic and foreign, have tried to access medical records and conduct communitywide surveys without informing anyone locally. They also acknowledged that most often they never are informed of the results of a study, nor see any impact from the research that is conducted. Their final request? "Please leave something concrete behind."

We fulfilled this request almost immediately. The diabetes clinic we saw on our first visit was a small room containing the metal frame of an old hospital bed and two wooden benches. Walls were covered with education posters that had been damaged by leaks from the roof. Patients waited to be seen outside in the hot sun with only a bench to provide rest. We raised concerns about moving some of the study equipment into this space, and the hospital administrator was able to provide space in an unused end of a patient ward. The space required renovation, needed cleaning and painting, but local workmen and carpenters were hired to create a space that included three small consultation rooms and a large waiting area. Another important feature was the creation of a large cement porch with a cover to provide a sheltered space for patients to gather.

ADAPT TO LANGUAGE, LITERACY, AND CULTURE

Development of the diabetes education curricula and research protocol was done both with a U.S. colleague, who was a registered nurse and a certified diabetes educator for over 30 years, and who had experience working in resource poor countries, and with Ugandan colleagues. Over the course of 3 years (2009 to 2011), we made several visits to provide study support and participate in mutual problem solving with the district hospital diabetes team.

The district diabetes team provided the day-to-day implementation of the project after the physician and nurse researcher partners conducted two all-day group education sessions and collected pre-intervention data. Participants who could speak and read English and who served as peer leaders attended the first session, in which the program was delivered in English. However, participants who attended the second education session were not required to speak English and had great difficulty understanding the spoken English. Since Ugandans were delivering the program, they were able to switch to speaking Luganda for the rest of the session. Because Ugandans were both the teachers and the learners, cultural gaps were minimized—but still persisted. Within Uganda, a country with over 50 spoken languages but whose official language is English, there are often language gaps between providers and patients; differences in how well a person knows English may be based on whether he or she lives in a rural or urban area. Low literacy was another challenge. Our physician colleagues noted that patients are not always truthful about their education level, because they fear being taken advantage of if a provider knows that they have little formal education. However, the major reason participants could not read the written materials in our study was their need for reading glasses. Administering all surveys in a group setting and reading the questions aloud in two languages, English and Luganda, was a workable but time-consuming solution.

Our research project introduced the concept of an activated patient who needs to know how to set behavioral goals; take medications; seek social and emotional support; and engage in the day-to-day self-management of diabetes. Furthermore, we used patient peers along with an interprofessional health care team to reinforce diabetes self-care support through ongoing education and care management. Our project was also able to fund a closed cell phone network so that participants could contact each other and the diabetes clinic at no charge. Cell phones are widely used in Africa, and in Uganda, but few people have enough money to pay for air time. The experience of a patient phoning a clinic nurse to ask about a health care issue was a first for most of the participants in the study.

After 4 months of intervention, the results showed a positive impact of peer support on glucose control, regular contact with other patients and the clinic by phone or in person, and a perception that peers were helpful in sharing goals for physical activity and eating, as well as for listening about feelings and experiences with diabetes. The success of this intervention depended on partnering with appropriate in-country resources and addressing a priority health need, as well as acknowledging the basic needs of the setting such as adequate shelter for a clinic and simple equipment (Baumann, 2011).

ENSURE SUSTAINABILITY

The challenge of any funded project is how to sustain it once the funding ends. Once the intervention was completed, I continued to work with my Ugandan colleagues to develop and deliver presentations about the study at international and local professional meetings, as well as to explore further funding. Two years after our project ended, I visited Uganda and met with my physician colleagues at Mulago, the diabetes clinic team, and several patients who had participated in the peer support study. The two physicians were able to obtain further funding from a UK-based nongovernmental organization to expand the peer support model to 10 other district hospital teams. This was a great step, since local leadership is critical to the ongoing success of translating research evidence to improve systems to care for adults with diabetes. My only regret was that they decided to drop many of the psychosocial measures from their research that are relevant to understanding how to improve the quality of life, not simply the biological outcomes of the intervention. The diabetes specialist nurse from Mulago has become quite skilled in providing diabetes education programs to public groups, nurses, and physicians.

The diabetes clinic team reported that they enjoyed working with informed patients who ask important questions and who are motivated to be part of their care because they feel better when their diabetes is better controlled. The clinic nurse on the diabetes team has instituted creative system changes to sustain some of the study elements: (1) patients are scheduled for 30-minute appointments every other month (from monthly) to provide enough time to address questions as well as self-care needs; (2) patients who participated in the peer project are scheduled at the clinic the same day so that they can continue to make contact with each other; (3) every diabetes clinic day, now twice a week, begins with a diabetes education session, held on the porch for patients waiting for their appointment that day and for members of the local diabetes club to meet. The foot care poster we developed continues to be used as an educational tool posted on clinic walls, and the bilingual diabetes educational booklets (English and Luganda) continue to be used for diabetes education.

Although there are successes to share in this work, the world is ever changing. The diabetes clinic nurse is likely to be promoted to chief nurse and will need to focus less on the diabetes clinic. Her promotion attests to her superb leadership skills and dedication to her patients. Furthermore, the entire district hospital facility is scheduled to be demolished, including the diabetes clinic we built, and relocated to a nearby site. Further, the diabetes specialist nurse from Mulago has been reassigned, due to hospital politics, and no longer works with patients with diabetes; however, she has increased her activities as a diabetes educator in the community. Hopefully, the positive experience with the diabetes self-management study and the tangible improvements in diabetes care will be incorporated into the future district hospital facilities and will be one of the many contributions to improving diabetes care in Uganda.

REFLECTIVE QUESTIONS

1. What plan would you develop to learn about how the health care system in another country, like Uganda, manages a specific health problem?
2. How would you communicate with a potential Ugandan partner your purposes/objectives, time, resources, role, and goals?
3. How is the leadership shared in this collaboration between researchers from the United States and Uganda?
4. What other strategies can be used to address language and literacy issues?
5. How would you establish the reliability and validity of written research instruments in this setting?
6. What critical elements of a project need to continue for sustainability to be achieved? How can threats to sustainability be overcome?

REFERENCES

Baumann, L. C. (2011). Insights on conducting research in low-resource settings: Examples from Vietnam and Uganda. *Translational Behavioral Medicine, 1*(2), 299–302. doi: 10.1007/ s13142-011-0040-4

Baumann, L. C., Blobner, D., Binh, T. V., & Lan, P. T. (March/April 2006). A training program for diabetes care in Vietnam. *Diabetes Educator, 32*, 189–194.

Baumann, L. C., Opio, C. K., Otim, M., Olson, L., & Ellison, S. (2010). Self-care beliefs and behaviors in Ugandan adults with type 2 diabetes. *Diabetes Educator, 36*(2), 293–300.

International Diabetes Federation. (2012). *Diabetes atlas* (5th ed.). Brussels, Belgium: International Diabetes Federation. www.idf.org/diabetesatlas/5e

CHAPTER 10

Maintaining Partnerships Through Leadership

Michele J. Upvall

The pace of change in health care has accelerated over the past 20 years. Change has always been a constant factor, but with new technologies and the realization of globalization we are seeing transformation in health care on a scale never seen before. Transformational change requires a new set of skills and a reconceptualization of leadership. Authoritative, hierarchal leadership ideas appropriate for the assembly lines of the industrial age are inappropriate in an age of transformation. Collaborating among teams, demonstrating outcomes and competencies, having the ability to synthesize complex ideas, and having skills that can be transferred to multiple settings are fundamental for today's health care provider regardless of country or clinical practice site (Porter-O'Grady & Malloch, 2011). These skill sets become particularly important in nursing as we confront challenges that include changing demographics, nurse migration, and a much needed emphasis on quality and competency that are without boundaries and require innovation for sustainable solutions (Gantz et al., 2012).

This chapter provides an alternative view of traditional leadership, describing assumptions of leadership in global health and how these assumptions, along with leadership skills, can be adapted fluidly among members of global health projects in order to maintain partnerships. Transformation is an outcome of global health partnerships, for both the guest and host partners at personal and professional levels, as well as within organizations. Partners, as members of a team, require leadership and ongoing assessment to fully realize the benefits of the transformational outcomes of collaboration. The essence of collaboration used within this context of team work extends beyond cooperation and simple support. Collaboration in this chapter denotes alignment of efforts among team members where power is shared and all members contribute their expert knowledge without the constraints of hierarchy. Partners are willing, even eager, and highly motivated members of the team (Henneman, Lee, & Cohen, 1995; Rosenberg, Hayes, McIntyre, & Neill, 2010).

AN OVERVIEW OF GLOBAL HEALTH NURSING LEADERSHIP

Leadership alone is a complex phenomenon, and, as any leader realizes, it is easier to describe a leader than to live out these leadership qualities and attributes daily. Leadership becomes even more complex in the context of global health where cultural differences, including communication processes, can be significant between guest and host partners. Defining global health leadership is elusive, but three core beliefs underlie development of global health nursing leadership as a process (Kim, Woith, Otten, & McElmurry, 2006). These core beliefs are not unique to nursing, but rather can be extrapolated to other health care providers and extend across practice settings:

- Leaders are born and can also be developed or "made"
- Leaders facilitate sustainable outcomes
- Leaders know themselves and inspire others to find their voice

Attributes of Global Health Nursing Leaders

Global health nursing leadership occurs within organizations and the highest levels of government, but the concept of leadership in global health nursing extends to nurses working within nongovernmental organizations or serving as volunteers on health care teams. Regardless of setting, there are certain attributes or qualities of leaders that enhance the potential for successful partnerships and sustainable outcomes. Kim, Woith, Otten, and McElmurry (2006) interviewed nurse leaders from eight countries, identifying competencies of global nurse leaders (see Box 10.1).

BOX 10.1 Competencies of Global Health Nursing Leaders

Competencies

Open-minded and flexible
Culturally aware and sensitive
Able to deal with complexity
Resilient, resourceful, optimistic, energetic
Honest and have integrity
Stable personal life and family support in formative years to help build self-confidence
Value-added technical or business skills; politically savvy
Conviction and passion

Source: Kim, Woith, Otten, and McElmurry, 2006.

These competencies are consistent with the theory of authentic leadership—that is, leadership that is considered transparent, encourages self-knowledge, and encompasses the attributes or competencies of resiliency, optimism, motivation, and self-efficacy (Wong & Laschinger, 2012). While Wong and Laschinger (2012) demonstrate the relationship between authentic leadership and empowerment among staff nurses, McMurray (2007) reminds us that it is important for us to know the self—our beliefs, how we feel empowered, and how we feel constrained. As leaders, it is also important to recognize that no one is consistent in his or her behavior (McMurray, 2007). No one operates at the highest level of behavior every day and in every circumstance and, as human beings, we all make mistakes.

The ability to forgive ourselves and others is another key attribute of global health nurse leaders that is often overlooked as we live out our leadership roles. Porter-O'Grady and Malloch (2011) refer to leadership vulnerability as "openness to others and new ideas" (p. 251). Vulnerability is seen from a position of strength, not weakness, as the vulnerable leader accepts both personal strengths and weaknesses and is able to be flexible in thinking. The vulnerable leader realizes limits and does not try to pretend otherwise for the sake of protecting ego. However, vulnerability does not imply a "woe is me" attitude or allow incompetence. Rather, the vulnerable leader promotes trust by encouraging dialogue among team members (Porter-O'Grady & Malloch, 2011). Ultimately, the leader in any setting helps others to progress and realize their potential (Ehrenfield & Nathan, 2010).

From Global to Local Nursing Leadership

Global health nursing leadership and the development of nursing as a profession is impacted by societal perceptions and expectations, as noted in previous and subsequent case studies. Stewart and Usher (2010) used critical ethnography to explore health care, organizational nursing leadership, and patient safety in Fiji. As part of their study they documented the influence of the nursing shortage and the other complexities of nursing practice, including ethnic tensions in Fiji. Senior nursing leaders and managers interviewed from the Ministry of Health discussed the impact of recent health care reform in which a clinical governance framework coupled with multidisciplinary education provided a sense of empowerment. Ultimately, this feeling of empowerment led to a more patient-centered approach. The nurse leaders reported more "walking around the wards" and "having an open door" (Stewart & Usher, 2010, p. 3156). These nurse leaders appeared sincere in their efforts to understand the challenges of the nurses who provide direct patient care, and they saw a connection between nurse working conditions and the ability to provide safe patient care.

This study of Fijian high-level nursing leaders is only one example of possibilities that can occur through health reform and a shared governance model. Although sustained results and challenges were not reported in the study, the potential exists for change to occur as nurse leaders at the national organizational level value leadership at the ward or local level. The distance between nurses engaged in front-line nursing and those within the Ministry of Health was perceived as shrinking, opening the door to nurse-to-nurse collaboration between the Ministry of Health and nurses in other organizations. When this occurs, the potential for ongoing policy change and thinking about health care from a transformational perspective is realized.

BOX 10.2

"The power of mission, the power of example, the power of inclusion, the power of collaboration can move us from where we are to where we are determined to be."

Source: Hesselbein, 2005, pp. 125–126.

A TEAM APPROACH TO EFFECTIVE GLOBAL HEALTH LEADERSHIP

The evolution of nursing from a hierarchal to a more team-centered approach can be noted in the above example of Fijian nurses. While the example provides more of an organizational perspective, the fluidity of leadership can be more easily illustrated through partnership teams.

Too often, though, teamwork is ignored when it should be promoted. Global health is a broad concept and, by its very nature, a complex one. Even the most "simple" projects contain elements of complexity and it is impossible for one individual to think of all the parameters and consequences when implementing a project plan. Issues pertaining to culture, socioeconomic differences, politics, and belief systems influence project planning. Promoting teamwork can begin with educating health care providers as members of a team throughout their curricula. The members of Education of Health Professionals for the 21st Century: A Global Independent Commission (Frenk et al., 2010) proposed nine instructional reforms for educating health care providers. One of the most significant reforms calls for:

> Promotion of interprofessional and transprofessional education that breaks down professional silos while enhancing collaborative and non-hierarchal relationships in effective teams. Alongside specific technical skills, interprofessional education should focus on . . . leadership and management capabilities (for efficient handling of scarce resources in conditions of uncertainty), and communication skills (for mobilization of all stakeholders, including patients and populations). (Frenk et al., 2010, p. 1951)

The commission goes further in its call for educational reform by encouraging interprofessional and transprofessional education from the time of admission into programs through graduation. Integrating the concept of health teams early on and throughout the educational journey allows for greater potential to increase the possibility of living the team concept throughout one's professional career.

Team Leadership Roles

Traditional teams have either a designated leader or a leader who emerges from the group. Sometimes no leadership at all is evident in a team. Strong leadership is required for teams to facilitate maximum outcomes and collaboration in global health. Critical team leadership roles include the following (Rosenberg, Hayes, McIntyre, & Neill, 2010, pp. 128–129):

- The convener: creates space for dialogue and manages the meeting
- The visionary: provides the inspiration for members to achieve goals
- The strategist: provides rational thinking for deliberate selection of strategic choices
- The team builder: promotes understanding of various team member perspectives, aligning ideas and persuading members

Rosenberg, Hayes, McIntyre, and Neill (2010) discovered in their interviews of global health leaders that while each of these team leadership roles is crucial to a team, few teams manage to have identified members demonstrating these roles. Complementary leadership denotes fluidity in leadership whereby team members take on the roles at different times during the work of the partnership. No one person, not even a designated leader, can fulfill all the roles successfully. If collaboration and true partnership are the goal of a team, then

> When partners begin to listen respectfully and openly share ideas, they develop an elasticity that allows one person to pull back and another to step forward, depending on the leadership needs of the moment. At such moments, as individuals cede leadership to other partners, they build trust and the bonds of close collaboration grow. (Rosenberg, Hayes, McIntyre, & Neill, 2010, pp. 128–129)

Trust within teams for sustaining partnerships is crucial when team members are meeting in a more traditional, face-to-face mode or even when meeting as a "virtual" team through technology such as Skype or other technology for long-distance communication. Indeed, trust has been cited as the most significant element of a successful virtual leadership team (Holland, Malvey, & Fottler, 2009).

The Role of the Project "Champion" on the Global Health Team

A leader who demonstrates ongoing commitment with an enthusiastic attitude and who values the perspective of the team members or partners can be called a "leadership champion."

This leadership role is considered pivotal to project sustainability (Leffers & Mitchell, 2011). Leadership champions support and may even strengthen sustainability of innovations at the institutional level (Johnson, Hays, Center, & Daley, 2004).

Specific leadership roles, considered external to the actual project team, that can be considered champion roles include the following (Rosenberg, Hayes, McIntyre, & Neill, 2010, pp. 137–139):

- The advocate: expresses passion for the project and may be the fundraiser
- The political influencer: cultivates relationships among those with power to promote a project
- The networker: demonstrates a significant "web of relationships" (p. 139) among a variety of individuals and groups to facilitate project goals

Advocacy, from encouragement of a project to even direct sponsorship and funding, is the foundation for all the above champion roles. Internal members of the project team can also be considered be leadership champions, especially the role of the visionary. However, for the project goals to be sustained, leadership champions can provide significant ongoing support even after a specific project has ended, as noted in the following chapter, dealing with ongoing project support.

ONGOING ASSESSMENT AND MONITORING OF PARTNERSHIPS

Partnerships require continual assessment to ensure project goals are being achieved. Partners may need to modify, add to, or even eliminate existing project goals. However, before specific project goals can be reviewed and revised, the partners should critically examine their relationships as partners and as leaders within the team. The likelihood of project sustainability lessens without a strong team. General assessment questions that team members should discuss to determine strengths of the partnership and opportunities for improvement are noted in Box 10.3.

BOX 10.3 Assessing the Partnership Team

- How well do we communicate? Are we listening to our stakeholders and each other?
- How do we negotiate disagreements and conflict?
- How are decisions made and communicated to all partners?
- What happens after partnership meetings? Is there adequate follow-through and attention to detail?
- Are we continuously learning and gathering new information to inform project goals?
- Are we staying within our budget parameters?
- What goals have we achieved at this point in the partnership?
- Are we celebrating our achievements?
- Are we sharing what we are learning and achieving through the project with each other and project stakeholders?

Source: Daulaire, 2005; Rosenberg, Hayes, McIntyre, and Neill, 2010.

Partners will need to determine specific points of time for assessing the partnership process. These times may center on a particular timeline or be attached to meeting specific goals within the project. Ongoing project monitoring is discussed in more detail in the next chapter, but it is important to emphasize the significance of developing assessment and monitoring plans from the very beginning of the partnership, including assessment of the partnership itself.

Effective Leadership Monitoring for Collaborative Succession Planning and Management

In a transformative, partnership model of global health nursing leadership, the role of leader is shared. No one individual is necessarily designated as "The Leader." Leadership roles will continue to emerge throughout the partnership as the need arises, and partners will assume leadership roles according to their personal and professional skills as well as experience. This partnership model of leadership, different from traditional models of leadership, requires a different perspective for thinking about succession planning and management. Expectations of "power over" those receiving resources (usually funding and/or knowledge expertise from high-income countries to low- and middle-income countries) are replaced by leadership collaboration.

Carriere, Muise, Cummings, and Newburn-Cook (2009) differentiate succession planning from succession management. They define succession planning as "a structured process involving the identification and preparation of a potential successor to assume a new role within an organization" (p. 549). Succession management is "a formalized process of role planning and leadership development to ensure the leadership pipeline is filled and the right talent is available when required" (p. 549). It is the latter definition of succession management that may best transfer to complementary, fluid leadership within partnerships. Formalizing the process can be challenging, but Rosenberg, Hayes, McIntyre, and Neill (2010) offer a "Leadership Checkup" (see Appendix 10.1) for ongoing assessment of leadership roles. This assessment tool includes all leadership roles, including champions who may be internal or external to the partnership. Similar to assessment of the partnership itself, timelines for addressing this leadership assessment should be agreed on by the partners at the beginning of the partnership.

CONCLUSION

True partnerships in global health nursing require new ways of thinking about leadership for strong collaboration and optimal sustainability. All partnership teams require the roles of convener, visionary, strategist, and team builder, as well as project champions. However, no partner necessarily maintains the same role(s) throughout the partnership. These leadership roles are fluid and emerge when required at various points during a global health project as a result of successful collaboration among the partners. Monitoring the partnership process, collaboration among stakeholders, and leadership roles at designated times during project implementation facilitates further growth of the partnership as a whole and individual partners. The following two case studies demonstrate the challenges involved in maintaining partnerships between academic institutions in different countries.

REFERENCES

Carriere, B. K., Muise, M., Cummings, G., & Newburn-Cook, C. (2009). Healthcare succession planning: An integrative review. *Journal of Nursing Administration, 19*(12), 548–555.

Daulaire, N. (2005). Leading for success. In W. H. Foege, N. Daulaire, R. E. Black, & C. E. Pearson (Eds.), *Global health leadership and management* (pp. 123–128). San Francisco, CA: Jossey-Bass.

Ehrenfield, M., & Nathan, M. B. (2010). Evolving leadership. In N. Gantz (Ed.), *101 global leadership lessons for nurses* (pp. 160–165). Indianapolis, IN: Sigma Theta Tau International.

Frenk, J., Chen, L., Bhutta, Z., Cohen, J., Crisp, N., Evans, T., & Serwadda, D. (2010). Health professionals for a new century: Transforming education to strengthen health systems in an interdependent world. *The Lancet, 376*, 1923–1958. doi: 10.1016/S0140-6736(10)61854-5

Gantz, N. R., Sherman, R., Jasper, M., Choo, C. G., Herrin-Griffith, D., & Harris, K. (2012). Global nurse leader perspectives on health systems and workforce challenges. *Journal of Nursing Management, 20*, 433–443. doi: 10.1111/j.1365-2834.2012.01393.x

Henneman, E. A., Lee, J. L., & Cohen, J. I. (1995). Collaboration: A concept analysis. *Journal of Advanced Nursing, 21*, 103–109.

Hesselbein, F. (2005). Leadership and management for improving global health. In W. H. Foege, N. Daulaire, R. E. Black, & C. E. Pearson (Eds.), *Global health leadership and management* (pp. 123–128). San Francisco, CA: Jossey-Bass.

Holland, J. B., Malvey, D., & Fottler, M. D. (2009). Health care globalization: A need for virtual leadership. *Health Care Manager, 28*(2), 117–123.

Johnson, K., Hays, C., Center, H., & Daley, C. (2004). Building capacity and sustainable prevention innovations: A sustainability planning model. *Evaluation and Program Planning, 27*, 135–149. doi: 10.1016/j.evalprogplan.2004.01.002

Kim, M. J., Woith, W., Otten, K., & McElmurry, J. (2006). Global nurse leaders: Lessons from the sages. *Advances in Nursing Science, 29*(1), 27–42.

Leffers, J., & Mitchell, E. (2011). Conceptual model for partnership and sustainability in global health. *Public Health Nursing, 28*(1), 91–102. doi: 10.1111/j.1525-1446.2010.00892.x

McMurray, A. (2007). Leadership in primary health care: An international perspective: *Contemporary Nurse, 26*, 30–36.

Porter-O'Grady, T., & Malloch, K. (2011). *Quantum leadership: Advancing innovation, transforming health care* (3rd ed.). Sudbury, MA: Jones & Bartlett Learning, LLC.

Rosenberg, M. L., Hayes, E. S., McIntyre, M. H., & Neill, N. (2010). *Real collaboration: What it takes for global health to succeed.* Berkeley, CA: University of California Press.

Stewart, L., & Usher, K. (2010). The impact of nursing leadership on patient safety in a developing country. *Journal of Clinical Nursing, 19*, 3152–3160. doi: 10.1111/j.1365-2702.2010.03285.x

Wong, C. A., & Laschinger, H. K. S. (2012). Authentic leadership, performance, and job satisfaction: The mediating role of empowerment. *Journal of Advanced Nursing, 69*(4), 947–959. doi: 10.1111/j.1365-2648.2012.06089

APPENDIX 10.1

Leadership Checkup

This tool can serve as a discussion guide to allow the partnership to reflect on how well the partners are filling leadership roles and what needs to be changed. All partners should participate in the discussion, not only the leaders.

	Poor	Good	Excellent
Sharing leadership			
How well are we filling gaps in leadership? Are all of the internal and external leadership functions being carried out?	☐	☐	☐
How well does the partnership's overall environment encourage people to voluntarily step up to leadership roles?	☐	☐	☐
How easily do people step down when their leadership role is no longer needed?	☐	☐	☐
How well are the leaders suppressing their egos and personal interests to work in the partnership's best interests?	☐	☐	☐
Convening			
How well are meetings planned?	☐	☐	☐
Is the facilitator able to create an open environment in which all members participate?	☐	☐	☐
Is needed information being communicated before and after meetings?	☐	☐	☐
Are follow-up actions clarified at meetings and monitored afterward?	☐	☐	☐
Communicating a vision			
Has one of the partners communicated a clear vision that other partners support?	☐	☐	☐
Do we have a clear goal and way(s) to measure progress against that vision?	☐	☐	☐
Shaping a strategy			
Is it clear how we will achieve the vision?	☐	☐	☐
Are changes needed in the strategy we have developed?	☐	☐	☐
Building a team			
Where are we along the spectrum of developing teamwork (recognition of differences, conflict, greater harmony, or accomplishment)?	☐	☐	☐
Are we becoming more cohesive?	☐	☐	☐
Advocating			
Do we have a partner with the ability to convey passion about our cause to external audiences or individuals?	☐	☐	☐
Is that partner actively serving as our spokesperson?	☐	☐	☐
Have we seen evidence that behaviors are changing as a result?	☐	☐	☐
Achieving political influence			
Is one of our partners able to tap into the right government leaders at the right time?	☐	☐	☐
In what government area do we need to exert more influence?	☐	☐	☐
Networking			
Are we taking advantage of the full networking capabilities of our partner group?	☐	☐	☐
Do we have a plan for networking among key stakeholder groups?	☐	☐	☐

Rosenberg, Hayes, McIntyre, and Neill (2010). Reprinted with permission, Copyright Clearance Center.

A Partnership Between Two Schools of Nursing

Marilyn Lotas
Marcia A. Petrini

Global health has become a major focus in nursing, growing out of the awareness of the extraordinarily rapid transformations in information, communication, health, and health services occurring throughout our global community. The community of global nurses is recognizing that, over the coming decades, nurses must be prepared to practice in an increasingly culturally diverse world. This is clearly demonstrated in the increasing focus on global health in nursing curricula at all levels. The effort of nurses and nursing organizations in international health includes research, service, and health capacity building. In this case study we describe the initiation and development of an 8-year partnership between two schools of nursing, one in China and one in the United States. The partnership began in 2005 after Dr. Marcia Petrini, dean of the HOPE School of Nursing, Wuhan University, Wuhan, China, was the keynote speaker at the Rozella Schlotfeldt Public Lecture at the Frances Payne Bolton School of Nursing (FPBSN), Case Western Reserve University (CWRU). During that visit Dr. Petrini talked about the goals for the development of the HOPE School of Nursing and its faculty and students over the coming years. This led to the first visit by a group of 10 administrators and faculty to FPBSN to learn how undergraduate nursing is taught in the United States both in the classroom and clinical settings. This first visit led to a comprehensive partnership that includes faculty development, curriculum development, faculty from FPBSN going to Wuhan University to teach graduate students in nursing administration and community health, and semester-long mutual student exchange.

CONTEXT: WUHAN UNIVERSITY AND HOPE SCHOOL OF NURSING

Wuhan University is a comprehensive national university directly under the administration of the Ministry of Education. The history of Wuhan University can be traced back to Ziqiang Institute, founded in 1893 by Zhang Zhidong, governor of Hubei Province and Hunan Province in the late Qing Dynasty. The institute changed its name several times before it was finally named Wuhan National University in 1928. It is one of the earliest comprehensive national universities in modern China. By the end of 1946, the university had established six colleges: the colleges of liberal arts, law, sciences, engineering, agriculture, and medicine.

During the past century, Wuhan University has built an elegant complex of primitive simplicity that beautifully blends the Chinese and Western architectural styles and is known as "the most beautiful university in China." Furthermore, Wuhan University's centennial humanistic contribution is expressed in its succinct motto: "Improve Oneself, Promote Perseverance, Seek Truth, and Make Innovations." Since its establishment, Wuhan University has graduated more than 300,000 professionals in various occupations, among whom are over 100 members of the Chinese Academy of Science and the Chinese Academy of Engineering. They have made significant contributions to nation building and social advancement. The achievements of Wuhan University have won it an extensive international reputation. In 1999, the world-renowned journal *Science* listed Wuhan University as one of the most prominent institutions of higher education in China. As a result, international exchanges and collaborative relationships with Wuhan University have been burgeoning in recent years. There are cooperative relationships with more than 300 universities and research institutes in over 40 countries and regions. Now, Wuhan University endeavors to shape itself into a world-class comprehensive research university.

In 2001, Wuhan University merged four single-mission universities in compliance with the regulations from the Ministry of Education. Before the early 1950s, Chinese universities were comprehensive universities, but when China was linked to the USSR, the educational system was changed, and universities became single-purpose. The Wuhan University merger included Wuhan University, Wuhan University of Hydraulic and Electrical Engineering, Wuhan Technical University of Surveying and Mapping, and Hubei Medical University, a return to a comprehensive university education for students.

In 2001, Wuhan University invited Project HOPE to assist in converting the school of nursing of the former Hubei Medical University from a 5-year baccalaureate program to a 4-year program based on the curriculum model of Wuhan University. This required a major revision of the curriculum from 348 credits to 150 credits, with one-third of the credits required university courses, one-third nursing courses, and one-third free electives. The five faculty initially assigned to the school were not fully qualified for university appointment, two having a baccalaureate degree and the other three having graduated from the *zhong zhuong* (nursing program entered by students after grade 9). The agreement with Project HOPE provided for hiring as dean a doctorally prepared nurse with experience in administration and development of university programs (baccalaureate, master's, and doctoral levels) in the United States and internationally and with clinical experience and a current license. Faculty development was needed to prepare the faculty to teach the incoming students, who often had more education than the faculty in the basic sciences and liberal arts. The curriculum was to promote critical thinking, clinical decision making, accountability, leadership, creativity, and the ability to be professional role models and to do clinical research and use transitional evidence-based nursing care in hospitals and clinical settings. Foreign textbooks, the Internet for recent journal articles, and research findings related to practice were used for theoretical references. Teaching strategies were adopted to comply with Wuhan University's standards by using interactive teaching methods to replace the traditional lecture and rote memorization from poorly written, obsolete texts full of misinformation and errors. The students were to learn to be self-directed learners, prepared for the future and the reality that nursing requires safe practice and lifelong learning.

The C. J. Huang Foundation, through Project HOPE, provided some financial support for the foreign dean, educational resources, and faculty development. The development of faculty was at locally designed workshops and through study in the United States, allowing the academic and clinical faculty to experience and observe nursing care and education in top universities and hospitals. The new curriculum concepts and content were hard for the faculty to visualize or teach prior to the study trips. They were able to see the nursing practice and clinical settings described in the texts and witness the independent roles of the nurses. They observed classes and developed a better understanding of how effective interactive teaching is and the importance of applying the knowledge in the clinical setting soon after. In China, the classic model of education is to teach all the didactic courses; then the last year of the program the students go to the hospital and are assigned to various units during a year rotation taught by the staff nurses. In the United States, the faculty observed the role of the academic faculty supervising the students in the clinical area.

The five faculty from 2003, when the first baccalaureate students were admitted, have increased to 22 in 2013. The number of students has increased from 28 to about 400 undergraduate students, 60 master's students, and 7 doctoral students, with approximately 7,000 continuing education students. The faculty relies on part-time clinical faculty who meet the requirements of clinical faculty for Wuhan University (master's degree, faculty development).

Description of CWRU and FPBSN: Home to approximately 10,000 students, CWRU is an independent research-oriented university with strengths in health care, including medicine, nursing, and dentistry; in engineering; in the arts and sciences; and in law, management, and social work. Founded in 1826 as the Western Reserve College, it evolved into the CWRU in 1967 through a merger with the Case Institute of Technology. The university's mission, to "improve people's lives through preeminent research, education and creative endeavor," highlights a commitment to "promote an inclusive culture of global citizenship."

For nearly 9 decades, the FPBSN has been a globally recognized leader in nursing education and innovation, impacting nursing education, research, and interprofessional scholarship and practice around the world. The educational programs of the school include the bachelor of science in nursing (BSN) degree, the graduate entry program for second-degree students, the master of science in nursing (MSN) degree, the doctorate in nursing practice (DNP), and the doctor of philosophy degree. FPBSN is home to a World Health Organization (WHO) Collaborating Center, one of 10 WHO Collaborating Centers in the United States and one of 38 in the world. The school has a long history of providing advanced degrees for international nurses and has an average of 55 international students each year. This year's students come from 18 countries. In addition, the school has provided consultation and short-term educational programs for multiple faculty groups, including 30 faculty and administrators from Wuhan University, over the past decade alone. This history of global involvement provided the context for FPBSN's participation in the comprehensive, institutional partnership with the HOPE School of Nursing.

Goals for the Collaboration: For any partnership to be successful and sustained over time, several elements must be in place, among them clearly delineated, congruent, and mutually accepted goals. In this partnership, the goals were modified by evolution throughout the process as some were achieved and new levels of activity became possible.

HOPE School of Nursing Goals: The goals for the collaboration for the HOPE School of Nursing were initially related to faculty development through a series of study tours. The study tours had objectives for the faculty to meet and arrangements were made by the WHO collaborating center of FPBSN.

A. Develop Wuhan faculty related to teaching methods other than lecture, specifically in the areas of teaching strategies used in the nursing laboratory in teaching fundamentals, simulation use, and clinical teaching through short-term study tours

B. Provide formal faculty development through pre- and post-doctoral programs for Wuhan faculty

C. Modify the HOPE School of Nursing curriculum to promote critical thinking, clinical decision making, accountability, leadership, creativity, and the ability to be professional role models, do clinical research, and use transitional evidence-based nursing care in the hospitals and clinical settings

D. Develop graduate level community health curriculum

Reciprocal FPBSN Goals: The goals of the FPBSN for the partnership were grounded in the institutional commitment to global outreach and the recognition of the importance of cross-cultural experiences in the education of our own students. These goals included the following:

- Support nursing educational capacity building through faculty development and curriculum consultation
- Provide opportunities for FPBSN students to increase their understanding of the impact of culture and community on health and health care delivery through a one-semester study experience in the HOPE School of Nursing
- Develop opportunities for cross-cultural research

ACTIVITIES OF THE COLLABORATION

Mutual Faculty Development

Activity in the first 2 years of the partnership focused on faculty development predominantly through short-term study tours. Initially, 10 faculty, including two clinical associate deans (both were nursing administrators from two key university hospitals in Wuhan), four clinical faculty (two from each hospital), the vice dean of the HOPE School, and three senior faculty, visited CWRU for 1 week. Over the next 5 years, for continuing faculty development, groups of four to six mixed academic and clinical faculty visited for 2-week tours. These short-term visits led to two Wuhan faculty engaging in year-long educational programs, one pre-doctoral and one post-doctoral. Since the initiation of the partnership, 30 faculty and 10 students from Wuhan and five faculty and six students from FPBSN have participated in cross-cultural educational experiences. In addition to the physical exchanges, there have been shared classes through the use of Polycom (video conferencing), with master's students from the two schools studying issues in community health nursing. Faculty from FPBSN have also traveled to Wuhan to teach graduate-level nursing theory and community health courses.

Curriculum Development

The Wuhan BSN curriculum was revised to reflect CWRU's early entry into nursing courses and clinical practice in the first year. In China the traditional curriculum requires the students to complete their academic work in the first 3 or 4 years and then spend 1 year rotating through the various services in the hospital for 10 months. Initially, Wuhan University had the students in theory and clinical practice during the students' last 2 years of nursing courses. After going to CWRU, the curriculum was revised so that the nursing courses began in the first year, with both theory and clinical practice throughout all 4 years.

The community health nursing has been expanded. Initially it was expanded to an entire semester, and now the class is split so that there are students all year in the community. In 2012, the undergraduate students began to do more activities in the communities, visit more in schools, and replicate what the faculty observed at CWRU, as well as continue to implement the programs that the graduate students did for their research. The community research projects were generated by master's students taught by one of the Case faculty who has been teaching students at the graduate level in community nursing and nursing theory for the past 5 years.

Other faculty have been teaching graduate-level courses and providing some guest lectures to the undergraduate students. Another activity created opportunities for master's students from Case and Wuhan to share several real-time classes in community health. This allowed the students to obtain perspectives on common public health issues and to be able to discuss them.

Two-Way Student Exchange

Beginning in 2010, the relationship between the schools expanded to include a two-way, one-semester student exchange. The exchange was designed to be an equal exchange of two senior students per year from each school studying for one semester at the other school. The academic programs of the students at each school were negotiated between the faculty of the two schools. After considerable discussion about a possible exchange, site visits were made by FPBSN faculty and staff to meet with HOPE faculty, visit clinical sites, and determine possible activities for the students. It was determined that the students would enroll in their parent school and pay tuition there, so that when they are in the other school, they pay their living expenses only. Credit from both institutions is accepted toward their degree requirements. Finally, with negotiations completed, an agreement was signed and in fall 2010, two students from each school exchanged places for the fall semester.

The goal for the exchange for FPBSN students was to experience community health care delivery in China and, in particular, to see Chinese community health care from the perspective of practitioners of traditional Chinese medicine and to gain insight into the Chinese health care delivery system. From the beginning, it was the expectation that they would attend classes with the HOPE School of Nursing students and spend 2 days per week working with the Qing Shan Community Health Clinic in Wuhan, China. This clinic is considered to be an outstanding example of traditional Chinese medicine. At the clinic, they worked with the clinic nursing staff observing traditional treatments such as cupping, massage, gua sha, moxibustion, and acupuncture. In addition, each group implemented a project focused on a select patient population being treated at the clinic as part of the CWRU capstone requirement.

The goals for the HOPE nursing students attending FPBSN included experiences with both community health and acute care with an overall goal of gaining understanding of the

U.S. health care delivery system. Students attend both the classroom and clinical components of second- or third-year adult health courses and participate in clinical work in the acute care setting along with the FPBSN students. They also complete coursework in public health nursing content and perform 150 hours of work in a combination of community health delivery settings. Students complete a community-based health care project most often focused on a selected patient population.

One of the challenges facing the HOPE School of Nursing and Dean Petrini was to develop the ongoing, local leadership of the school in preparation for the withdrawal of the Project HOPE support.

ACHIEVEMENTS, CHALLENGES, AND LESSONS LEARNED

Impact on Faculty and Institutions

After visiting FPBSN for these study opportunities, the faculty changed the curriculum, modeling the sequence of courses on the FPBSN curriculum. The faculty also learned about the many other services in which nurses work in the United States, such as hospice, flight nursing, school nursing, and community nursing. The faculty visited a variety of hospitals during the study tours so that they could observe nursing in the different clinical areas and see the various roles of the nurse not known in China. The person in charge of the undergraduate program (known in China as the faculty secretary for the undergraduate program), after visiting Case, agreed to make revisions in the curriculum sequence and content. It should be noted that a primary objective of the study tours was not just to expose the faculty and administrators to a different model of nursing and nursing education, but also to excite and motivate them to want to modify the content and the process of educating students currently used in the HOPE curriculum. Significant change became possible only when a critical mass of faculty and administrators had been exposed to new ideas and were ready to incorporate those ideas into the HOPE program. In this way, the impetus for the changes evolved from the faculty as a whole rather than the changes being imposed from above, with the administrative role being the facilitation, evaluation, and monitoring of the changes. The revisions have made a great improvement in the progress and attitude of the students. They become active in nursing courses in the first year and go to the clinical area for practice along with their classes, and they find that they enjoy working with the patients and families.

In addition there have been many changes in the manner in which they teach. The two university hospitals have modified their administration and practice after their visits. There have been many changes in the clinical setting in the administration, patient teaching, involvement of families, and in patient care. The Chinese government now provides scholarships to faculty to study abroad for 6 months to 1 year. In addition, the Chinese government provides 1-year scholarships for PhD students to study overseas. In 2013, the Chinese government added 5-month scholarships for undergraduate students. In fall 2013, there were four students studying at Case, two sponsored by the school and two sponsored by the national government.

Impact on Students

Presented with a challenge of living in a strange environment with strangers provides growth for all involved. While data about student perceptions of their experiences have not been systematically collected, considerable anecdotal evidence is available. FPBSN students have identified their experience in China as "life changing," "overwhelming," and "not always easy but incredible." As one student from Case commented, "China was not my first choice, but I feel so much a part of this community now I do not want to leave and I hope to return soon and work."

The Wuhan students report that the educational demands in the United States are greater than in China, which, until they went to the United States, they thought were great. They have also expressed satisfaction knowing that, while they have to work hard, they are able to "keep up with" their American colleagues. Several students have asked about the possibility of doing graduate work in the United States.

The director of the community health center where two students studied traditional medicine techniques for patients recovering from strokes wanted to hire them. He said, "they have been excellent students and we have been students, too. We have learned so much from them."

Challenges for the HOPE School of Nursing

Language: Throughout the process, we have encountered many challenges, some anticipated and some not. One anticipated challenge with the student exchange program was that none of the FPBSN students spoke Chinese. While many of the HOPE School of Nursing classes are conducted in English and most of the faculty and many students spoke English, patients in the clinical settings did not. Since one of the goals of the student exchange was to learn about health care delivery in China, this was a major barrier. The HOPE School of Nursing faculty addressed the issue by having the FPBSN students partnered with a HOPE School of Nursing student in the clinical area. A related challenge for the HOPE School of Nursing students at CWRU was that, while they spoke conversational English, the medical terminology used in the United States was less familiar. This was usually corrected over time through a medical terminology course and time spent in the clinical setting.

The cost of housing for the Chinese students in the United States is also a challenge. While the cost of tuition is eased as a concern by having students on both sides of the exchange pay tuition to their home school as usual, housing in a private U.S. institution can be an ongoing issue. This has been addressed by finding acceptable housing for the students outside of the university system.

Leadership: Another challenge is finding a leader who meets the criteria of Wuhan University with an academic BS, MS, and PhD, research grants, and clinical and teaching experience who can be appointed and continue to develop the faculty and school. Chinese advanced education for nurses only was initiated with one program in 1983 and 11 in 1984 for the baccalaureate programs; the MS programs were approved in 1992 for Beijing University, but it was several years before others were initiated; and the PhD programs for nurses were first introduced in 2005. The first baccalaureate graduates were in 1989, the first master's graduates were after the mid-1990s, and PhDs have only been in the past few years. The number of PhD nurses are few in the country. Chinese nurses who have studied abroad for advanced education often do not have an academic background, since they graduated from nonbaccalaureate academic programs for their initial nursing education and then were not able to continue in academic sequence. Graduation from foreign universities without the basic academic baccalaureate program initiated after the national exam disqualifies potential candidates.

The exchange program is now entering its fifth year, and ongoing leadership, institutionalization, and sustainability have emerged as primary concerns. Both universities have a commitment to international outreach and have developed some infrastructure that will support the programs of the schools. Within the schools of nursing, however, the issue of ongoing leadership and commitment is significant as administrators and faculty within the programs change, as well as program priorities. The exchange program has been incorporated into the curriculum of both programs supporting its institutionalization. It will be essential over the next 2 to 3 years, however, to transition the leadership of the exchange to other administrators and faculty and to maintain faculty development activity that will educate and motivate new generations of faculty to sustain it.

Lessons Learned

Given the opportunity to work in an environment different than their own, undergraduate and graduate students and faculty can all learn about another culture in ways that can enhance their provision of care in their own culture. Learning about other cultures is an ongoing process and will continue through the partnership.

A major lesson learned was the importance of developing the evaluation of a process during the period of initial planning. While the activities of the partnership were generally well thought through, we did not create a comprehensive evaluation process for the partnership outcomes. Some evaluation of individual activities was completed, such as student evaluations of the educational activities, and some retrospective evaluation is being planned. Yet we would have had a much richer and more complete evaluation had we made that part of the initial planning. One specific example is that while we do have some data related to student satisfaction with the educational activities, we have no data on whether having these international experiences impacted their ongoing professional development in any way. In addition, while we are able to identify specific achievements of the collaboration, data documenting the institutional impact on either side of the partnership have not been systematically collected.

FUTURE PLANS FOR ONGOING PARTNERSHIP

Future plans for the partnership include continuing the educational outreach, program evaluation, and developing a program of research evolving out of the work of the partnership. Specifically, Wuhan University has learned that the Chinese government will sponsor MS students to study abroad; the plan is to obtain some of these funds to send graduate students abroad to enhance their education and in turn improve the quality of the MS program. This strategy will help develop ongoing and future leadership for the school.

Developing programs of research by both faculty and students is also part of future planning. Specifically, studies need to be developed that provide evidence to identify best practices in clinical settings and the impact of culture on practice and outcome. Joint publications of activities of both research and the programs will be encouraged. Each student who participates in an exchange should be able to produce at least one article for publication in an international science citation index (SCI), and the Chinese students should, in addition, publish in a top Chinese journal. Finally, we plan to identify models and develop instruments to measure outcomes of international partnerships such as this one.

CONCLUSION

This program has greatly enhanced nursing education in HOPE School of Nursing of Wuhan University. It has set new standards for education and practice by those who have participated. A director of nursing commented, "We have made some changes, and more are planned, but change is a slow process." At the same time, the FPBSN faculty and students who have participated have been enriched and changed by the experience. It has been like dropping a pebble in a pond as the ripples have reached out beyond these two schools. The students touched by this program are working across both China and the United States, introducing new ideas and new ways to care for patients and families. The impact is greater than was perhaps originally anticipated.

REFLECTIVE QUESTIONS

1. One of the characteristics of this partnership is the awareness of the contribution each partner is making to the other. How does this change the activity, the outcomes, and the sustainability of the relationship as compared to an international outreach activity wherein one partner is clearly the "giver" of benefit and the other the recipient?
2. Sustainability of an international program is dependent on its integration into the overall mission of the school or institution and on the ability of the current leadership/administration to effectively transition the leadership of the program to the next generation. What steps are essential in making such a transition?
3. This partnership has promoted major changes in nursing curriculum, teaching strategies, and models of nursing care. What are the essential steps in creating such substantive change?
4. What are the characteristics of the individuals involved in an academic exchange that make it successful?
5. How can the resources and richness of international exchange programs be shared and stimulate faculty, students, and administration in the participating institutions?

The Voluntary Medical Male Circumcision Project: The Role of the Nurse Leader and Jhpiego Technical Advisor

Leah J. Hart
Peter Johnson
Geoffrey Menego

CONTEXT: KENYA[1]

The east Africa country of Kenya shares its borders with Tanzania to the south, Uganda and southern Sudan to the west, Somalia and the Indian Ocean to the east, and Ethiopia to the north. Approximately 62% of its young people are younger than 25 years of age in an estimated population of over 44 million (Central Intelligence Agency, 2013).

In Kenya, 6.3% of adults between the ages of 15 and 49 are HIV positive. In 2009, 1.4 million Kenyans were infected; approximately 80,000 die each year from conditions related to the disease. Prevalence of HIV varies widely, from 0.9% in the northeastern province to 13.9% in Nyanza. Other than Nairobi (with a 7% prevalence rate taken as its own entity), Nyanza and the western provinces have the highest prevalence rates, at 13.9% and 6.6%, respectively. From 2003 to 2009, the number of men and women receiving HIV testing and counseling tripled in Kenya. Also, more than half of pregnant women accepted an HIV test and subsequent counseling from 2007 to 2009 (KSPA, 2010).

Jhpiego, an affiliate of Johns Hopkins University, is the lead partner in a project known as APHIA*plus* (AIDS Population and Health Integrated Assistance): **P**eople-driven and client-centered, **L**eadership at all levels, **U**niversal access to services, **S**ustainability. The project was initiated in January 2011, funded by the United States Agency for International Development (USAID) in Kenya, and supports the Ministry of Health (MOH) of Kenya to improve health outcomes and impact through sustainable country-led programs and partnership. The programs implemented by the project include voluntary medical male circumcision (VMMC), HIV testing and counseling (HTC), maternal/child and neonatal health (MCNH), family planning (FP), HIV care and treatment, and social determinants of health, among others. This case study focuses on the VMMC.

PARTNERSHIP FOR KENYA MALE CIRCUMCISION PROJECT

A partnership between Jhpiego, PATH, EGPAF, World Vision, Broadreach, and Mildmay facilitates the voluntary circumcisions of 20 million men between the ages of 15 and 49 in eastern and southern Africa by 2016 for HIV prevention.

Rationale for Voluntary Medical Male Circumcision

Male circumcision is an important intervention that is increasingly being incorporated into national HIV prevention programs, especially in settings where HIV prevalence is high and the prevalence of male circumcision is low, such as in parts of Nyanza and the western provinces in Kenya. VMMC has been shown to reduce men's risk of acquiring HIV through heterosexual intercourse by as much as 60%. In order to protect the spread of HIV among women, VMMC in noninfected men reduces the likelihood of infection in women, because HIV-negative men cannot infect their partners. Study models project that if circumcision rates reach a level of 80% for men, an equal decline in infection rates in women will occur over the following 15 years (PEPFAR, n.d.).

Further, studies show that in addition to being somewhat protected against acquiring the HIV virus, circumcised men are less likely to acquire a number of sexually transmitted infections (STIs). Reduced rates of STIs also benefit women as prevalence rates fall in countries where VMMC attains high coverage rates. A further benefit to women is protection against human papillomavirus (HPV), which is associated with cervical cancer in women. As a result of the likely reduction in HIV infections and cervical cancer in women, billions of U.S. dollars could be saved in treatment costs.

Project Goals

The VMMC program supports 29 health facilities in the western region of Kenya to provide free, high-quality VMMC services. The aim is to circumcise 80% of uncircumcised men aged 15 to 49 in eight districts in Nyanza and four in the western provinces. In line with national VMMC guidelines, the project supports integration of VMMC services into existing health services delivery systems, such as voluntary counseling and testing, family planning, antenatal care services, outpatient, and sexually transmitted infection clinics. This is done through static health facility service via outreach and campaigning during school holidays. Specific project goals include:

- Strengthen and expand VMMC static service delivery by capacity building health care workers through training, mentorship, and site orientation.
- Improve and maintain quality of services through provision of equipment, instruments, educational materials, and job aids (such as the circumcision procedure checklist).
- Reach men above age 25 with VMMC services through innovative recruitment techniques.
- Perform post–male circumcision (MC) follow-up with the support of automated SMS reminders (10 messages from day 1 to 6 weeks).
- Support the Ministry of Health (MOH) to help it capture MC data through routine health information systems.
- Expand the number of sites supporting VMMC at both facility and community levels.
- Support and strengthen VMMC leadership and coordination at the national, provincial/county, and district levels.
- Medicalize traditional circumcision in traditionally circumcising communities.
- Support early infant male circumcision (EIMC).

Role of Nurses

Nurses provide the majority of health services at all levels of health care delivery in this target area of Kenya (see Table 10.1). In small facilities, especially in the rural areas of the country, nurses hold the highest level of the technical expertise in terms of providing treatment of minor ailments, dispensing of drugs, nursing patients, maternal and child health services, among many other services—in addition to management of the facilities.

TABLE 10.1 Providers of VMMC Services

Cadre of health care worker	Number of providers	Provider types (%)
Nurses and midwives	84	75.6
Clinical officers	26	23.4
Medical officer	1	1

Although the Jhpiego/APHI*plus* project began in 2011, VMMC began in Kenya in 2008 as an HIV prevention strategy. Initially, it was challenging to reach potential clients due to personnel shortages. At that time, only medical doctors and clinical officers (assistant medical officers) were allowed to perform circumcisions. The scope of practice for Kenyan nurses did not cover VMMC. In June 2009, the government of Kenya decided to allow nurses to perform circumcisions after undergoing training, since they were the majority of the skilled personnel in health facilities. The Nyanza Reproductive Health Society collaborated to train nurses to perform VMMC surgery (Curran et al., 2011).

Geoffrey Menego serves as the technical advisor for the Jhpiego/APHI*plus* VMMC project in Kenya. He holds a nursing degree and a master's degree in community health and development (MCHD) from the University of the Great Lakes/Tropical Institute of Community Health and Development and brings expertise in community health and development and community health nursing. As technical advisor his role is to:

- Provide technical leadership, coordination, and supervision for all VMMC activities for the APHIA*plus* Western Kenya Project, and ensure maximum integration of project activities across and within technical areas.
- Ensure that Jhpiego's scope of work for the APHIA*plus* Western Kenya Project is carried out to the fullest extent possible and to the highest possible degree of quality.
- Lead the process of developing work plans and activity budgets for all VMMC activities for the project.
- Provide all necessary support to ensure the successful implementation of project activities, including through technical oversight, work planning, budgeting, reconciliation of finances, and reporting.
- Supervise the work of all Jhpiego staff contributing to the success of VMMC activities for the APHIA*plus* Western Kenya Project.

Results

In the Jhpiego-led VMMC program, 74,390 male circumcisions have been performed in the past 2½ years, with target goals exceeded for 2011 and 2012 (see Table 10.2). The project is expected to exceed its 2013 target goals as well. Of these procedures, 80% were performed by nurses, who form 84% of the surgical teams.

Through Geoffrey Menego's leadership, surgical teams have been trained along with mentorship of technical staff, orientations, and on-the-job training of staff. Presentations and coordination at the local, national, and international levels have also been convened and championed by Geoffrey.

CHALLENGES

There are challenges for the success of VMMC programs in Africa, particularly because of the need for support at the administrative levels in the host country. Political priorities for planning and implementation of the MC programs can facilitate or slow the progress

TABLE 10.2 Number of Men Receiving Services

Year	Target	Number circumcised
2011	12,500	16,345
2012	30,000	35,214
2013	40,000	27,831 (as of August 2013)
TOTAL	**82,500**	**74,390**

of the program (Reed et al., 2012). Other specific challenges include project delays that are incurred due to administrative factors that lead to delayed procurement of essential equipment required for service delivery. Having local project champions such as Geoffrey Menego coordinate activities helps with these administrative challenges. Additionally, policies that reduce access to pharmaceuticals required for MC service delivery can delay operations due to the lack of necessary medications.

Other administrative challenges include factors that occur at the local treatment facility. First, delays can occur in the timely flow of data from the local treatment facility to the Ministry of Health level. Second, some facilities lack adequate space for VMMC delivery.

LESSONS LEARNED

There are aspects of the VMMC project that were particularly effective. For one, allowing the MOH to take the lead and coordinate VMMC service delivery has ensured ownership of the program at all ministry levels, as well as assurance of sustainability. Community health workers were effective community mobilizers and helped link many men to VMMC services. The strategy known as MOVE (Model of Optimizing Volume and Efficiency) during campaigns enabled the program to reach many men and attain set targets. Jhpiego staff, known for their technical leadership and training expertise in terms of high-quality VMMC service delivery, met the MOH/WHO-recommended standards. The opportunity for Jhpiego to successfully provide VMMC trainings and static facility delivery of services from the campaign approach has provided visibility for the organization at the national, provincial, and district levels.

Most relevant to global nursing, nurses and midwives provided the majority of VMMC services, leading to the success of the APHIA*plus* VMMC project implementation, as well as meeting the demand for future service delivery.

REFLECTIVE QUESTIONS

1. The process of sensitizing community leaders to the benefits of VMMC took several months. Does this surprise you? Why or why not?
2. Do you agree with the need for universal HIV testing before conducting VMMC? What are the advantages and potential disadvantages?
3. VMMC reduces HIV risk for men (directly) and for women (indirectly). In Kenya, the prevalence of HIV in women is about twice the prevalence in men (Kenya National Coordinating Agency for Population and Development, 2010). To reduce transmission of HIV in the entire Kenyan population, what other strategies besides VMMC would you recommend be scaled up?
4. Early resumption of sexual intercourse can potentially increase the risk of HIV transmission to female partners. What counseling would you recommend that VMMC service providers offer men and their partners to reduce partner risk?

5. Men seeking VMMC may come with a variety of sexual and reproductive health concerns. What other sexual and reproductive health education and counseling topics might be addressed before and after VMMC?

NOTE

1. This case study was funded by the U.S. Agency for International Development under the APHIA Plus project, in collaboration with the Kenya Ministry of Health.

REFERENCES

Central Intelligence Agency. (2013). *The World Factbook, 2013–14*. Washington, DC: Author.

Curran, K., Njeuhmeli, E., Mirelman, A., Dickson, K., Adamu, T., Cherutich, P., . . . Stanton, D. (2011). Voluntary medical male circumcision: Strategies for meeting human resource needs of scale-up in southern and eastern Africa. *PLOSMedicine*. www.plosmedicine.org/article/info%3Adoi%2F10.1371%2Fjournal.pmed.1001129

Kenya National Coordinating Agency for Population and Development. (2010). Kenya Service Provision Assessment Survey.

PEPFAR. (n.d.). PEPFAR's best practices for voluntary medical male circumcision site operations. Author.

Reed, J. R., Njeuhmeli, E., Thomas, A. G., Bacon, M. C., Bailey, R., Cherutich, P., . . . Bock, N. (2012). Voluntary medical male circumcision: An HIV prevention for PEPFAR. *Journal of Acquired Immune Deficiency Syndrome, 60*(3), S88–S95. doi: 10.1097/QAI.0b013e31825cac4e

CHAPTER 11

Ongoing Project Support

Leah J. Hart
Peter Johnson

> Give a person a fish and that person will eat for a day. Teach a person to fish and that person will eat for a lifetime.

This chapter is written from the perspective of nurses engaged in international health work from within a nonprofit/nongovernmental organization (NP/NGO). Global health work in the NP/NGO world often revolves around grant cycles. For long-lasting, positive change to be wrought for a target group, a global health nurse must maintain a long-term perspective and realistically assess whether activities will continue to make a difference after the grant money is spent.

Of course, a nurse can volunteer or work internationally short term without planning ongoing project support at the individual level when serving with an organization that has a strong partnership built into its model of care. Sustaining partnerships at the organizational level is essential to ethical and responsible global health care. Volunteering on a medical mission that performs surgeries in one place, one time, for example, may be fulfilling and exciting, and will undoubtedly affect the lives of those people who benefit from the surgery. However, this type of intervention is distinct from projects that seek to create long-lasting positive effects. The outcomes achieved by the nurse contributing to the short-term project, while significant, are unlikely to directly lead to any significant long-term effects on health or health systems.

In the NP/NGO world, wherein program managers are responsible for reporting the results of the work accomplished using grant funds, a "one-time" intervention is not an option. Furthermore, it may be more fulfilling to work on projects that have a long-term vision. If not, you may leave a place where you put your heart and soul into an effort and come back to find things are exactly as they were before the work was started.

To uphold professional and ethical standards for global health nursing, project implementers must be realistic about the goals of a project, considering time and resources available. Part of this consideration should focus on ongoing project support (Crigger, 2008). Ongoing project support is a crucial part of any global health venture that involves any hope for long-term, sustainable effects. Thus, ongoing support must be considered during the planning phase of a project. Developing a specific strategy for ongoing support at the inception of a global health endeavor will involve defining the overall life span and specific stages of the project and budgeting for appropriate resources and personnel to support all stages, even those when minimal contact is planned with the target country or population.

Jhpiego: An Affiliate of Johns Hopkins University

Jhpiego organization relies on about 35 local offices staffed by professionals from within the countries in which they are located. Clinical experts at the headquarters offices (Baltimore and Washington, DC) provide strategic support during short-term visits and ongoing project support.

Jhpiego strengthens the capacity of locally hired public health and health professionals in multiple program efforts over a period of time. Relationships are established this way with governments, ministries of health and education, and local clinical experts. The work also benefits from a deep understanding of the local health care system, culture, and language(s), as well as the various challenges and opportunities relevant to the local context.

THE "LAY OF THE LAND" IN GLOBAL HEALTH

For success in program implementation, including the ongoing support phase, understanding the various influential partners involved in global health work is vital. A typical landscape of partners will include the following:

- Local* office of an international NP/NGO
- Local* NGO
- Faith-based organization
- Local* university
- Government agency (such as the Ministry of Health or suboffices)
- Professional associations (such as the nursing association)
- Regulatory bodies (a nursing council, for example)

*The word "local," in this sense, refers to the international setting.

Prior to beginning project work, it is wise to "do your research." Inquire about the current players in the health field, about any tensions or particular strong partnerships that exist, and about those influential organizational leaders who may be instrumental to a project's success or failure.

Don't Go It Alone

A long-term program that will require ongoing support will by definition *not* be a one-person show. It is worth mentioning not only the international players, but also the team of program implementers, from an NP/NGO perspective:

- Programming experts
- Finance
- Proposal development team
- Monitoring and evaluation specialists
- Public health and medical field experts

Defining Project Goals

All global health programs should have a clearly articulated mission and goals, and nurses who participate in global health projects must clearly understand them to be effective partners. In particular for grant-based work, a project implementer should always have the written goals and objectives of the project that was funded in mind. A question that a global health nurse operating in the NP/NGO sector should consider is *Who is funding this, and what deliverables do they expect as a result of the funding?* Project operations should all relate to these deliverables, as well as to the overall goals of the project.

PLANNING FOR SUCCESSFUL PROJECTS AND ONGOING PROJECT SUPPORT

An important question to ask before spending valuable resources to conduct global health work is *What local capacity exists to continue this work when the initiation phase is over?* In other words, is it possible to keep things going with remote ongoing project support? If not, engage with local stakeholders to shore up capacity as necessary (or be ready to let the project go). This process may involve training and capacity building to improve written language skills, computer skills, and organizational structure or setting up incentive structures to encourage professionalism. If the project plan is overly ambitious, too complicated, or out of touch with the local context, no amount of ongoing project support will keep things on track. Aligning expectations with reality at every phase of a project will help bypass avoidable failures and result in long-term sustainability and lasting effects.

To understand effective ongoing project support, it may be helpful to think of what project support (and capacity building work in general) is not. To promote local ownership of projects, it may be that you, the ongoing project support contact, will not directly create deliverables. It is more meaningful and helpful in the end if you review, edit, and generally support the production of a deliverable (such as a research plan, a program report, or a publication) rather than draft it yourself.

Relationship Building

Nurses who are interested in global health work are likely a self-selected group of people who are interested in learning about other parts of the world and experiencing other languages, cultures, and people through travel. As noted in previous chapters, to be an effective partner in global health work, the nurse must also be prepared to enter into a partnership that joins with host country partners in respectful, reciprocal, and ongoing relationships. On-the-ground support of a project in the global context will indeed involve all the fun, excitement, challenges, and—at times—discomfort of most international travel. Still, one of the most rewarding parts of working in an international NP/NGO community is building relationships with people from all over the world.

Above and Beyond

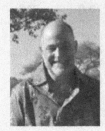

You can take relationship building so seriously that it can lead to running a marathon! At the urging of a major development donor, Peter Johnson, director of the Global Learning Office, ran a marathon in Gaborone, the capital city of Botswana, to raise money for a school. The money raised was primarily donated by U.S. midwives. The school that received the funds is located in the home village of a Jhpiego office staff member who has become a friend of Peter's through their shared global health work in Botswana and the region.

To provide effective ongoing project support after an in-country visit to a global health project, you will need to effectively establish connections during your visit(s). You can do so by avoiding the following pitfalls:

- Working with too few stakeholders or stakeholders who are not representative of the majority (not part of the mainstream)—you'll meet resistance when they leave
- Promising more than you can deliver
- Providing what *you* think people need instead of what they (actually) need
- Providing what people want without undergoing a process of appreciative inquiry (AI)

- Forgetting to see the big picture: addressing one part of the health system (training) while supplies/equipment remain absent
- Spending all your time with one key person on the ground—it's important to garner diversity in your partnerships
- Forgetting to seek out nursing colleagues—be prepared to work with a variety of professionals in global health, but do make a sincere effort to strengthen the global partnership of nurses

---

A Prime Example of What Happens When . . .

A donor provided funds to start a midwifery education program in a place where gaps existed in terms of meeting the needs of pregnant women. The program was housed in a School of Public Health and was run by high-quality educators with vast midwifery experience. As graduates of the program were produced, it became clear that a vital factor had been overlooked in planning the intervention to address the needs of mothers and babies. There was no law in existence to govern practice of midwives. The donors and implementers of the education program had not engaged with lawmakers, councils of health professionals, and professional associations to ensure that graduates of the midwifery program would be able to legally practice. Now, the scope of practice for those graduates (there are more than 40, to date) is limited by the regulatory environment. This is a prime example of a well-designed, well-meaning intervention that relied on too few stakeholders.

Cross-Cultural Relationship Building

This topic has been addressed in earlier chapters. Still, it is worth mentioning that ongoing project support will require a keen ability to build relationships transculturally. The primary method for building an appreciation for a culture different than one's own is to understand one's own culture. Cultural self-awareness is indispensable to building relationships with those who may hold different beliefs and values from yours (Bramwell & Irvin, 2009).

In light of the inevitable differences between you and those you are supporting, you must listen carefully to your partners on the ground. Double-check the alignment of your understanding of the project progress with your colleagues' by asking clarifying questions at every turn. Seek to understand your differences as well as to celebrate them.

It can be just as important to find common ground with your in-country partners. When working with nurses, ask about their experiences as nurses. Finding a common passion for the work you do will be a compelling force for achievement of project goals. This can be done formally or informally. For example, when engaged in a workshop or training with a group of nurses, consider beginning the training with an exercise to get to know your audience and their experience. Request that participants share a particularly memorable patient or community with which they have worked. This can be the basis of a "getting to know you" exercise or a method of identifying strengths and weaknesses of the health care system where these nurses practice. Be sure to participate in the storytelling yourself. You may be surprised at the similarities of nursing stories from around the world, even with drastic differences in available resources for caring for patients and communities.

STAYING IN TOUCH

Scheduling Ongoing Project Support

Planning meetings, trainings, research activities such as data collection or analysis, and other major events often determines the travel schedule associated with in-country support of global health initiatives. In between these trips, it is important to stay in touch.

Consider proactively pursuing phone, Skype, or e-mail communication and be sure to send any follow-up deliverables promptly after a trip. Besides providing means of communication necessary to keeping things moving, using the various methods here described will document your efforts at ongoing project support.

Operational Tools

Be sure to use tools, including documents for tracking project progress, that have been established while working with stakeholders in country. If new and unfamiliar management systems are imposed remotely, there is likely to be a disconnect between those promoting the tool and those who are unfamiliar with it.

An example of a tool for remote project support may be as simple as an activity matrix e-mailed as a Word document. Table 11.1 presents a rough outline of an action plan matrix following up a program activity.

Technology and Media

Visits to countries, whether or not they are global health–focused, are expensive. It is therefore responsible and prudent for program managers to determine how to best stay connected between trips. Technology has changed the way the world communicates and operates, and global health is no exception (Lewis et al., 2012).

mHealth

- Cell phones: calling
  While in country, it is strongly recommended that you acquire a local SIM card. This requires an unlocked phone (talk to your carrier about the process of unlocking a phone for use outside the United States). Alternatively, arrange to borrow a local cell phone from a partner while you are visiting. It is critical that you be able to be in phone contact with your partners to maximize the time spent face to face. When considering whether to stay connected by phone after returning home, consider the local context. Although cell phones have become ubiquitous worldwide in terms of numbers of phones/population, there may be patterns of phone ownership and use that will influence how effective a device the phone is for communication related to ongoing project support (WHO, 2011). For example, it may be easy to connect with project leaders who stay in an urban area but more difficult to connect directly with rural health care providers, who may not have consistent cell phone service. The types of

TABLE 11.1 Draft Program Activity and Schedule Matrix

Action item	Who's responsible?	Due date	Notes/Progress
Compiling results	Local staff		Completed
Data entry	Local staff		Completed
Data analysis	Local staff with headquarters (HQ) support		Completed
Report writing	Local staff with HQ support		Drafting in progress
Results dissemination meeting	Local staff and HQ staff		Communicating with stakeholders with regard to availability and scheduling of dissemination meeting

phone and phone plans available may also be a factor. Many international cell phone companies do not charge for incoming calls, for example, ensuring that people are willing to pick up all calls, without concern for cost. From the U.S. side of things, of course, international cell phone calls or international plans with no roaming can be quite expensive.

- Cell phones: texting (known internationally as "SMS")
  In terms of local communication, sending an SMS is a highly reliable and appropriate form of communication. Internationally, it may be difficult and expensive to find carriers that include international text messaging as part of regular plans (Zurovac et al., 2011).

- Tablets and smartphones
  These are becoming increasingly popular, even in very poor and rural settings, worldwide (Vital Wave Consulting, 2009). Applications for Android/Windows machines provide an exciting window of opportunity for providing remote training, practice reminders, or even alternative ways to stay in touch, such as "Whatsapp" (www.whatsapp.com/android).

eHealth

- Skype
  This method of connecting for free with anyone who has Internet access is an invaluable resource for keeping in touch. Aspects of a free Skype account include the following:

  - Video and voice calls to anyone else signed up for Skype: This is a good venue for regularly scheduled check-ins.
  - Instant messaging: For very brief exchanges, or for "just saying hello," instant messaging via Skype is preferable to e-mail.
  - Screen sharing and file sharing: You can send files via Skype as an attachment as if by an e-mail carrier. Even more useful is a live screen capture. When you screen share, the person on the receiving end of the call can see your screen and your mouse. You can jointly review and edit documents with colleagues remotely using this helpful feature.

  By paying a monthly fee, additional features are available:

  - International calls to mobile phones and landlines (unlimited minutes): This is helpful for staying in touch not only with colleagues, but also with friends and family while traveling.
  - Text messages: For those who have smartphone devices running the Skype app, this is often a cheaper alternative to international text plans with cell phone carriers.
  - Group conference calls for up to 10 people (www.skype.com/en/what-is-skype).

- E-mail
  E-mail is a tool that should be approached with some caution. First, it can be difficult to interpret cultural nuances on both ends, leading to potential miscommunications or unfortunate relationship dynamics. Second, e-mail volume can be a deterrent to reading, let alone responding, to e-mails. Keeping e-mails brief and focused will improve response rates from local partners and reduce the potential for misunderstanding. Depending on the nature of your relationship with the colleague on the ground, it may be appropriate to reach out for non-work-related events, such as holidays, family events, and just saying, "I'm thinking about you—hope you're doing well."

- Webinar meetings
  - Web-based presentations are a preferred alternative to e-mailed presentations in terms of knowledge transfer and engagement of recipients in question-and-answer sessions.
  - Consider holding webinar meetings at times that would be during normal business hours for the target location, which may mean very early or late hours for you, the presenter.
  - Keep in mind the different levels of technology infrastructure and user comfort level when hosting a webinar presentation or meeting. Avoid creating any barriers, such as password-protected presentations or large files to be shared during the presentation (including videos that are not yet streamed/downloaded).

The Power of People

Human capital is the most valuable resource a project has. The previous chapter addresses local leaders and champions who can be instrumental to the success of global health interventions. These same champions can be an important source of ongoing project support by providing follow-up training, addressing questions, and touching base more regularly with less attendant cost.

Regional Champions

From Zambia and Kenya, respectively, Lastina Lwatula and Rosemary Kamunya are nurse-midwives who are two of Jhpiego's most powerful advocates, mobilizers, trainers, and nurses. In the past 5 years, they have conducted scores of trainings, reaching hundreds of local leaders on topics such as:

- Assessing local capacity
- Enhancing training capacity
- Strengthening nursing education
- Improving quality
- Improving reproductive health service delivery
- Strengthening nursing association
- Supporting nursing policy

They have provided trainings in their home countries as well as in many other regions, among these Uganda, Botswana, Swaziland, Lesotho, Tanzania, Ghana, and Ethiopia.

WITHDRAWING ONGOING PROJECT SUPPORT

It may become obvious that ongoing project support is insufficient to keep a project alive. There may be schedule delays for major events or a lack of responsiveness to efforts to keep in touch. If this is the case, be proactive in requesting a conference call with appropriate players to assess the health of the project and to evaluate what further project support is needed that is not currently being provided. Maintaining professional, respectful communication is always important but is especially critical at times when there may be tension between the local implementers and those providing ongoing project support. See Table 11.2 for potential threats to project implementation and suggested responses.

   If there is a long-term established pattern of nonresponsiveness, lack of engagement, and stakeholder disinterest in a certain location, it may prompt the difficult decision to discontinue project support. Efforts should be made to avoid this, of course, but at times it is

TABLE 11.2 Assessing and Responding to Project Threats

Concerning pattern	How to address
Decreasing or sporadic communication	Remain proactive in your communications and promptly reply to responses.
Unresponsiveness to project deliverables	Request confirmation of the receipt of the deliverable, along with specific feedback. Provide a formal evaluation form and ask for it to be returned for "official" feedback.
Increasing side communication	Remain professional in your communications: Do not write things that leave the impression that you are personally frustrated with the project. Clearly restate the goals of the project and encourage all players to recommit to the goals or to voice specific barriers that are preventing progress. Encourage a meeting in which all partners are invited to participate.
Long delays in implementation	Reassess the capacity of the implementers. It may be that further capacity building is necessary before the project can move forward. Continue to be proactive in your communications, and redouble your relationship-building efforts. Consider requesting an in-person visit.

the most responsible and logical option in light of limitations of time and resources. Before withdrawing support, every effort should be made to communicate the wish to revitalize the project. Make at least three offers to travel to meet with stakeholders in person and discuss together what could be done to improve project vitality. If the offers are refused or ignored, then make it clear that project support will be withdrawn if responsiveness and engagement remain low. Be prepared to set clear, redefined goals, timelines, and limits to get a project back on track or to define an end point should that be necessary.

Ongoing Project Support as a Means of Program Evaluation

Ongoing project support often involves monitoring and evaluation that can potentially be used to answer research questions. As you develop plans for ongoing project support, consider aligning the monitoring and evaluation indicators to the research agenda of nurse scholars engaging in global nursing efforts.

Evaluation is an important aspect of all project-based work—not only for improved project performance, but also to demonstrate results for funders. Use the original goal and purpose of the grant funding as a benchmark for whether the ongoing project support was effective. It may be that the end product of a project does not match the deliverable, as it was written in a work plan. However, it might be that the process, or the end product, was still helpful. Examine with the team: What went well? What could have been improved? What needs adjusting for future projects? Communicate these things, along with successes, to the funder when you present results.

CONCLUSION

The availability of technology reduces the likelihood that partnerships will end when the visiting team departs. Whether for months or years, providing ongoing project support can be a challenging yet rewarding process. The tools contained in this chapter are some ways to build relationships, to stay connected, and to monitor your success in your endeavor to provide ongoing project support.

REFERENCES

Bramwell, O., & Irvin, S. (2009). Cultural awareness in intercultural mentoring: A model for enhancing mentoring relationships. *International Journal of Leadership Studies, 5*(1), 37–50.

Crigger, N. (2008). Towards a viable and just global nursing ethics. *Nursing Ethics, 15*(1), 17–27.

Lewis, T., Synowiec, C., Lagomarsino, G., & Schweitzer, J. (2012). E-health in low- and middle-income countries: Findings from the Center for Health Market Innovations. *Bulletin of the World Health Organization, 90,* 332–340. doi: 10.2471/BLT.11.099820; www.who.int/bulletin/volumes/90/5/11-099820/en

Vital Wave Consulting: UN Foundation-Vodafone Foundation Partnership. (2009). mHealth for development: The opportunity of mobile technology for healthcare in the developing world.

WHO. (2011). mHealth: New horizons for health through mobile technologies: Second global survey on eHealth. www.who.int/goe/publications/goe_mhealth_web.pdf

Zurovac, D., Sudoi, R., Akhwale, W., Ndiritu, M., Hamer, D., Rowe, A., & Snow, R. (2011). The effect of mobile phone text-message reminders on Kenyan health workers' adherence to malaria treatment guidelines: A cluster randomised trial. *The Lancet, 378,* 795–803.

Interprofessional Partnerships With a Telehealth Project in Waslala, Nicaragua

Ruth McDermott-Levy
Miguel Angel Estopinan

CONTEXT: NICARAGUA

Nicaragua is the poorest country in Central America and the second poorest country in the Western hemisphere (Central Intelligence Agency, 2013). Nicaraguans living in the city have access to doctors, nurses, and health services, but those living in rural communities, such as the communities surrounding Waslala, receive primary health care at health outpost clinics staffed by physicians and nurses still in their first year of practice. Additionally, the travel time to the hospital for more complex health problems can be as long as 8 hours and includes walking and traveling by horse or truck (Singh, Kulkarni, Keech, McDermott-Levy, & Kligler, 2011). Within the rural communities, volunteer community health workers (CHWs) who have received basic health training in common diseases serve as the first link to the health care system. For the most part, Waslala's CHWs' highest level of education is the 8th grade, with most CHWs having a 4th-grade or lower formal education. With their basic health training, the CHWs must make health recommendations to the members of their communities.

Waslala was among the regions where the 1980s Nicaraguan Contra–Sandinista war was fought (Water for Waslala, n.d.). U.S. participation and support of the Contras during the war has influenced the perception of people from the United States in the currently Sandinista-governed region. Villanova University College of Nursing and College of Engineering have been working within the Waslala region since 2004. The early programs involved water access and water hygiene. (See Water for Waslala at www.waterforwaslala.org.) Initially U.S. workers and Nicaraguan organizations got to know each other and worked on building mutual trust. As the relationship between the university, the local Catholic parish, and community organizations in Waslala developed, an opportunity presented itself to introduce cell phones into the CHWs' toolkit to support the health of the remote, rural communities. Introduction of cell phones supported the health of the people in the region in two ways: Equipped with the cell phones, the CHWs could (a) have a real-time health consultation with a nurse or physician in Waslala and (b) record patient information via SMS, generating an electronic health record (EHR). The EHR provided a previously unavailable way of gathering health data in the region.

A TEAM APPROACH

To develop and maintain a sustainable telehealth project, an interprofessional team approach was necessary. The first team members included faculty from Villanova University College of Nursing, College of Engineering, and School of Business, along with representatives of the local community development nongovernmental organization (NGO) (Asociación de Desarrollo Integral y Sostenible, ADIS). The history of successful programs between all constituencies and the trusting relationships that had formed facilitated the implementation of a new project in the region. The faculty worked with the in-country public health providers through the Catholic parish health program to do the following:

- Address the health problems
- Identify the health information to be recorded, including the software for recording the EHR data
- Develop a solar-powered method of providing energy to cell phones and computer systems
- Develop a project timeline
- Secure funding for the project

The initial project funding came from a National Collegiate Inventors and Innovators Alliance Sustainable Vision grant (see www.magpi.net/Notes/Funding/National-Collegiate-Inventors-and-Innovators-Alliance-Sustainable-Vision-Grants) toward developing the first phase of the project.

In addition to serving the community of Waslala, the telehealth project included an educational component of program development, technology implementation, and software development in an underresourced region. Thus nursing, engineering, and business students were included in all aspects of the project. This enhanced our work as the students easily participated in creative and innovative approaches to conceptualizing, implementing, and troubleshooting all aspects of the project—a new experience for both the in-country team members and the faculty. In addition, at the time there was very little in the literature regarding the use of cell phones with CHWs in this capacity. The students offered valuable and creative ideas that were untethered to previous assumptions. Their input and their willingness to take risks helped move the project forward.

It was also important to engage the CHWs as partners in this project. On the telehealth exploratory visit in May 2011, a qualitative descriptive study of the CHWs' learning and resource needs was conducted to gain an understanding of the CHWs' perceptions of the health problems in their communities (McDermott-Levy & Weatherbie, 2013). This

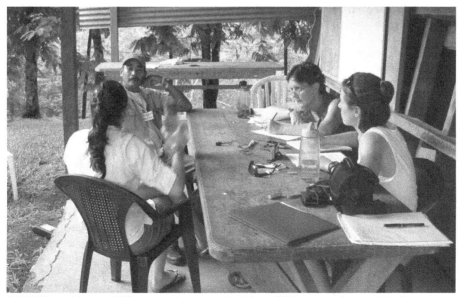

Ruth McDermott-Levy and Villanova students consult with local CHWs.   *Source*: R. McDermott-Levy

information, along with the inclusion of the CHWs in problem solving and process evaluation for the project, has established the partnership between the CHWs and the other team members. In a follow-up study in May 2013, the CHWs reported that having cell phones and contact with health care professionals increased their confidence, increased the respect garnered from their communities, and enabled them to recognize themselves as important members of the telehealth project team (McDermott-Levy & Fitzpatrick, 2013) (see Table 11.3).

WORKING ACROSS DISCIPLINES

Working in an ongoing international project that relies on technology has stretched the roles of all team members. A variety of challenges have been addressed during this project. The first was working across disciplines: Each discipline has its own body of knowledge and vocabulary. Within this group of nurses, engineers, and businesspeople, the same word can have different meanings. For example, in nursing the word *scale* is a noun: a tool for measuring a parameter (such as weight), a health indicator (depression scale), or a tool for measuring a variable to be tested (acculturation scale). But our colleagues in business and engineering use *scale* as a verb: to indicate growing or developing a product or innovation to its fullest capacity. Frequently in discussions, we found that we needed to stop to be sure we all understood how a word was being used and whether we were all using the same definition. In a conference on working across disciplines sponsored by the Institute of Medicine, Dr. Patricia Werhane (2013) from DePaul University described boundaries that are formed between disciplines and the value within and between the boundaries of each discipline. Dr. Werhane recommended using "Creole" in interprofessional communication as she described a blend of languages from each discipline forming a shared language to promote interprofessional work. In addition to the language of a particular discipline, many people see the role of a nurse only as providing care in the hospital. For many outside of the profession, nursing is defined as a series of skills. Early in the project, we needed to expand the idea of nursing for our colleagues beyond the boundaries of a hospital to include public health activities of surveillance and community interventions.

WORKING ACROSS CULTURES

The second area that needed to be addressed was work across cultures. Most of the members of the U.S. team had been working in Nicaragua for some time, but they had limited Spanish-language facility. From the nursing perspective, the projects were primarily health education and limited to week-long visits. The telehealth project promised to be a long-term project that would require frequent contact and many visits to Waslala. Although the faculty members have attempted to learn Spanish, frequently they have focused their efforts on project development and sustainability. The U.S. team travels with Villanova students fluent in both English and Spanish as interpreters. Currently, a Villanova engineering graduate student lives in Waslala as a program coordinator. He has become fluent in Spanish and serves as an interpreter for electronic and online live communications. He also has served as a cultural broker in identifying situations that may have cultural implications for the Nicaraguan or U.S. team members. His cultural brokering has involved national holidays, interaction with community leaders, and personal safety considerations for those working in Waslala. The team members of both cultures have acknowledged that when there appear to be barriers related to culture, we must focus on our common goals of supporting CHWs and the people of Waslala. This has helped promote the success of the telehealth program.

One valuable way of immersing the U.S. team members into the culture and the realities of life for the CHWs was sponsoring overnight stays in rural communities along with home visits to ill community members. Most communities do not have electricity or water in their homes. An opportunity to experience first-hand living without the amenities of modern life has helped the team members from the United States appreciate the CHWs' realities and value their work.

TABLE 11.3 Important Factors in an Interprofessional/International Project

Trust
Between partners: Take time to listen to each group's needs (across disciplines, across organizations).
Between disciplines: Recognize the expertise of each discipline, clarify expectations and roles.

Language
Between cultures: Learn the language or use bilingual interpreters.
Between disciplines: Ask questions to clarify, and be sure the other members understand terms.

Cultural Bridging
Between teams: Acknowledge history, focus on common goals.
Student team members: Support global health opportunities, support student interaction, include time to
  share cultures.

Because the consistent U.S. team members were faculty and had teaching responsibilities, it became evident that we needed in-country technical and nursing experts as the telehealth program grew to include more communities. The Villanova University engineering faculty had been working with faculty at Universidad Nacional de Ingeniería (UNI: National University of Engineering) in Managua to develop sustainable engineering courses. Including UNI faculty and students in the Waslala telehealth project was a natural progression. Villanova nursing faculty reached out to nursing faculty at Universidad Nacional Autónoma de Nicaragua (UNAN: National Autonomous University of Nicaragua) in Matagalpa, Nicaragua. An UNAN faculty member sent a senior nursing student from Waslala with the Villanova team working in Waslala. The group had opportunities to share the project and discuss how the UNAN nursing students could participate in the project. Currently, students and faculty from Villanova, UNI, and UNAN collaborate with the local community development NGO (ADIS) and the CHWs in program development and evaluation. Including in-country faculty and students from nursing and engineering backgrounds has also provided a greater cultural context of the project since the Nicaraguan nursing students are well versed in the Nicaraguan protocols for disease prevention and management. Collaborating with U.S. and Nicaraguan nursing students and faculty has also helped both schools meet global health curricular goals. Additionally, the Nicaraguan engineering faculty and students are aware of the technical resources that are available locally for supporting a telehealth project. When the entire team is in Waslala, we try to have a social activity for the U.S. and Nicaraguan students that includes sampling local cuisine, enjoying local music, and dancing. This allows the students to share cultures beyond professional practice while having fun together. The faculty has been known to dance a bit as well. In light of the history between the two countries, coming together to work toward common goals and have some fun provides an opportunity to ease the past history of conflict between our countries while looking toward the future.

WORKING WITH TECHNOLOGY IN A DEVELOPING COUNTRY

Nurses rely on technology in many aspects of their work, from entering patient assessment data into a computer to managing a ventilated patient. It is not often that nurses have the opportunity to be part of developing technology that will be used in patient care. The nursing faculty and students needed to share with the engineering group important health parameters and ways that health information is recorded. This required the nursing group to meet frequently with the engineers and clearly state the health indicators without using confusing medical jargon. Because we all had worked closely together, each group was willing to ask questions to be sure its members understood what the members of the other discipline were trying to communicate.

To implement a project using cell phones, the CHWs had to be taught to enter the health data of the people in their communities. Many of the CHWs had never texted or used a cell phone before. Initially, the engineers, as the program designers, tried to teach the CHWs

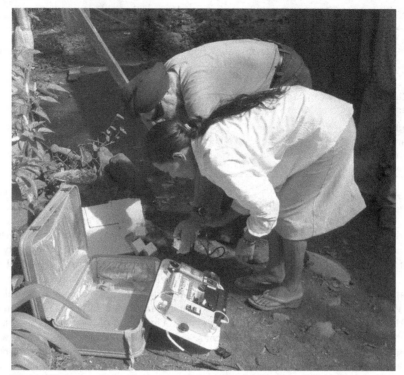

Waslala/Villanova partners share communication technology.   *Source*: R. McDermott-Levy

how to use the phones. We all soon realized that our nurses were more prepared for teaching patients and others to use technology, because they have to teach people to use devices such as glucometers and home oxygen. To the engineers' relief, the nurses took over the role of teaching the CHWs how to enter patient data. Although it was not without challenges, we learned that there are some skills that are best left to the discipline with the expertise in a specific area.

OPPORTUNITIES FOR GROWTH

The telehealth project has been a rewarding professional, educational, and service experience for all team members. Students and faculty have had opportunities to conduct research, publish, and present at national conferences. We have relied on our previous relationships and built on that trust and mutual respect to establish a project that has garnered the attention of the Nicaraguan Ministry of Health as a model for bridging gaps in health care access in remote areas of Nicaragua. As the program has grown, we have discovered that being the "on-call nurse" and telephone triage is a new role for the nurse responding to the CHWs' calls. As more communities come online in the telehealth project, we will need more nurses or physicians to respond to the CHWs' emergency calls. We have started recruiting U.S. and Nicaraguan graduate nursing students to collaborate with the Waslala on-call nurses in developing decision trees for telephone triage. The decision trees will provide algorithms for the nurse to aid in making decisions in triaging emergency problems.

We have also seen opportunities for collaborative research with our in-country faculty. We are working to develop research projects that include simulations and validation with CHWs' skills and trainings. This will support the project but also will support evidence-based practice in a developing country. Collaborative research will promote U.S. and Nicaraguan faculty development of cross-cultural research skills. By working across cultures, the faculty and students have the opportunity to understand the complexity of global health issues.

REFLECTIVE QUESTIONS

1. What words are used in nursing practice that have different meanings for other disciplines?
2. What is the benefit of recording health data of people in a remote, rural community?
3. How would you manage staying overnight in a community with no electricity, bathrooms, or running water? How would first aid be provided in such a community?
4. What cultural practice would you share with a Nicaraguan nursing student?
5. What tool or equipment used in nursing practice would you have liked to have had a role in developing? How would you change or modify that tool or equipment?

REFERENCES

Central Intelligence Agency. (2013). *The world factbook: Nicaragua.* https://www.cia.gov/library/publications/the-world-factbook/geos/nu.html

McDermott-Levy, R., & Fitzpatrick, T. R. (2013). Community health worker use of cell phones in a telehealth project. Unpublished raw data.

McDermott-Levy, R., & Weatherbie, K. (2013). Health promoters' perceptions of their communities' health needs, knowledge, and resource needs in rural Nicaragua. *Public Health Nursing, 30*(2), 94–105. doi: 10.1111/j.1525-1446.2012.01047.x

Singh, P., Kulkarni, S., Keech, E., McDermott-Levy, R., & Kligler, J. (2011). Making health care more accessible to rural communities in Waslala, Nicaragua, using low-cost telecommunications. *NCIIA, Catalyzing Innovation,* March, 1–7. nciia.org/sites/default/files/u7/Singh_1.pdf

Water for Waslala. (n.d.). Our background. www.waterforwaslala.org/about/background

Werhane, P. (2013). Business ethics and management professionalism: What can be learned for transdisciplinary professionalism for health. In *Establishing transdisciplinary professionalism for health,* conducted at the meeting of Institute of Medicine of the National Academies, Washington, DC.

Using Technology to Support an Ongoing Partnership for Nursing Education in Uganda

Jeanne M. Leffers
Speciosa M. Mbabali
Rose Chalo Nabirye
Scovia Nalugo Mbalinda

Health Volunteers Overseas (HVO) offers several programs for nurse volunteers, including programs in nursing education, oncology, and nurse anesthesia. As noted in Case Study 1.1, "Selecting an International Project Site: Health Volunteers Overseas," countries that participate in partnered nursing programs request nursing partners for their specific needs and priorities. Since the majority of HVO volunteers can stay about 3 to 6 weeks for any assignment, the need for continuity is essential to partnership and sustainability. This case study highlights how ongoing support can be built using technology. Sustaining the partnership between HVO and the nursing education program in Kampala, Uganda, facilitates the mission and goals of the sponsoring organization.

HVO sponsored a number of medical and health programs from as early as the 1980s, but there was not a nursing program specifically for nursing education. In early 2000, Mrs. Speciosa Mbabali, then head of the Department of Nursing at Makerere University, approached HVO to request a nursing partnership in Uganda. Specifically, Makerere University had just begun a baccalaureate nursing program with some support from Case Western Reserve University in the United States. At that time, there were few nurses in Kampala whose nursing education extended beyond the diploma or baccalaureate level. It was clear that over the course of program development, having other nurses come to assist the faculty at Makerere as they built their program would build capacity for academic success. Two nurses with expertise in global health nursing, Julia Plotnick and Marie O'Toole, made an initial HVO assessment visit in 2001 to determine goals for the nursing collaboration. In response to the health needs of Uganda, which has a high infant and child mortality rate, the goal was to prioritize support for pediatric nursing both at Makerere University and at Mulago National Referral and Teaching Hospital. The nursing education program was launched in 2001. Since that time HVO has responded to requests from a variety of other country nurse leaders and has completed assessments and begun programs in India, Cambodia, Tanzania, Honduras, Bolivia, and Vietnam, with ongoing assessments in other countries.

CONTEXT: UGANDA

Uganda is a landlocked country located in east Africa, bordered by Kenya to the east, Tanzania to the south, Rwanda to the southwest, the Democratic Republic of the Congo to the west, and South Sudan to the north (Index Mundi, 2013). Uganda is comprised of

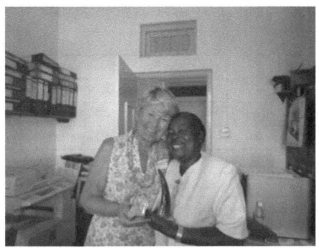

Jeanne Leffers (left) with Speciosa Mbambali at Makerere University Department of Nursing.

many ethnic groups of people. The Baganda (16.9%) are the most predominant, followed by Banyankole (9.5%), Basoga (8.4%), and Bakiga (6.9%). The country has an area of 241,035 square kilometers and an estimated population of 35 million people and is administratively divided into 112 districts (Index Mundi, 2013).

Uganda was originally a British Protectorate and gained independence from Britain in 1962. Uganda has been quite unstable politically and has had many governments since its independence, with current president Yoweri Kaguta Museveni the longest serving president, who has served since 1986.

Uganda is largely an agricultural country, with approximately 87% of its population living in rural areas (Global Health Initiative, 2011). Due to economic instability, the country remains one of the financially poorest in the world, with almost 40% of the population living on less than $1.25 per day (World Bank, 2012).

Health

Life expectancy in Uganda is 54 and 57 years for males and females, respectively. Uganda, like most countries in sub-Saharan Africa, has a high burden of communicable disease morbidity and mortality, but reflects patterns worldwide to shift to significant increases in noncommunicable disease morbidity (WHO, 2013). Communicable diseases such as malaria and HIV/AIDs continue to require resources for prevention and treatment and continue to contribute to morbidity and mortality. Children are particularly at risk for mortality owing to many factors. First, Uganda's fertility rate is among the highest in the world, with 6.7 births per woman. However, the maternal mortality rate is high (435 per 100,000), largely owing to hemorrhage and sepsis often resulting from the lack of a skilled birth attendant (Ministry of Health, 2010) (see Table 11.4). Second, with the large percentage of the population located in rural areas, access to health care is more limited. Third, poverty impacts food availability, basic sanitation measures, and prevention strategies.

Uganda was the site of the first reported case of HIV/AIDs in humans, which occurred in Masaka, Uganda, in 1982/1983 (Kiweewa, 2008). The morbidity rate was reported to be more than 30% of Ugandan residents infected with the virus during the 1980s, attributed largely to the mobility of truck transporters who passed the virus among women across east Africa as well as to the lack of prevention strategies. However, due to the efforts of the governmental administration, the rates fell to 6.4 % by the end of 2008 (Kelly, 2008). Uganda's success was the most effective response to the AIDS epidemic of any African country.

TABLE 11.4 Uganda Health Indicators

Health indicator	Rate reported 12/2011
Maternal mortality	435 per 100,000 births
Infant mortality	76 deaths per 1,000 live births
Newborn mortality	29 deaths per 1,000 live births
Under-5 mortality	137 deaths per 1,000 live births
Childhood immunization	46% immunized
Malnutrition (underweight and stunted growth)	38%
HIV/AIDS prevalence	Adults 6.4 % Children 0.7%
TB prevalence	426/100,000 population/year

Although reports challenge the statistics (Kiweewa, 2008), with the arrival of anti-retrovirals, there was a shift from high mortality to prevention and treatment strategies. Of particular importance to children are the PMTCT (Prevention of Mother to Child Transmission) programs and early prophylaxis for children born infected with HIV. See Table 11.5 for reference to leading causes of death in children.

Health Care System

Uganda's health care system is based on health services that range from rural community or village health teams and health centers II, III, IV at the parish, subcounty, and county levels, respectively, to district, regional, and (two) national hospitals. Although 80% of the population lives in rural areas, the hospitals are mainly found in urban areas, and the only two national hospitals are in Kampala, the capital city of Uganda. The health centers and hospitals may be public, owned and run by the government; private not-for-profit (PNFP), owned and run mainly by faith-based organizations; and private for-profit, owned and run by individuals or organizations. However, most health workers are found in urban hospitals, leaving the biggest percentage of the population without skilled attendants. Only US$33 is spent per capita on health, lower than the Africa regional average. In addition, the country ranks lower than its regional neighbors on public financing for health spending—22.6% of total health expenditures—affecting the country's ability to deliver the Uganda National Minimum Health Care Package (UNMHCP) to all (Ministry of Health, 2011).

Uganda depends on funding from donors such as the Global Fund to Fight AIDS, Tuberculosis, and Malaria (Global Fund) and the U.S. Agency for Internationl Development (USAID) to maintain services (Ministry of Health, 2011). A recent report of the U.S. government supporting the government of Uganda's health priorities is President Obama's Global Health

TABLE 11.5 Leading Causes of Death in Children Younger Than Age 5 in Uganda

Malaria	25%
Neonatal diseases	23%
Pneumonia	19%
Diarrhea	17%

BOX 11.1 Global Health Initiative Priorities

GHI Principles in Practice

Focus on women, girls, and gender equality by making maternal and reproductive health the central focus of GHI in Uganda and emphasizing investments in the health care system components that most directly impact the provision of maternal, neonatal, and reproductive health services.

Encourage country ownership and invest in country-led plans by building the capacity of the government of Uganda to achieve the health care systems strengthening objectives outlined in the HSSIP.

Build sustainability through health systems strengthening by concentrating on addressing Uganda's major health care systems weaknesses.

Increase impact through strategic coordination and integration by focusing efforts on a select set of districts.

Source: Global Health Initiative, 2011.

Initiative (GHI) (Global Health Initiative, 2011). The priority of this partnership is addressing high maternal and child mortality by improving access to health services, increasing health care system capacity, and strengthening the Ministry of Health's village health team (see Box 11.1).

Mulago Hospital

Mulago Hospital is the largest government hospital in Uganda, with 1,500 beds. Established in the early 1900s, the "new" Mulago Hospital was built in 1962. As the national referral and teaching hospital, it is the location of specialty medical and nursing services and training programs. Despite its national prominence, the lack of national funding for health care limits the effective treatment for what is expected care in many higher income countries. People of means are more likely to access care at privately run hospitals, where various cardiac, orthopedic, and other specialty surgical and medical services are available.

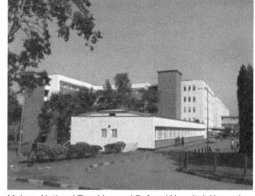

Mulago National Teaching and Referral Hospital, Kampala, Uganda.

Makerere University

Makerere University was founded in 1922 and for many years was considered the premier university of east Africa. The medical school at Makerere was founded in 1924 and currently has 13 academic departments. Until the mid-1990s, the only education for nurses in Uganda was at the enrolled and registered levels, comparable to licensure and diploma programs, respectively, in the United States. Nurse leaders sought to move the profession forward through the development of a baccalaureate program for nursing, which started in 1993 at Makerere University. In order to build the program, it was necessary to collaborate with nursing programs internationally.

RELATIONSHIP BEGINNINGS IN KAMPALA

The HVO nursing program in Kampala developed with nurses serving not only as pediatric educators at Makerere University and Mulago Hospital, but also in other specialties. To assist the administrative staff of HVO in their work with the application process and partnership work for nursing education, each program has a volunteer coordinator. From the beginning of the partnership until 2008, Julia Plotnik served as the nursing coordinator for HVO volunteers in Uganda.

Jeanne's Perspective

This is a role I assumed in 2009 after participating in two volunteer service experiences. My first trip occurred in 2008, during a sabbatical semester when I elected to spend 6 weeks in Kampala as a HVO volunteer. Prior to that time, my global health experience has been limited to work with smaller nongovernmental organizations (NGOs) such as Intercultural Nursing, Inc., and other programs whose work took me to Guatemala, Honduras, and the Dominican Republic to provide nursing services. My HVO experience was my first experience as an educator and educational consultant. Prior to my sabbatical experience, I talked to three nurses who had served with HVO in Kampala; read trip report summaries posted on the HVO volunteer resources site, KnowNET; and began e-mail correspondence with the department chair of the Makarere University nursing program. Internet communication has proved a highly effective way to sustain the HVO partnership.

During my first visit to Uganda, I had been scheduled to teach in the community health and pediatric nursing courses as well as mentor junior faculty at Makerere University and nurses at Mulago Hospital. I arrived in Uganda with teaching materials prepared and saved to my laptop computer as well as to portable flash drive devices. Remarkably, in a city where electric services are often unavailable for up to 12 hours or more each day, Makarere University had a nursing computer laboratory located at the Makerere Medical School and a portable LCD projector to be used in the classroom. In addition, in the guesthouse where I stayed across from Mulago Hospital, there was Internet service available when we had electricity. This allowed me to revise and improve all materials on the

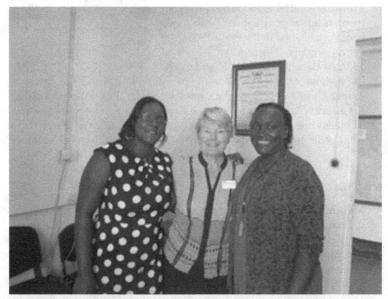

Left to right: Scovia Nalugo Mbalinda, Jeanne Leffers, Rose Chalo Nabirye at the Makerere University Department of Nursing.

computer while in Kampala and prior to printing or presentation. This was particularly helpful as I adapted the teaching materials to the culture and specific nursing practice context in Uganda. Additionally, as nurses serving in any role in global health recognize, it is imperative that we remain flexible and adaptable to changing circumstances. As anticipated, I found many situations when it was necessary to make adaptations to my planned work at both Makerere University and Mulago Hospital. On arrival, I was asked to create new presentations and new curriculum tools, and also, because of my experience as a graduate program director at my home university, to prepare a proposal for a Master's Program in Nursing for Makerere University's nursing department. The use of the Internet became invaluable in accessing documents, manuscripts, and journal articles through the online library access to my home university. I was able to communicate with faculty colleagues back in Massachusetts to seek assistance with materials that they were willing to share with my Ugandan colleagues. This international access to information while working in Uganda continued to be a much-needed resource on my return visits in 2009 and 2012.

CONTINUING COLLABORATION

Jeanne's Perspective

On my return home from Uganda I was able to continue communication with Makerere University colleagues using the Internet, e-mail, telephone, and Skype to sustain collaboration. In this way I was able to maintain my personal connection with the faculty at Makerere University and assist them as they revised and moved the master of science in nursing proposal forward. In addition, when a U.S. public health nursing colleague of mine, Dr. Sara Groves of Johns Hopkins University, took on a long-term assignment to work with the Johns Hopkins University/Makerere University collaborative Gates Foundation grant in the spring of 2009, I was able to assist her as she prepared for her experience and communicate with her while she was in Uganda. Likewise, when I was unable to return to Uganda between 2009 and January 2012, Sara was able to reciprocate for me by sending information about the extensive and most valuable collaborative work she completed during her stay. Collaboration among nurses who work globally in the same location is important for consistency, partnership, and sustainability.

Currently in Mbarara, Uganda, Sara continues her collaboration and relies upon cell phone and Skype contact to continue the partnership with Makerere University faculty.

Assuming the role of HVO nursing coordinator for Uganda required me to continue contact with the administration at the Department of Nursing at Makerere and the on-site Ugandan HVO coordinator for all HVO programs. Using the Internet as a communication tool, as well as telephone and Skype, allowed me to continue collaboration, reassess needs, and match HVO volunteers to appropriate programs. Currently, approximately 8 to 10 HVO nurse volunteers work in Uganda each year, bringing skills in academic and clinical teaching, professional development, and curriculum development. Their specialties have extended from the original focus on pediatrics to include neonatal intensive care, diabetes, critical care, neurology, and medical surgical nursing, as well as pediatrics. My role requires me to spend considerable time in communication with each volunteer prior to the visit in Uganda as well as during the initial phase of his or her collaborative assignment. By doing so, I am able to extend the partnership between HVO nurses and our partners in Uganda.

In addition, I serve on the Nursing Education Steering Committee for HVO where we advise the HVO administration about the current and proposed nursing education programs and offer guidance to gain support for expressed needs by our respective program partners. Such support requires not only HVO administrative support but also outreach to potential nurse volunteers in requested specialty areas. Additionally, I personally try to reach out to national organizations in the United States to find possible nurses who will meet the Makerere University nursing program's needs.

Rose's Perspective

I started working with HVO personnel when I took over headship of the Department of Nursing from Mrs. Mbabali in 2005. I was introduced to the then HVO coordinator Josephine Buruchara. Communication between the department and the HVO coordinator was mainly by telephone. By then, there were very few computers in the department of nursing, and the use of technology was very limited. Very few students had e-mail accounts. Moreover, the faculty and the few students who had e-mail accounts used them for private messages. However, I left the department in 2006 to go to the United States to pursue my PhD. By the time I returned in 2010, the use of e-mails both by faculty and students was very common, and communication was very easy between students and faculty. Faculty started using the Internet to send coursework assignments, class schedules, and other important notices to students.

Likewise, it was easy to communicate with the HVO coordinators by e-mail or Skype if there was need. This has eased planning for the HVO visits, because we can now send course outlines early enough for the preparation of schedules before arrival in Uganda. The Internet has also enabled more interaction between the students and HVOs even after they have left the country, because students can send questions to the HVOs and get responses. Indeed HVO volunteers and other visiting faculty have helped supervise students' research work by use of the Internet and Skype. We have benefited from webinars, video, Skype, and telephone conferencing.

In 2012, during her visit, Nancy Anderson created transcultural nursing on a Facebook page and the students and faculty from Uganda and the United States discussed interesting topics and shared their clinical experiences. It is quite amazing how the students in Uganda have caught up with the information age!

Although we are sometimes limited by the poor electricity supply or low bandwidth, it has been a very wonderful experience for both students and faculty and we will always look out for new advances in technology from our colleagues, the HVO volunteers.

EXAMPLES OF ONLINE TECHNOLOGY RESOURCES

Since the development of the World Wide Web and search engines in the mid-1990s, access to information and communication has dramatically altered the development and sharing

TABLE 11.6 Considerations for Online Communication

Language and communication	Privacy concerns	Proper use for online platforms
Consider formality and respectful language	Health Insurance Portability and Accountability Act (HIPAA)	License agreements for users
Review messages prior to sending for issues that relate to respect for cultural differences	Confidentiality	Copyrights
Respect professional boundaries and sharing of personal information	Consent to share information	Trademarks
		Users must conduct themselves in a respectful manner and abide by the rules of use for posting content or information.
		Proper citations of material and permission for use

of knowledge. Nurses can use a variety of technological applications to advance global health. A caveat to using such public communication resources is the need to be aware of issues of privacy, appropriate use, and legality (see Table 11.6).

Skype

Skype is a service where users can communicate with family, friends, or professional colleagues using either voice or voice and camera using Skype service, telephones, and webcams for real-time communication. Developed in 2003, this service provides users with the experience of face-to-face communication across miles. While many global health workers use Skype to communicate with family and friends while away from home serving in other countries, the service is also useful for communication between nurse partners to sustain partnerships and provide ongoing support.

Social Networking Tools

Facebook, Twitter, and LinkedIn have all emerged since and are used by millions of people worldwide to communicate often in real time. I find that I communicate with nursing and community partners from my global health experiences on a regular basis using the more informal social networking techniques. However, with all such public communication strategies nurses must maintain professional, ethical, and respectful communication using such networking tools.

Webinars

Web conferencing technology tools, commonly referred to as webinars, are a resource allowing groups to conference across distant locations. They facilitate real-time online meetings, workshops, trainings, or educational presentations, allowing group communication wherein participants can view the same visual materials simultaneously, communicate by text message visible on the screen, and ask questions using text messages or audio/video chat. Creating a webinar requires technological support, but a distinct advantage of their use is the ability to access a webinar from any computer that has Internet access.

Online Communication Platforms and Listservs

The use of communication platforms where the user can access targeted topics can serve as a resource for making connections for nurses worldwide. These can be of help to partners from host country and visiting programs alike in order to address common interests and challenges.

The Global Alliance for Nursing and Midwifery offers communities of practice to facilitate communication between 3,359 members in 161 countries. Nurses can sign on and get e-mail updates from the listserv at https://knowledge-gateway.org/ganm. In addition to the regular communication about topics of interest to nursing and midwifery, at the website members can log in to view achieved discussions, access the library of posted resources, and search for specific topics.

Global Health Delivery (GHD) Online (www.ghdonline.org) is part of the Global Health Delivery Project of Harvard University and is an online collaboration platform that connects global health professionals and creates opportunities for communication and exchange of ideas and resources through various virtual communities. GHD online was begun in 2008 and now has 8,500 members representing more than 2,500 organizations in 170 countries. Their mission is to "to improve the delivery of health care worldwide, especially in areas with limited resources, by fostering the exchange of knowledge and critical information in expert-led, thematic, communities" (Global Health Delivery Project, 2013). Membership is free thanks to the support of Harvard Medical School and Brigham and Women's Hospital. The project is supported by advisors, team members, and 40 health care expert moderators representing medicine, public health, and nursing. Members share their expertise, questions, and insight through communication in 10 public virtual communities including Global Health Nursing & Midwifery, Health IT, and Innovating Health Care Delivery, as well as communities that focus on HIV/AIDs, TB, malaria, and noncommunicable diseases. Other resources include a blog and information reminding the participants to follow the terms of use, privacy policy, and applicable intellectual property and access to information laws. In addition, translation is available into Arabic, French, Haitian Creole, Spanish, and Russian.

Internet Resources

- PubMed: www.ncbi.nlm.nih.gov/pubmed
- Medline Plus: www.nlm.nih.gov/medlineplus
- World Health Organization Global Health Library: www.globalhealthlibrary.net/php/index.php
- Hesperian Health Guides are produced by the Hesperian to support knowledge for communities and health workers. The most commonly known book is *Where There Is No Doctor* by David Werner (Werner, 2013). Their open copyright policy and free downloads of books translated into many languages facilitates the distribution of educational materials to people across the globe. Visit their website at http://hesperian.org/books-and-resources/digital-commons
- *The Lancet* has a global health collection that offers open access to users who register. It is a collection of research, commentaries, and authoritative reviews that address health issues in low- and middle-income countries. Users can access and register at www.TheLancet.com
- UNICEF provides a variety of resources and reports relevant to international health at www.unicef.org
- The World Health Organization is a resource for health topics, data, statistics and reports of WHO programs and projects at www.who.int/en

REFLECTIVE QUESTIONS

1. Consider differences in communication between personal, face-to-face conversations and those that occur virtually using technology. How might you alter your conversation when using electronic media?
2. Identify a global setting where you have worked or plan to work. What cultural differences between that setting and your home setting must you consider when communicating electronically?
3. You might have observed violations of privacy, intellectual property, or respectful communication when using electronic media. What steps can you consider when joining a platform for global health or sustaining communication with international partners?

REFERENCES

Global Health Delivery Project. (2013). About Us. http://www.ghdonline.org/about

Global Health Initiative: Uganda. (2011). A strategy for accelerating reductions in maternal land neonatal mortality. U.S. Mission Uganda. Interagency Health Team. www.ghi.gov/documents/organization/184707.pdf

Index Mundi. (2013). Uganda demographics profile. www.indexmundi.com/uganda/demographics_profile.html

Kelly, A. (2008, December 1). Background: HIV/AIDs in Uganda. *The Guardian.* www.theguardian.com/katine/2008/dec/01/world-aids-day-uganda

Kiweewa, J. M. (2008). Uganda's HIV/AIDs success story: Reviewing the evidence. *Journal of Development and Social Transformation, 5,* 53–61. www.maxwell.syr.edu/uploadedFiles/moynihan/dst/Kiweewa.pdf?n=6688

Ministry of Health. (2010). Health sector strategic plan III, 2010/11–2014/15. www.health.go.ug/docs/HSSP_III_2010.pdf

Ministry of Health. (2011). Uganda health assessment. http://health.go.ug/docs/hsa.pdf

Werner, D. (2013). *Where there is no doctor.* Berkeley, CA: Hesperian.

World Bank (2012). *Poverty headcount ratio at $1.25 a day.* http://data.worldbank.org/indicator/SI.POV.DDAY

World Health Organization. (2013). Countries: Uganda. http://www.who.int/countries/uga/en

CHAPTER 12

Sustainability of International Nursing Programs

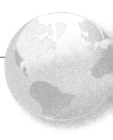

Mary E. Riner
Marion E. Broome

Around the globe many academic nursing and service organizations are developing programs across national borders to engage in global health improvement. They have made commitments to host communities to develop service, education, and research programs in countries with emerging economies and inadequate educational resources, as well as in more developed countries with significant health and education resources. Many faculty members are engaging in binational or even multinational collaborative research. These outreach and engagement programs provide opportunities for nurses, students, and faculty to increase their participation in global health and collaboratively address key health problems such as maternal and infant mortality, AIDS, malaria, and diabetes with their global partners.

To develop a sustainable global health agenda, academic and service organizations must make it a priority to develop and allocate the required human and fiscal resources. This requires a strong mission statement from senior leaders that communicates this priority to internal and external audiences (Memmott et al., 2010; Riner, 2011). It also includes strategic planning for effective identification and development of partners and programs. Engaging in careful planning allows partnerships to develop sustainable programs that can make a difference in the health of local populations.

Achieving the benefits from this type of institutional commitment requires building capacity over time as partnerships are initiated, developed, sustained, and, when needed, ended. Building capacity in global health needs to be strategic and goal-oriented, address the needs of both partners, and evolve over the course of the partnership. A previous chapter on capacity building explores these global health needs in greater detail.

There are social-political dimensions to global health partnerships. "Genuine" north–south partnerships (Crossley & Holmes, 2001) call for ensuring that the needs of both partners are being addressed and the relationship is bidirectional. This does not mean that the benefits are always equal, but rather that resources are used in an equivalent manner in meeting goals valued by the partners.

DEFINITIONS OF SUSTAINABLE PARTNERSHIPS

Although there are many definitions of sustainability related to new program adoption, one of the simplest and most straightforward descriptions of it as a global term is "the continuation process that encompasses a diversity of forms that the process may take" (Shediac-Rizkallah & Bone, 1998, p. 92). This generic conceptual definition is grounded in the idea of continuation. This allows room for growth, evolution, transformation throughout time, and changing local conditions and partner participation.

Adopting an operational definition of a sustainable partnership can provide an anchor by which to develop goals and work plans, garner resources, and evaluate progress and outcomes. Within the context of quality improvement, sustainability has been defined "as the capacity to collaborate, to make developmental progress in realizing partnership objectives, and to secure a stable financial base" (Edwards et al., 2007, p. 38).

Descriptions of sustainability have been developed by international health and development organizations. The World Health Organization (WHO) conducted a sustainability evaluation project for the African Programme for Onchocerciasis Control. For that parasite control project, sustainability was defined as "the ability of a project to continue to function effectively, for the foreseeable future, with high treatment coverage, integrated into available health care services, with strong community ownership using resources mobilized by the community and government" (WHO, 2004, p. 5). The Centers for Disease Control and Prevention's health communities program defined sustainability as "a community's ongoing capacity and resolve to work together to establish, advance, and maintain effective strategies that continuously improve health and quality of life for all" (Centers for Disease Control, n.d., p. 8).

SUSTAINABILITY AS A WAY OF BEING IN AN ONGOING RELATIONSHIP

From the perspective of global citizenship, building the mutual capacity of partners allows the development of strong relationships that are mutually beneficial. When members of the partnership expect to contribute and to receive benefits over time, there is cause for investing energy broadly. Energy can be invested in learning about and appreciating one another's organizations; the political, social, and economic climate; and the dynamics of country-level relationships. With time, partners can understand the nuances of the dynamics shaping the partnership, both internal and external to the formal partnership.

Individuals are the basic building block of partnerships, and individuals involved in partnerships benefit from opportunities for personal development. When these persons have opportunities for personal and career growth, they are more likely to stay engaged in the partnerships. Just as the partnership's needs change over time, so, too, do the individual's needs evolve. Effective partnerships allow for this individual development and understand how it affects the partnerships.

Sustainability creates the capacity for partnerships to "unlock" value retained within single organizations (Barnes & Phillips, 2000, p. 182). This can lead to achieving more significant contributions to the mission of the partner organizations. It can also result in identifying new practical and research projects, as well as development of second-generation projects that evolve out of the primary mission of the partnership, dissemination activities, and funding awards.

PLANNING FOR SUSTAINABILITY

Sustainability of global health programs requires planning in order to achieve outcomes that address change and innovation that continues after the visiting partners depart or the funding ends. Effective programs require program or project design factors that have been clearly defined, negotiated, adequately funded, and considered needs for training (Shediac-Rizkallah & Bone, 1998); include capacity building factors; and plan for sustainable innovations (Johnson, Hays, Center, & Daley, 2004).

Capacity building factors include structures and formal linkages, champions or leaders who engage stakeholders, administrative policies, adequate resources, and expertise to sustain innovations or program interventions (Johnson, Hays, Center, & Daley, 2004). Attributes for sustainable innovations include the alignment between the program and the needs of the stakeholders, effective relationships, and ownership across stakeholder partners (Johnson, Hays, Center, & Daley, 2004).

THREATS TO SUSTAINING PROGRAMS

Threats to sustaining partnerships need to be identified and addressed for success in host country ownership to occur (discussed in the next chapter). One threat is project financing. In low- and middle-income countries (LMICs), most projects depend on donor funding, which often targets a specific problem for a population. Donor funding can define the scope of work and the length of time available, as well as shape the political realities of where and how the work gets done and who will do it. Donor funding can be temporary and when withdrawn leaves challenges to sustainability of the program (Edwards & Roelofs, 2006; Shediac-Rizkallah & Bone, 1998).

Another threat to sustainability of programs can be the duration of the project. Short-term projects often do not provide adequate time to address sustainability factors and can lead to failures in transfer of ownership, continuation of interventions or innovations, or improvement in health outcomes.

As organizations adopt innovations and effective approaches are diffused into other parts of the system, the changes need to be permanent. Uneven support for training on the innovation by both partners is a threat to sustainability (Edwards & Roelofs, 2006). The lack of training can be essential to develop capacity, leadership, and expertise among host country partners for new innovations developed by the program and partnership. Lack of adequate funding or time for training can undo the successes of the partnership. In addition, new partnerships developed during changing local environments or leaders can present a need to innovate amid a shifting political landscape (Edwards & Roelofs, 2006). Without a careful assessment of the organizational and the broader community environment, programs can lack the support needed to sustain them (Shediac-Rizkallah & Bone, 1998).

Butt, Markle-Reid, and Browne (2008) found that partnerships frequently fail when they are complex to administer, are time-consuming to establish, require investment of scarce resources, and have a potential for loss of decision-making control. When complexity of the program or complexity of developing necessary relationships begins to become a burden, then the costs may be viewed as outweighing the benefits, threatening any chance for sustainability.

SUPPORT FOR SUSTAINABILITY

Developing strong and transparent partnerships, managing planned transition points, and engaging local champions in leading integration efforts are important for sustaining programs (Edwards & Roelofs, 2006). A conceptual model of sustainability grounded in Rogers's diffusion-of-innovation work identified five important elements: establishing an identity through goal setting, developing an infrastructure involving people and technical and financial resources, creating tangible and intangible incentives, providing incremental opportunities for participation, and integrating change into the regular business (Edwards et al., 2007). Tangible incentives are more measurable, such as an increase in the number of patients treated and a decrease in complications following hospitalization, while intangible incentives are less visible but can include higher prestige or reputation. These factors can promote sustainability once the formal program or funding ends. These elements of diffusion of innovation occur within sustainable relationships. Relationships can be thought of in terms of a life cycle in that they have stages of development, establishment, and maintenance.

Life Cycle of Relationship Development

Through developing relationships, nurses can set goals that develop an identity for their partnership with nurses around the world. This can lead to furthering nursing knowledge as well as development of practice (Sochan, 2008). As nurses from disparate organizations, communities, and countries develop personal and organizational relationships, they may effect societal change locally in how nursing contributes to the health care enterprise. For example, collaborative relationships have fostered capacity building in nursing organizations, research partnerships, and development of educational programs.

In order to avoid the possibility of colonialism or imperialism, both partners need to focus on the benefits they are receiving from the relationship and outcomes. To avoid developing an unbalanced partnership in terms of giving and receiving, Allen and Ogilvie (2004) recommend focusing on reciprocal, mutual benefits of interinstitutional activities. Creating intangible and tangible incentives throughout the partnership facilitates investment and sustainability.

Establishing and maintaining positive relationships among the key stakeholders needs to be an objective of the partnership. In order to engage in effective international education partnerships, all partners need to be able to effectively communicate within the team. They must demonstrate respect for cultural differences, recognize and learn from both diversity and similarity, agree to common goals early in the development process, work hard at maintaining a sense of humor, and engage in face-to-face opportunities to get to know colleagues (Kuehn et al., 2005).

Relationship Development Stage

Successful navigation of the early interaction stage can lead to a strong partnership. Communication, trust, and a shared vision are critical elements of a successful partnership. They are foundational and must be addressed when the relationship is in the formative stages and the goals are being established (Kuehn et al., 2005; Larson, 2003; Riner & Becklenburg, 2001). These relationship elements may affect sustainability with improved health outcomes, continuation of program activities and innovation, and host country ownership as illustrated in the conceptual model of partnership by Leffers and Mitchell (2011).

Problems may occur in later stages if the formative stage is not effectively negotiated. These problems can include low levels of internal commitment, failure to identify the key roles and responsibilities of partners, failure to establish "win/win" relationships, or departure of key personnel (Heffernan & Poole, 2004).

Established Stage

Initial favorable development of relationships can lead to achievement of program goals and also opportunities to further develop the program—that is, tailor it to meet new needs or include more groups. The latter occurred in a multicountry demonstration project in which, in year 1, three European countries were included in a leadership development program. In years 2 and 3, nurse leaders from Central American and Caribbean countries were also included (Wright, Cloonan, Leonhardy, & Wright, 2005).

As individuals develop effective working relationships a track record of working together is established. This can lead to opportunities for questioning approaches and sharing ideas that can result in expanding perspectives about how to further develop the partnership (Wright, Cloonan, Leonhardy, & Wright, 2005).

Maintenance Stage

The goal at this stage is to maintain relationships with individuals from the partnership over time and circumstances, although some partnerships may be formally dissolved. Some partnerships are intended to be ongoing, with no defined time limit. In these types of partnerships, the relationships and people engaged in the partnerships will change over time. New people will be added and others will leave the partnership due to job changes or promotions, retirements, and death. If the program was dependent on external funding, when the funding ends there can be a tendency for contacts to become less frequent, which presents the possibility of diminished relationships.

Formal partnerships may end with achievement of project outcomes and some programs may have intentional goals of being sustained by the host country partner with the formal partnership dissolved. When this is the case, the relationships may change in nature, but be sustained in new or different ways. Nurses from the partnerships may meet at global conferences or become partners in assisting another agency to adopt a new program. Technology, as discussed in previous chapters, is also a viable way of maintaining the relationship.

STRATEGIES TO ENSURE SUSTAINABILITY

Cultural humility is an essential orientation to the continued success of any program. It has been described as a lifelong process of self-reflection and self-critique (Tervalon & Murray-Garcia, 1998), as well as a way of being in a respectful partnership in which differences and similarities are explored and each individual's values, priorities, and goals are respected (Hunt, 2005). Cultural humility, for example, allowed a partnership between a community hospital in the Dominican Republic and a U.S. school of nursing to be developed and sustained in the face of the vast differences in resources between the countries (Foster, 2009).

Strategies to ensure internal commitment to the partnership are important to implement. They can include clearly identifying the responsibilities of each partner, structuring the relationship as a "win/win," identifying key personnel, and knowledge sharing to occur over time to prevent deterioration if staff turnover occurs (Heffernan & Poole, 2004). Additional sustainability actions include continual focus on assessing and enhancing, when necessary, the partners' ability to collaborate, level of trust, communication, credibility, enthusiasm, and excitement; planning for and maintaining relationships among key stakeholders; and implementing, evaluating, and, when necessary, reassessing and modifying plans (Johnson, Hays, Center, & Daley, 2004).

EVALUATION OF SUSTAINABILITY

Different skills, resources, and perspectives are needed for moving from development to maintenance of an international program partnership. When these aspects are addressed at the outset of the program, the naturally occurring evolution of a program is anticipated, thereby increasing the likelihood of sustainability.

Programs evolve over time as initial goals are reached, new resources are garnered, new individuals join the partnership or current ones leave, and the processes for engagement change. Although these changes can threaten the existence of a program, flexible thinking, partnership reassessment, and re-envisioning the purpose and process can lead to even more significant work being accomplished.

Shediac-Rizkallah and Bone (1998) developed a set of guidelines for sustainability planning that can be used at many stages of program evolution to assess effectiveness (see Box 12.1). These elements are comprehensive and allow users to tailor their assessment based on the relevance of the element. The categories include project design and implementation, organizational setting, and community environment.

Aspects of sustainability associated with the success of one community-based onchocerciasis parasite control program in Africa included integration with routine health care services, adequate availability of resources to support the work, efficiency in terms of cost-effectiveness, use of simple, uncomplicated routines and procedures, acceptance by health staff and inclusion in routine activity, and community ownership. By addressing all these factors, this project functioned effectively (WHO, 2004). Box 12.2 provides useful websites with additional information on evaluation.

BOX 12.1 Guidelines for Sustainability Planning

Project design and implementation factors:

1. *Project negotiation process.* Are project approaches and goals discussed with recipient community members as equal partners? Are the needs of the community driving the program, or are those of external donor agencies and technical experts? Is a negotiation or consensus-building process in place to reach a compromise for addressing everyone's (including donors, community, technical experts) needs?
2. *Project effectiveness.* Is the project (perceived as) effective? Is it visible? What are the (desirable and undesirable) secondary effects of the program?
3. *Project duration.* What is the project's grant period (number of years in operation)? Is it a new project, or is it an existing program that is acquiring additional funds?
4. *Project financing.* What are the sources of funds for the program (internal, external, a mixture)? What are the community's local resources? Can the community afford the program (e.g., is it able to pay maintenance and recurrent costs)? How much are community members willing/able to pay for services? What strategies are in place to facilitate gradual financial self-sufficiency?
5. *Project type.* What type of project is it (e.g., preventative vs. curative)?
6. *Training.* Does the project have a training component (professional or paraprofessional)?

Factors within the organization setting:

7. *Institutional strength.* What organization will be implementing the program? How mature (developed, stable, resourceful) is this organization? Is it likely to provide a strong organizational base for the program?
8. *Integration with existing programs/services.* Is the program vertical (categorical), or is it horizontal (comprehensive or integrated)? Are goals, objectives, and approaches prespecified, or are they adapted to the local population and setting and over time? Is the program compatible with the mission and activities of its host organization? Is the implementing organization the recipient of program funds or is there an intermediary organization?
9. *Program champion/leadership.* Is there a program champion? What are his or her attributes? If there is no champion, can one be identified/nurtured so that he or she may serve as an advocate for the continuation of the program? Is the program endorsed from the top? How well is it supported?

Factors in the broader community environment:

10. *Socioeconomic and political considerations.* How favorable is the general socioeconomic and political environment for the sustainability of the program to be a realistic goal?
11. *Community participation.* What is the level of community participation? What is the depth (amount) of involvement? What is the range of involvement (types of activities)?

Shediac-Rizkallah and Bone (1998). Reprinted with permission, Oxford University Press.

BOX 12.2 Suggested Websites

1. Case study and tools used to conduct an evaluation of the sustainability of a community-directed treatment program for onchocerciasis control. World Health Organization (2004). Guidelines for Conducting an Evaluation of the Sustainability of CDTI Projects. www.who.int/apoc/publications/guidelinesevalsustainabilitycorrectedversionsept04.pdf
2. Academic Program in Sustainable International Development. http://heller.brandeis.edu/academic/sid/index.html
3. American Indian Development Associates. (2001). Program sustainability: Developing strategies for maintaining programs over the long term. www.aidainc.net/Publications/Sustainability.pdf
4. U.S. Agency for International Development. www.usaid.gov/what-we-do/global-health

CONCLUSION

Developing international programs through partnerships with colleagues in other countries as well as within one's own national borders with culturally diverse groups is a worthy endeavor. The opportunity to grow and learn from each other while improving nursing education and nursing practice is invaluable from an individual and organizational perspective. It allows individuals to grow intellectually, emotionally, and culturally. It allows institutions to expand their capacity to engage in promoting the health and well-being of individuals in countries with inadequate resources. This privilege must be exercised respectfully and responsibly.

REFERENCES

Allen, M., & Ogilvie, I. (2004). Internationalization of higher education: Potentials and pitfalls for nursing education. *International Nursing Review, 51*, 73–80.

Barnes, N. J., & Phillips, P. S. (2000). Higher education partnerships: Creating new value in the environment sector. *International Journal of Sustainability in Higher Education, 1*(2), 182–190.

Butt, G., Markle-Reid, M., & Browne, G. (2008). Interprofessional partnerships in chronic illness care: A conceptual model for measuring partnership effectiveness. *International Journal of Integrated Care, 8*.

Centers for Disease Control and Prevention. (n.d.). A sustainability planning guide for healthy communities. www.cdc.gov/healthycommunitiesprogram/pdf/sustainability_guide.pdf

Crossley, M., & Holmes, K. (2001). Challenges for educational research: International development, partnerships and capacity building in small states. *Oxford Review of Education, 27*(3), 395–409.

Edwards, J. C., Feldman, P. H., Sangl, J., Polakoff, D., Stern, G., & Casey, D. (2007). Sustainability of partnership projects: A conceptual framework and checklist. *Joint Commission Journal on Quality and Patient Safety, 33*(12), 37–47.

Edwards, N. C., & Roelofs, S. M. (2006). Sustainability: The elusive dimension of international health projects. *Canadian Journal of Public Health, 97*(1), 45–98.

Foster, J. (2009). Cultural humility and the importance of long-term relationships in international partnerships. *Journal of Obstetrical, Gynecological and Neonatal Nursing, 38*, 100–107. doi: 10.1111/j.1552-6909.2008.00313.x

Heffernan, T., & Poole, D. (2004). "Catch me I'm falling": Key factors in the deterioration of offshore education partnerships. *Journal of Higher Education Policy and Management, 60*, 75–90.

Hunt, L. (2005). Beyond cultural competence: Applying humility to cultural setting. In G. Henderson, S. Estroll, L. Churchill, N. King, J. Oberlander, & R. Strauss (Eds.), *The social medicine reader* (Vol. II, pp. 133–136). Durham, NC: Duke University Press.

Johnson, K., Hays, C., Center, H., & Daley, C. (2004). Building capacity and sustainable prevention innovations: A sustainability planning model. *Evaluation and Programs Planning, 27*, 135–149.

Kuehn, A. F., Chircop, A., & Downe-Wamboldt, B. (2005). Exploring nursing roles across North American borders. *Journal of Continuing Education in Nursing, 36*(4), 153–162.

Larson, E. (2003). Minimizing disincentives for collaborative research. *Nursing Outlook, 51*(6), 267–271.

Leffers, J., & Mitchell, E. (2011). Conceptual model for partnership and sustainability in global health. *Public Health Nursing, 28*(1), 91–102. doi: 10.1111/j.1525-1446.2010.00892.x

Memmott, R. J., Coverston, C. R., Heise, B. A., Williams, M., Maughan, E. D., Kohl, J., & Palmer, S. (2010). Practical considerations in establishing sustainable international nursing experiences. *Nursing Education Perspectives, 31*(5), 298–302.

Riner, M. E. (2011). Globally engage nursing education: An academic program model. *Nursing Outlook, 59*(6), 308–317.

Riner, M. E., & Becklenburg, A. (2001). Partnering with a sister city organization for an international service-leaning experience. *Journal of Transcultural Nursing, 12*(3), 234–240.

Shediac-Rizkallah, M. C., & Bone, L. R. (1998). Planning for the sustainability of community-based health programs: Conceptual frameworks and future directions for research, practice and policy. *Health Education Research Theory & Practice, 13*(1), 87–108.

Sochan, A. (2008). Relationship building through the development of international nursing curricula: A literature review. *International Council of Nurses, 55*(20), 192–204.

Tervalon, M., & Murray-Garcia, J. (1998). Cultural humility versus cultural competence: A critical distinction in defining physician training outcomes in multicultural education. *Journal of Health Care for the Poor and Underserved, 9*(2), 117–125.

World Health Organization (2004). Guidelines for conducting an evaluation of the sustainability of CDTI projects. www.who.int/apoc/publications/guidelinesevalsustainabilitycorrected-versionsept04.pdf

Wright, S., Cloonan, P., Leonhardy, K., & Wright, G. (2005). An international programme in nursing and midwifery: Building capacity for the new millennium. *International Nursing Review, 52*, 18–23.

Sustaining Public Nursing Education in Liberia

Mary E. Riner
Marion E. Broome

CONTEXT: LIBERIA

The country of Liberia, in west Africa, is 43,000 square miles in size and is bounded by the Atlantic Ocean and Sierra Leone on the west, Guinea to the north, and Cote d'Ivoire to the east. The country was founded in 1822 by the American Colonization Society, which hoped to settle freed slaves in west Africa, and has never been a colony of any other country. The form of government is considered a constitutional republic, with a chief of state elected by the people (President Ellen Sirleaf, 2005–present). The country is also governed by a national assembly featuring both a house of representatives and a senate. The current population is 4.1 million (www.africa.upenn.edu/Country_Specific/Liberi.html). The English-speaking Americo-Liberians, descendants of former American slaves, only make up 5% of the population, with the indigenous Liberian population comprising 16 different ethnic groups.

In 1971, while in his sixth term as president, William S. Tubman died and was succeeded by his long-term associate, Vice President William Tolbert. Tolbert was ousted in a military coup in 1980, and after 9 years of corruption, brutality, and civil war, there was another rebellion in 1989 by Charles Taylor. In 1997, a "free" election was held, and during the next 5 years Charles Taylor bankrupted the country. In 2012 an international court convicted Taylor of aiding and abetting war crimes (www.infoplease.com/world/countries/liberia). During the 20 years of civil war and conflict, 200,000 civilians were killed, hundreds of thousands more became refugees, and many of the professionals in the country relocated to the United States. In 2006, President Ellen Sirleaf, elected to the first of two terms as president, began the lengthy process of restoring the country's badly damaged infrastructure.

BUILDING NURSING EDUCATION IN LIBERIA

John F. Kennedy Medical Center (JFKMC) is the largest medical complex in the city of Monrovia and, indeed, in the country of Liberia. The general administrator (GA) of JFKMC has responsibility for oversight of all educational and training programs in the Tubman National Institute of Medical Arts (TNIMA). TNIMA was opened in 1945 through the cooperation of the Liberia National Public Health Service (now the Ministry of Health and Social Welfare) and the U.S. mission (www.TNIMA.org/about us.html). TNIMA now offers a variety of health professions programs (e.g., physician's assistant, x-ray technician), but began with the merging of the professional and practical nursing programs. TNIMA remained open throughout the political conflict and continued to educate nurses

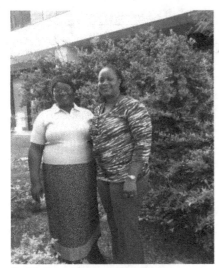

Cynthia Bondoe, registered midwife, and Ada Brow Wraynee, registered nurse, at the Tubman National Institute of Medical Arts in Liberia.

and other allied health professionals. In 2010, the Indiana University School of Nursing became involved at the request of one of their alumni, Wvannie Scott-McDonald, RN, PhD, general administrator of the JFKMC, who was a graduate of the doctoral program at Indiana University in the 1990s. Dr. Scott McDonald had been appointed the GA for JFKMC in 2008.

The extended conflict had a serious impact on nursing education in Liberia. Although several private schools of nursing continued operations, with intermittent closings when the conflict was too bad, TNIMA remained in continuous operation. However, its educational resources, including library resources, technology, and clinical resources, were all affected to one degree or another. Faculty workloads increased during these years, and class schedules were often interrupted.

At the beginning of the partnership between the Indiana University School of Nursing and JFKMC/TNIMA in 2010 to 2011, there was one primary goal for this collaboration: to provide a series of leadership workshops for nurses who were ward managers and supervisors at the JFKMC. However, in 2011 Indiana University received a U.S. Agency for International Development (USAID) grant to rebuild the health and life sciences programs at the University of Liberia (www.universityliberia.org). Nursing was included as part of that project, and the decision was made to expand the partnership to develop the first public bachelor's of science in nursing program. The long-range purpose of both of these goals was to build leadership capacity in nurses who are current and future leaders of Liberian nursing by establishing the first public RN-to-BSN program at the University of Liberia (UL) and strengthening the practice and leadership abilities of the clinical managers.

Goal 1: Developing Clinical Management and Leadership Skills for Nurse Leaders

As we stated in the foregoing chapter, to achieve the benefits of such a partnership the type of institutional commitment on both sides is critical. To build capacity over time, relationships must be developed with individuals across both settings, and these relationships must be based on trust, transparency, and common goals, as well as a commitment to learning from each other in order to improve health care for citizens of the host country. Hence Dr. Wvannie Scott-McDonald and the two authors decided that interaction between the nurse clinical leaders and the authors needed to be fairly frequent and that it should allow for sustained interaction over more than one visit.

Therefore, in 2010, at the inception of the partnership, two week-long workshops were held over a period of 6 months. Three nurse leaders from the United States, the authors and a colleague from the University of Massachusetts, worked with 12 clinical managers from the wards and clinics at JFKMC and Mother–Baby Hospital. These managers were selected to attend by Dr. Scott-McDonald. Early on, the two authors decided to use a problem-based, participant-centered approach to engage in values clarification and to develop goals for the workshop. In the workshop, they used examples from practice that had been challenges for them, including physician–nurse communication and equipment supply and maintenance. After the first workshop the participants were eager to use the strategies they had discussed and looked forward to sharing their successes at the next workshop. During the first workshop we stressed the importance of nurses to the organization. Dr. Scott-McDonald's week-long participation also demonstrated her commitment to the program and to the participants.

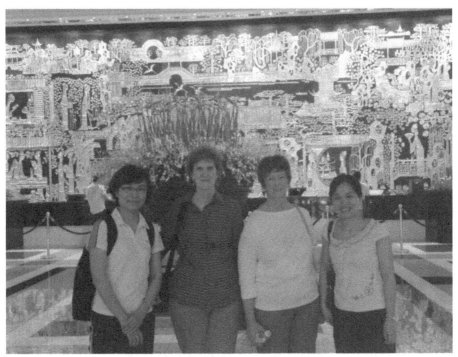

Zhao Juanjuan from Sun Yat-sen University in Guangzhou, China; Marion Broome and Mary Riner from Indiana University; and Ma Zhang from Sun Yat-sen University.

Participants developed and shared their own goals for the two workshops, and these goals guided the content and learning activities:

- When and how to take initiative
- Improve as a leader in order to influence the behavior of colleagues
- Team building
- Skills for dealing with staff and difficult situations
- Motivating staff to provide high-quality care
- Skills for difficult decisions and policy issues
- How to work with all team members: sharing views
- How to integrate outside health members into master plan
- How to take responsibility and accountability
- Improve nursing environment, patient care
- Understand various leadership styles: strategic thinking
- Create master schedule for workers

We emphasized that patients came to a hospital for nursing care and that the hospital was "the nurses' house," and thus the nurses needed to set the tone for care safety, quality, and accountability. One of the most gratifying conversations when we returned for the second workshop was the participants' invitation to tour "their house"—which we immediately accepted. Another was seeing that the 12 values identified in the values clarification exercise (see Table 12.1) had been listed on placards and hung in each ward.

Other content/activities in the workshops included the following:

- Values clarification (see Table 12.1 for values identified)
- Leadership model (Kouzes & Posner, 2007)
- Leadership self-assessment

- Team building
- Team leadership
- Conflict resolution
- Precepting students (part of the nurse manager role at JFKMC)
- Evaluation of performance strategies

As mentioned in the foregoing chapter, programs that are sustainable are built on the precept that individuals are the basic building block of partnerships and that individuals involved in the partnerships benefit from opportunities for personal development. These nurse managers were given opportunities for personal and career growth, and it was clear to them that the GA, Dr. Wvannie Scott-McDonald, believed in them and their ability to grow and flourish as leaders.

Goal 2: Development of the First Public BSN Program in Liberia

Building capacity in global health needs to be strategic and goal-oriented, address the needs of both partners, and evolve over the course of the partnership. After the relationship-building and leadership workshops were underway, the opportunity to develop the first public bachelor of science in nursing (BSN) in the country arose when a USAID grant was awarded to Indiana University (Reafsynder & Dennis, 2010) to rebuild the health and life sciences programs at the UL.

After careful assessment of the resources existing already at TNIMA and JFKMC and the UL, we recommended that initially we build the BSN program as an RN-to-BSN program. There was strong support for this program from both UL president Emmett Dennis and Dr. Scott-McDonald. Meetings were held with the board of nursing (www. Facebook/Liberian Board of Nursing and Midwifery) to discuss the plans. We met with faculty at TNIMA and conducted an evidence-based practice research workshop to review the document that harmonized nursing education programs in west Africa and to solicit their ideas about their own development needs. This would enable us to plan future education and training grounded in their needs and goals and build capacity for the new RN-BSN at UL.

Another major goal of the USAID grant that was related to capacity building was developing faculty from Liberia through studies for a MSN degree in nursing education. We anticipated that if these nurse educators from Liberia (with BSN degrees) could study with faculty in the United States who were known for their pedagogical expertise in both classroom and clinical education, then they, in turn, could lead the new BSN program at the UL. We believed (and they agreed) that exposing faculty leaders from Liberia to contemporary education concepts and practices in the United States (including simulation

TABLE 12.1 Values Clarification Outcomes

The following leadership values were identified by the participants of the workshop in spring 2011.
- Learning
- Excellence
- Achievement
- Determination
- Evaluation
- Respect
- Supportive
- Honesty
- Integrity
- Productivity

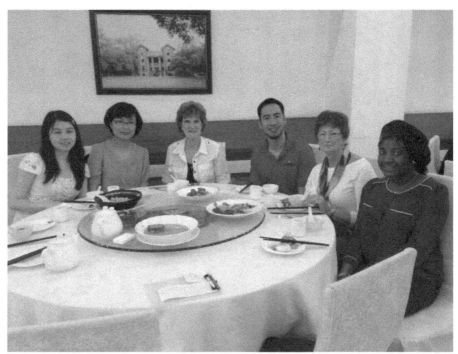

Ma Xiang, master's nursing student; Zhao Juanjuan from Sun Yat-sen University
in Guangzhou, China; Marion Broome; Shuennhau Chang, nursing student;
Mary Riner; and Kemi Olofinkua from Indiana University.

technology and online education) would best prepare them for the future. As the country rebuilt the school of medicine at the UL and as the JFKMC continued to evolve its medical practice using contemporary technology (such as for imaging and surgical procedures), it became clear to the authors that faculty for the future needed to gain knowledge and skills that were not currently available in Liberia and that could better prepare nurses for the future. After having opportunities to observe, learn, and practice in a progressive health care environment in a Western country, the Liberian faculty could then develop an adaptive curriculum that would build courses and skills based on what the needs of Liberia were (e.g., the high maternal–infant mortality rates). Therefore, a decision was made to bring the two academic directors of the midwifery program and the nursing programs from TNIMA to Indiana University to study for 18 months of course and clinical education. They would then finish their education practicum and evidence-based project (i.e., developing the RN-BSN curriculum working with Dr. Riner, who would be on a funded Fulbright sabbatical in fall 2013).

The authors worked with faculty at TNIMA to identify their needs in the following areas for faculty development:

- New course development and how best to teach
- More audio/visual resources, including computers and projectors
- Successful teaching strategies, including engaging students in writing on the board and discussion, varying teaching methods during the class, recap of previous lecture, giving pretests for challenging subjects such as math, having a blueprint for the class session, using students for tutoring in small groups
- Ethical issues associated with teaching
- Simulation: case writing and debriefing
- Strategies for how to keep up with current practice in the discipline

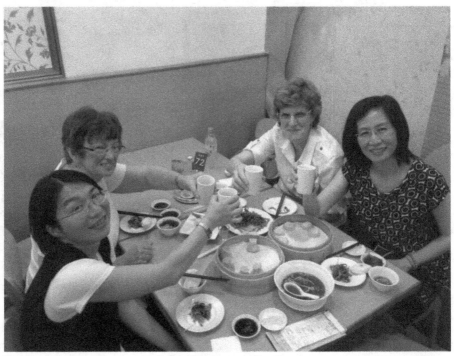

Mary Riner and Marion Broome with Shiow-Ching Shun and Yeur-Hur.

- Basic life-saving skills certification needed
- Test design and item construction, how to write and evaluate multiple choice and essay questions

CHALLENGES DURING THE PROCESS AND EVOLUTION OF THE PARTNERSHIP

As was discussed in the foregoing chapter, any diffusion of innovation (in this case the RN-BSN program) requires five important elements, according to Rogers: establishing an identity through goal setting, developing an infrastructure involving people and technical and financial resources, creating tangible and intangible incentives, providing incremental opportunities for participation, and integrating change into the regular business (Edwards, Feldman, Sangl, Polakoff, Stern, & Casey, 2007). In this section we focus on highlighting some of the challenges that arose related to the fourth and fifth elements.

Because the second primary goal of this partnership evolved with the initiation of funding from USAID, an increase in the number of partners invested in sustaining and setting goals for the partnership occurred. The decision making related to what kind of program (i.e., BSN completion for nursing or midwifery) was in constant flux, and the processes and outcomes were not always within the sole purview of the original partners. There remains a great need to address high rates of maternal–infant mortality. In general, nurse midwives are paid less than hospital nurses and so often choose to return to school for a BSN in nursing and not midwifery, so there is a clear need for more baccalaureate-prepared nurse midwives in the country. Most midwives who do choose to obtain a bachelor's degree complete 3 additional years in nursing. Therefore, the authors found themselves having to significantly revise the plans for the RN-BSN program, placing the focus on a BS in midwifery to gain the support of other BS programs in the country as well as the Ministry of Health. Consistent with Rogers's diffusion of innovation theory, we adapted to that need for a change in original plans by hiring a consultant from a U.S. school who was a nurse-midwife and who had worked in Liberia in the rural counties for years. The master's student, who was the director of the TNIMA program in midwifery, also was a valuable resource to the team in the time of change.

CONCLUSION

We and our Liberian partners at TNIMA remain convinced that a public option for completion of baccalaureate degrees in both nursing and midwifery is essential in order to prepare the future workforce to meet the needs of the citizens of Liberia. Therefore, continued focus on building relationships with broad constituencies in health care in the country will be critical to sustaining the program, which was designed to build clinical leaders and nurse educators for the future health care system of the country.

REFLECTIVE QUESTIONS

1. What particular strengths would you bring to a group that is working to build its members' confidence and skills as leaders?
2. When your goals for a project are reformed and reframed by a larger group, how do you feel? How do you respond to the larger group?
3. In light of your understanding of Liberia, what strategies would you use to help the two students acculturate while master's students?

SUGGESTED WEBSITES

www.africa.upenn.edu/Country_Specific/Liberi.html
www.infoplease.com/world/countries/liberia
www.TNIMA.org/aboutus.html
www.universityliberia.org

REFERENCES

Edwards, J. C., Feldman, P. H., Sangl, J., Polakoff, D., Stern, G., & Casey, D. (2007). Sustainability of partnership projects: A conceptual framework and checklist. *Joint Commission Journal on Quality and Patient Safety, 33*(12), 37–47.

Kouzes, J. M., & Posner, B. Z. (2007). *The leadership challenge* (4th ed.). San Francisco, CA: Jossey-Bass.

Reafsynder, C., & Dennis, E. (2011). Center for Excellence in Health and Life Sciences (CEHLS) at the University of Liberia (UL). Funded by the U.S. Agency for International Development Through Higher Education for Development (HED).

CHAPTER 13

Host Country Ownership

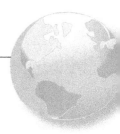

Michele J. Upvall

In Chapter 12 issues of sustainability were discussed in terms of the partnership and planning processes. Ending formal, funded partnerships with mutual respect can be considered the final phase of sustainability, a final step to the maintenance stage previously discussed by Riner and Broome. True partnership with eventual host country ownership can be measured only in years of effort, not in weeks or months. Partnership leading to ownership is a definitive outcome of sustainability (Leffers & Mitchell, 2011). Our goals in global health include meeting the needs of society and achieving global equity while confronting rapid social change and political challenges. At the organizational level, achieving these lofty goals requires multidisciplinary teams who are willing to invest their energy and skills (Rosenberg, Hayes, McIntyre, & Neill, 2010). The nurse, as a member of the team, must also maintain awareness of his or her individual contribution to the transfer of ownership.

Clinics, health care programs, and educational programs in low- and middle-income countries (LMICs) may begin with intense support from the partners, but as the host partners learn from their guest partners, ownership evolves naturally. Dissolution of a true partnership may never need occur, considering the opportunities for ongoing communication through e-mail, Skype, and free texting apps available globally. Partnerships can continue long after specific project goals are achieved with full ownership of the project assumed by the partner, agency, or government. Professional association with the partners may continue, and perhaps new projects may be developed long after the original project is transferred to a partner. Partners can continue to help each other develop professionally.

COMPLETING THE PARTNERSHIP JOURNEY

Not all partnerships end with positive outcomes—previous chapters have discussed threats to partnerships. It is possible that as targets and goals are achieved, the partners may become complacent and threats to the partnership may go unrecognized. Partnerships that complete the full journey have common elements as they continue to move toward the final goal. Box 13.1 contains the essential elements described by Rosenberg, Hayes, McIntyre, and Neill (2010).

Sustaining momentum and having the ability to adapt to changing circumstances is crucial for all phases of the partnership. Often partners believe that once communication issues are confronted and goals mutually set, there is no further need to be concerned with organizational or cultural issues. However, these issues can occur any time, up to the very end of the partnership, and it is important to be vigilant and flexible throughout the process. Strategies for achieving goals may need to change over time, as may the goals themselves.

The second element moving toward project ownership, transfer of control and giving credit, depends on how the partnership was structured from its inception. Individual guest

---

BOX 13.1 Key Elements of the Last Mile in the Partnership Pathway

- Adapting approach to sustain momentum
- Transferring control in a supportive way
- Capturing and communicating lessons learned
- Dissolving the partnership when the goal is achieved

Source: Rosenberg, Hayes, McIntyre, and Neill, 2010, p. 146.

---

partners must continually evaluate the partnership process to assess and identify the extent to which ownership and control of the project is taking place. Each partner should share in the evaluation process and provide feedback in preparation for ownership. It is expected that shared responsibilities and those primary to one member or members of a team will need to be assumed by fewer people. Funding is particularly vulnerable at this point, and without planning for future funding, projects may cease to exist altogether. Being sure that all partners receive credit for their efforts can be a motivating factor in ensuring continuation of the project once the partnership ends. Community members may recognize the remaining partner as a role model, and giving credit will enhance their community status.

Communicating lessons learned throughout the partnership is the third element for successful transfer of ownership. Disseminating information through the media, including social media such as blogging, as well as public reports, newspaper and journal articles, conferences, and workshops, will allow other partnerships and projects to grow. Ideas will be stimulated with the potential of ongoing development and improvement of partnerships.

Finally, Rosenberg, Hayes, McIntyre, and Neill (2010) discuss the actual dissolving of the partnership. Questions partners may ask in guiding the process of dissolution include (p. 23):

- Has the partnership reached its goal?
- What impact has the partnership had on global health?
- What, if any, would be added if the partnership continued?
- What loose ends (final communications, final credit giving, dissemination of lessons learned) need to be tied up?
- What actions and what target date are appropriate for dissolving the partnership?

The authors (Rosenberg, Hayes, McIntyre, & Neill, 2010) recognize that there may be a sense of sadness or a feeling of letdown as the partnership nears its end. So much energy, time, and resources may have been invested in the partnership that after it is over, decompression occurs. They recommend that partners completely terminate the relationship once a project is "owned" by the partner, as confusion can occur, not to mention wasting of resources. A firm ending of the partnership for a particular project may be necessary and feasible, but should not preclude a partnership with the same individuals or agency for the future.

BOX 13.2

"We were used to working in the field with so many wonderful people, sharing meals, and sharing problems, sharing a real camaraderie, and developing deep friendships. . . . The joy was in the trip rather than in the arrival."

Source: Henderson, 2007, p. 5, as cited in Rosenberg, Hayes, McIntyre, and Neill, 2010, p. 155.

EVIDENCE OF LOCAL OWNERSHIP

Eradication of smallpox is often cited as an example of success in global health, and Rosenberg, Hayes, McIntyre, and Neil (2010) discuss the successes and potential perils to this campaign while describing their partnership pathway model. The ongoing efforts of multilateral and bilateral agencies working with national governments, nongovernmental agencies (NGOs), and private partnerships to manage the HIV/AIDS epidemic illustrates a more current example of both success and failure in the process of local ownership.

Negative effects of funding from agencies such as the World Bank and other multilateral agencies have been documented, including destabilization of entire health systems (Parker, 2002). In effect, such agencies have been considered "neocolonialists," replacing the direct rule of the colonialist order with economic dependence. However, the AIDS program in Brazil funded by the World Bank offers a glimpse into promoting long-term sustainability and is often promoted as a model for AIDS programs in other countries with few resources. Initiated in 1993 with funding from the World Bank, the Brazilian AIDS program successfully implemented policies to prevent the spread of HIV and provided antiretroviral therapy (ART) access to all those already affected by AIDS. Community mobilization at the local level, involvement of NGOs, and decentralization of policy with power given to the local municipalities have helped mitigate the AIDS epidemic in Brazil (LeLoup, Fleury, Camargo, & Larouze, 2010).

The World Bank worked with the Brazilian Ministry of Health over a 20-year period addressing AIDS beginning with macro-level, countrywide efforts and then influencing local health program policy. In Swaziland, southern Africa, the opposite circumstance occurred when two physicians from the UK National Health Service (NHS) returned to a rural hospital where they had previously worked in the 1990s. Shocked at the impact HIV/AIDS was having on the local population, they developed a partnership with the hospital over a 10-year period. The partnership at first improved tuberculosis (TB) and epilepsy services, and a few years later the partnership led to linking the TB program to other rural health centers. An integrated primary, secondary, and tertiary care approach to TB was the result, and community health workers were then associated with the centers. Previously, these community health workers were independent of the health care system, leading to fragmentation. A chronic disease management for epilepsy was the next program to be developed followed by HIV education and ART. Novel approaches to reaching patients in every corner of the region were developed, and these efforts were supported by the regional health officials as well as the Ministry of Health. Clearly, the impact of small initiatives begun at one hospital affected the health of the Swazi nation, mitigating devastation from both communicable and chronic diseases (Wright, Walley, Philip, Petros, & Ford, 2010).

ONGOING CHALLENGES FOR OWNERSHIP

Challenges to partnerships occur at the individual project level, but the partnership may never reach fruition or ownership due to threats of a more general nature: lack of human resources to carry out the work and inadequate translation of national health policy into the local health sector during times of shifting economies. These issues may be out of the control of the partners, but the effects strongly impact nursing partnerships.

Nursing Self-Sufficiency/Migration

The ability of a country to fulfill its domestic human resource needs in meeting the health care demands of its country can be considered a measure of self-sufficiency. If a country does not have an adequate supply of nurses or nursing staff are unevenly distributed—that is, most are working in urban areas, while rural providers are scarce—the overall health indicators of the country will suffer. Little and Buchan (2007) provide examples of countries (Iran, Australia, Oman, Malawi) and regions (Caribbean) that were deliberate in workforce

---

BOX 13.3 Indicators of Self-Sufficiency

---

1. Proportion of the stock of international and educated nurses in a country at any one point in time
2. Proportion of the annual nurse inflow that is internationally educated
3. Number of qualified nurse applicants that are turned away from schools of nursing each year
4. Number of funded educational nursing seats as compared to the number required
5. Percentage of nurses who are licensed but not employed in nursing as compared to other countries
6. Annual outflow of nurses from employed in nursing to employed in nonnursing in a country
7. Percentage of nurses of working age who let their licenses expire

Source: Little and Buchan, 2007, p. 18.

---

planning and thus managed to stem the tide of migration and increase the numbers of their existing workforce. These countries/regions achieved success through their ability to collaborate with many partners, including international partners, government support, short- and long-term workforce planning, significant increases in training programs, decreased reliance on importing workers from other countries, and economic investment (Little & Buchan, 2007, p. 9).

Measuring self-sufficiency is a long-term and complex phenomenon. Self-sufficiency indicators described by Little and Buchan (2007) (see Box 13.3) range from the static measure of the raw number of nurses in a country at one time to retention of nurses or nurses who allow their licenses to expire.

These indicators should be considered in context of the country and its circumstances. Tracking statistics in government offices can be a problem in any country, compounded by a possible lack of a registration office or an inability to track expired licenses. Nurses may not have the funds to renew their licenses, and hospitals and clinics may not require that a renewed license be on file. Nurses may also seek employment in the private sector and may not be counted in government statistics, thus contributing to the complexity.

Migration of nurses from country to country or even to different geographic regions within the country is a significant force affecting self-sufficiency. Even countries considered the source of nurses for migration, such as the Philippines and India, may experience deleterious effects to their health care system due to rapid turnover of jobs as nurses leave the country as soon as they obtain the required experience for migration (Littlejohn, Campbell, Collins-McNeil, & Khayile, 2012). Nurses migrate for a variety of reasons, sometimes called the "push–pull factors" of migration. Kingma (2006) documents reasons nurses migrate: adventure, financial considerations, lack of career opportunity and advancement at home, quality of life in the home country (including personal safety), and advanced educational opportunities. The phenomenon of physicians migrating and subsequently not being licensed in their new country has led to the development of special programs to educate these physicians about the role of nursing.

While nurse migration ebbs and flows according to changing political and social climates across the world, increasing nursing's self-sufficiency through educational capacity-building efforts offers opportunities for partnerships leading to host country ownership. The most current example in the United States is the partnership with the Peace Corps and SEED, formerly the Global Health Service Corps, to develop nursing and physician capacity in Malawi, Tanzania, and Uganda (www.peacecorps.gov/response/globalhealth/). Program volunteers serve for 1 year with the option to renew for a second. The first group of volunteer nurses and physicians in the program left for their respective host countries in July 2013.

Shifting Economies

The downturns and upward shifts of the global economy affect the health care of nations in unpredictable ways. Countries experiencing recession find themselves unable to provide the same level of funding for partnerships as they had in the past. At the opposite extreme are countries with growing economies that, in a reversal of roles, have now become donors rather than recipients of funding. Russia is a prominent example of this phenomenon, but Russia's own health statistics, especially those related to TB and HIV/AIDS, indicate that Russia may not be ready to go it alone. A regional program is being developed by the UN to facilitate Russia's becoming a "knowledge hub" for other, nearby countries (Clark, 2013).

A counter argument for the recipient to donor phenomenon questions the moral authority of longstanding high-income countries to provide funding and other resources for partnerships. For example, the United States invests more resources into health than any other country in the world, but outcomes within the United States are no better, or may even be worse, than in other countries. But what of a country such as Angola, the second-largest oil producer in Africa and an exporter of diamonds and minerals (Costa Mendes et al., 2013)? Although economically one of the richest countries in Africa, it ranks 148 of 169 on the UN Human Development Index of 2011 (http://globaledge.msu.edu/countries/angola/economy). How long will it take a resource-rich country such as Angola to obtain self-sufficiency in its health workforce? When will country ownership of health care ever be feasible? Another serious threat is withdrawal of funding before ownership occurs. Host countries may not be able to replace these lost funds, and partnership sustainability may be thwarted.

LOOKING AHEAD

Host country ownership of partnership projects is dependent on the complex forces of politics and economy and the motivation of governments and individuals who implement health policy. Whether a partner assumes ownership may be influenced by forces totally out of the control of the partners and their immediate project concerns. Nurses can play a significant role in facilitating ownership, but a literature review of international partnerships demonstrates that more effort is needed to develop collaborative relationships to the point at which donor support is eventually no longer needed (George & Meadows-Oliver, 2013). Human and financial resources are crucial to ongoing sustainability after the partnership ends.

Professional associations can be a support for nurses struggling with education and resource deficiencies. Kenner and Boykova (2012) chronicle the development of the Council of International Neonatal Nurses (COINN) and Kenner's personal journal of establishing the specialty of neonatal nursing in the United States into a force for impacting global health. These professional associations provide ongoing support at local levels yet facilitate ownership of individual programs and projects.

A stellar example of host country ownership is that of the Aga Khan University School of Nursing (AKUSON) in Karachi, Pakistan, already highlighted in a previous case study. The nursing faculty from AKUSON represent the highest level of achievement for host country ownership as they develop nurse educators in government schools of nursing within Pakistan; develop new programs throughout east Africa, Tajikistan, and Syria; join internationally recognized associations such as Sigma Theta Tau International; and conduct, publish, and present research findings at local and international conferences.

The two case studies that follow this chapter offer a detailed look into ownership within an academic institution in Vietnam and a children's hospital in Cambodia. In both of these examples, Health Volunteers Overseas (HVO) played a prominent role in developing nursing capacity, but it was the motivation of local nurses that expanded initial program goals and promoted ownership from within the institutions.

SUGGESTED WEBSITES

Center for Global Health and Diplomacy site focusing on private–public partnerships. www.ghdnews.com/index.php/global-health-partnerships-and-solutions/public-private-partnerships

Global Health Institute research center concerned with global health governance and diplomacy. http://graduateinstitute.ch/globalhealth

Official site for the International Centre on Nurse Migration. www.intlnursemigration.org

International Council of Nurses position paper on nurse migration. www.icn.ch/images/stories/documents/publications/position_statements/C06_Nurse_Retention_Migration.pdf

Quick fact sheet on nursing self-sufficiency from the ICN Center International Centre on Migration. www.twna.org.tw/frontend/un16_commission/webPages_4/ICN%20Monthly%20Mailing/2007/May%20&%20June/3.pdf

REFERENCES

Clark, F. (2013). The changing face of aid in Russia. *The Lancet, 382,* 113–114.

Costa Mendes, I. A., Marchi-Alves, L. M., Mazzo, A, Nogueira, M. S., Trevizan, M. A., deGodoy, S., . . . Arena Ventura, C. A. (2013). Healthcare context and nursing workforce in a main city of Angola. *International Nursing Review, 60*(1), 37–44. doi: 10.1111\j.1466-7657.2012.01039.x

George, E. K., & Meadows-Oliver, M. (2013). Searching for collaboration in international nursing partnerships: A literature review. *International Nursing Review, 60,* 31–36.

Henderson, D. A. (2007, October 26). Smallpox eradication: Memories and milestones. *CDC Connects,* 5.

Kenner, C., & Boykova, M. (2012). Global health and neonatal nursing: A personal journey. *Maternal Child Nursing, 37*(5), 317–324.

Kingma, M. (2006). *Nurses on the move: Migration and the global health care economy.* Ithaca, NY: Cornell University Press.

Leffers, J., & Mitchell, E. (2011). Conceptual model for partnership and sustainability in global health. *Public Health Nursing, 28*(1), 91–102. doi: 10.1111/j.1525-1446.2010.00892.x

Le Loup, G., Fleury, S., Camargo, K., & Larouze, B. (2010). International institutions, global health initiatives and the challenge of sustainability: Lessons from the Brazilian AIDS programme. *Tropical Medicine and International Health, 15*(1), 5–10.

Little, L., & Buchan, J. (2007). *Nursing self sufficiency/sustainability in the global context.* Geneva, Switzerland: International Centre on Nurse Migration. www.intlnursemigration.org/sections/research/commissioned.shtml

Littlejohn, L., Campbell, J., Collins-McNeil, J., & Khayile, T. (2012). Nursing shortage: A comparative analysis. *International Journal of Nursing, 1*(1), 22–27. www.ijnonline.com/index.php/ijn/article/view/21

Parker, R. (2002). The global HIV/AIDS pandemic, structural inequalities, and the politics of international health. *American Journal of Public Health, 92,* 343–346.

Rosenberg, M. L., Hayes, E. S., McIntyre, M. H., & Neill, N. (2010). *Real collaboration: What it takes for global health to succeed.* Berkeley, CA: University of California Press.

Wright, J., Walley, J., Philip, A., Petros, H., & Ford, H. (2010). Research into practice: 10 years of international public health partnership between the UK and Swaziland. *Journal of Public Health, 32*(2), 277–282. doi: 10.1093/pubmed/fedp129

A Collaborative Project in Remote Villages in Central Vietnam

Jill B. Derstine
Pamela Hoyt-Hudson

CONTEXT: VIETNAM

When flying into Vietnam, as if by magic, vast patches of green appear on the ground, which, as the plane begins to circle, become rice paddies. Square after square of green rice paddies. This is somewhat deceiving because, once on the ground, you see that there are cities that teem with people.

Tour groups visit these crowded cities but rarely get to see the small villages that surround them, dotting the countryside. People have worked hard to rebuild their nation and preserve its resources since the end of the Vietnam War in 1975. The health care system consisted of traditional practice influenced by the Russian system for hospital care. On the lifting of the American embargo on Vietnam in the early 1990s, American and other foreign nongovernmental organizations (NGOs) arrived and began to initiate newer, more modern practices.

Although a formal health system has been traditionally nonexistent or rudimentary, the Vietnamese government set goals for the period from 2000 to 2010, "which include improving the health of all people, preventing disease, combining modern medicine with traditional medicine and socializing health care" (Smith, Fitzpatrick, & Hoyt-Hudson, 2011, p. 199).

This case study describes a collaborative project between two nursing programs, a foundation, and a nongovernmental organization (NGO) that was designed to bring about health changes in the communes of Nam Dong Province near the city of Hue, Vietnam. The Dreyfus Health Foundation (DHF) of the Rogosin Institute in New York (Smith et al., 2011, pp. 17, 18) and Health Volunteers Overseas (HVO) worked together with department of nursing faculty from Temple University at the School of Nursing at Hue University of Medicine and Pharmacy in Hue, Vietnam.

A prior partnership between DHF and Temple University served as a catalyst for the project launched in Vietnam in 2004. In 2002, the DHF and the department of nursing faculty from Temple University partnered in a community-based initiative to improve the health and well-being of inner-city residents in Philadelphia. This collaborative work led to a series of conversations between the authors: Derstine, who was then the chair of the nursing department at Temple University, and Hoyt-Hudson, global nursing coordinator at DHF (see Box 13.4). Building on their shared interest in global nursing and public health, the authors began to identify points of intersection in their respective work and to explore the possibilities for a collaborative global initiative. Derstine's work in Vietnam since the 1990s in cooperation with HVO and Hue University provided a strong base for this new partnership. DHF had officially launched its global nursing program in 2002 and was considering

BOX 13.4 Memories of the Beginning Collaboration

In October 2002, I had the good fortune to meet Dr. Jill Derstine, who was chair of the nursing department at Temple at the time. We shared our mutual interest in global nursing and I learned of Jill's work in Vietnam. Jill expressed interest in the Problem Solving for Better Health Nursing (PSBHN) program and felt that it would be both applicable and useful to nurses and nursing students in Vietnam. Following the initial meeting, I agreed to do an assessment visit with Jill at Hue University in Vietnam during my routine spring visit to Asia. In March 2003, Jill and I met with Dr. Tran Duc Thai, who was chair of the department of nursing at Hue University at that time. Dr. Thai had previously attended an international nursing conference and was already familiar with the DHF and its problem-solving model. He immediately expressed enthusiasm and willingness to expand the collaborative efforts to include the PSBHN program. During the assessment visit, we discussed the programmatic approach and timeline for the launch at Hue University. We decided that it would be best to integrate the PSBHN model into the community health course work with the third-level nursing students. This would be the most likely point of intersection, as the students would then implement their PSBHN projects in the field as part of the coursework. We did encounter one challenge during the planning phase, which included the structure of the workshop. Historically, DHF encourages individuals to work through the PSBH process and implement their own projects so that they each take ownership of the work. However, Dr. Thai felt strongly that the students would need to work in small groups with the goal of three to five projects emerging from the PSBH workshop. We agreed to honor Dr. Thai's recommendation so that the new pilot was set up for success. I was pleasantly surprised by the ease with which we all came to this decision and the positive and collaborative spirit that was in the air. I had a wonderful first visit to Hue, Vietnam, and was particularly touched by the Vietnamese people's kind and gentle way of being. I still remember watching the young school children joyfully playing during recess in their blue uniforms with the girls in white bows and the boys in ties. I recognized the song "Ring Around the Rosie" despite my inability to understand the Vietnamese language. It is a fond memory that will be with me forever. I also was very encouraged by the leadership and flexibility exhibited by the HVO members and the involved nursing faculty at Temple University. I felt quite confident that we were off to a good programmatic start and the collaborative work would lead to something fruitful. (Pamela Hoyt-Hudson, personal communication, June 2013)

expansion to new countries, such as Vietnam. The timing was right to consider a collaborative project, but the authors recognized the importance of engaging Hue University and HVO in the exploratory dialogue. The proposed project needed to be relevant to local needs, as well as feasible from all viewpoints. Derstine and Hoyt-Hudson conducted a joint assessment visit in Hue, Vietnam, at Hue University in March 2003 to further discuss collaborative project potential with Hue University School of Nursing faculty and key HVO personnel.

Collaboration in health care is not a new trend, and it is one of the hallmarks of successful implementation of teaching abroad sponsored by health care institutions and other interested parties (Crow & Thuc, 2011; Potempa, Phancharoenworakul, Glass, Chasombat, & Cody, 2009; Wang, Collins, Vergis, Gerein, & Macq, 2007; Weinstein, 2004). Collaborative relationships affect and improve patient outcomes and ideally embrace cultural sensitivity (Weinstein, 2004). What makes this collaboration unique is that it includes university nursing programs, an NGO, and a foundation. These agencies worked together seamlessly throughout the planning, implementation, and evaluation of this successful project.

Dr. Derstine, a faculty member at Temple University, had been participating in various projects with HVO since 1994 and at the time was working in Hue in rehabilitation and nursing curriculum. Derstine's ongoing work with HVO, as well as her existing relationships in Hue, further catalyzed the broader collaborative project with DHF. The chair of the nursing department at Hue University, Tran Duc Thai, fully embraced the idea of a joint project.

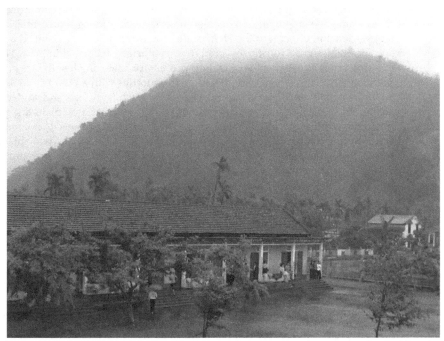

Village school in rural Vietnam.   *Credit*: J. Derstine

HVO

HVO is "dedicated to improving the availability and quality of health care in developing countries through the training and education of local health care providers" (Health Volunteers Overseas, 2007, cover page). The present nursing project described in this chapter actually evolved from a rehabilitation project, funded by the U.S. Agency for International Development (USAID) and implemented by HVO, which included nurse educators participating with other rehabilitation professionals teaching rehabilitation to Vietnamese nurses in Hanoi and Ho Chi Minh City. In this series of workshops, nurse educators worked with Vietnamese rehabilitation nurses to teach them the role of the nurse on the rehabilitation team. As a direct result of these rehabilitation workshops, the participating Vietnamese nurses requested up-to-date information on nursing curricula (O'Toole, Melli, Moore, & Derstine, 1996). The USAID grant received additional funding to continue the project by linking up three universities from the United States with three nursing schools in Vietnam with the purpose of expanding the scope of the curricula to include rehabilitation nursing. Under the auspices of HVO, the Hue University School of Nursing and the Temple University Department of Nursing in Philadelphia developed a partnership in 2003. Several workshops conducted by Temple University faculty were supported as an extension of the original USAID project, but due to increased local need and interest, and with rehabilitation outcomes having been met, it became necessary to seek additional collaborative support. The DHF was able to facilitate steps forward by sponsoring a Problem Solving for Better Health Nursing (PSBHN) workshop for Hue nursing faculty and all third-year nursing students in conjunction with the community health curriculum at the school of nursing.

DHF

In 1989, DHF developed a program, Problem Solving for Better Health (PSBH), which has since been implemented in more than 30 countries. The program engages communities in an action-oriented process to solve local health problems. As PSBH expanded globally,

DHF recognized that nurses were critical to the success of these community-based initiatives. Dame Sheila Quinn, an esteemed international nursing figure, and Dr. Barry Smith, a physician and director at the DHF of the Rogosin Institute, envisioned a PSBH program specifically designed for nurses. PSBHN was officially launched in 2002. This global nursing program is a cost-effective, practical process for achieving health care goals for targeted populations. PSBHN has been piloted in 15 countries with a broad cross-section of nurses and nursing students. The program is based on teaching nurses and student nurses a five-step problem-solving framework that they use to develop action plans and projects in their home communities or work environments. The nurse-led projects do not require significant seed funding to execute and are often implemented using locally available resources. This problem-solving process is familiar to nurses as it is the basis of their nursing education, and yet it is an innovative approach that leads to personal action and social responsibility for improving local health conditions.

The PSBH five-step framework (www.dhfglobal.org/who/pdf/psbh_handbook.pdf) is introduced over the course of a 2- to 3-day workshop held in a variety of settings, including academic institutions and health care facilities.

The five-step process includes:

1. Defining the problem, including the *nature*, *size*, *cause*, and *contributing factors*
2. Prioritizing the problem (identifying a piece of the problem that one can realistically solve)
3. Defining a solution (asking a "Good Question"); the "Good Question" includes the following dimensions: Will doing *what*, with *whom*, *where*, and for *how long*, achieve the *desired objective*?
4. Creating an action plan, including the *why*, *what*, *how*, and plans for *evaluation*
5. Taking action

Participants are encouraged to use available resources, including information and funding, to address the problems they have identified. Each participant leaves the workshop with a clearly defined problem, a "Good Question," and a practical action plan. Most importantly, participants return to their communities with a renewed commitment to impact health and quality of life (Dreyfus Health Foundation, n.d., p. 6).

DHF created a global network to decentralize the operating and management structure of this program. National coordinators organize the basic workshop training as well as the follow-up and monitoring process. During the workshop training each participant develops an action plan to address a relevant health problem that he or she wants to solve. After the workshop training, the participant executes the project in his or her work environment or home community. The local team works with the participants during the implementation phase to assist with project follow-up and monitoring. Each project requires an evaluation tool so that impact and outcomes can be measured. Thousands of nurse-led projects have been implemented in hospital and community settings as a result of this global nursing effort. Many projects have been sustained, expanded, and replicated in other hospitals and communities, resulting in policy impact. Preliminary data from the DHF global nursing initiative indicate that the problem-solving process has increased the skill set and professional confidence of the nurses and enhanced their leadership potential. Most of the student nurses say that nursing education has been positively influenced in those countries where the program was integrated into nursing curricula (China, Dominican Republic, Ghana, India, Indonesia, Poland, United States, and Vietnam) (Hoyt-Hudson, 2007).

FIRST STEPS TOWARD COLLABORATION

The initial Dreyfus workshop was held during the week of March 7, 2004, and involved two DHF facilitators, two Temple nursing faculty, and various members of HVO who were support personnel for HVO's projects in Vietnam. Prior to the PBSH program launch, Hue nursing faculty escorted the workshop facilitators to several villages in Nam Dong province to view the potential sites where students would complete their projects.

Program Plan for Initial Dreyfus Problem-Solving Workshop

The workshop was held during the week of March 7, 2004. In attendance were 38 nursing students, six Hue University nursing faculty, two DHF facilitators, and two Temple University nursing faculty.

The objectives of the workshop were to:

- Conduct a 2½-day workshop titled "Problem Solving for Better Health—Nursing™" for the nursing program at Hue University College of Medicine and Pharmacy.
- Encourage each participant to bring a community health problem that he or she would like to solve.
- Help the workshop participant develop and complete a plan of action to solve the problem by the end of the workshop.
- Integrate the projects into the nursing curriculum as part of the community health course.
- Help participants use available community resources to implement their projects.
- Conduct a 1-day follow-up workshop 6 months after the first workshop.
- Visit the project periodically (DHF facilitators).

DHF provided a small amount of money to be used for available resources to support the project. In addition, DHF provided the school funds to cover lunch and breaks and provided folders, worksheets, and PSBH handbooks for all participants. Finally, DHF reimbursed the school for translation of the handbook into Vietnamese prior to the workshop. It was a long-range goal that the PSBH program become a self-funded yearly event as well as a permanent part of the curriculum.

THE WORKSHOPS

The initial workshop proceeded on schedule (see Box 13.5). There was a noticeable level of excitement and enthusiasm among the students. The authors were pleased and surprised that the students came to the workshop with ideas for problems: It was obvious that the faculty had prepared them for the workshop. The students and facilitators divided into small groups with one or two facilitators for each group. Breaking down the problem into a manageable project proved to be the most challenging aspect for the students. As the workshop progressed and students began to see their projects take shape within the PSBH model, they realized that they were going to have actual results.

Topics generated at this first workshop included:

- Sanitation issues at a village that took care of its garbage by disposing it into the surrounding jungle.
- Malnutrition among children younger than 5 years of age.
- Lack of knowledge about immunization, including its importance and its side effects and how to treat them.
- Need for improvement in the skills of assistant nurses at Hue University Hospital for transferring patients. This problem was developed by two faculty members who noted the recurring evidence of patient falls in the hospital.

The team returned in May 2005 to evaluate the projects and to conduct a new workshop with the new third-level class. DHF provided funding, and the long-term goal was discussed to support achieving the first goal of inclusion of the program into the curriculum.

BOX 13.5 Daily Workshop Activities

Workshop Activities

Day 1 (8:30 a.m.–5:30 p.m.)

Formal opening ceremony, two or three plenary sessions, several small group sessions, lunch break, two coffee breaks. Each student comes to the workshop with one problem related to the community health course. Students organize into three groups with one Hue University faculty member in each group. Each group decides on one health problem that reflects their community health coursework.

Day 2

Set up as day 1, but facilitators work with the students in small group sessions to develop action plans for their problems.

Day 3

Students finalize plan of action and be ready for implementation. All PSBH action plans to be presented at the closing ceremony. DHF certificates will be given to the students.

A core of trained Hue University nursing faculty were to be trained to continue the work and integrate the program into the curriculum. In this second workshop, nursing faculty acted as the facilitators with the help and guidance of the two Temple University nursing facilitators and one DHF facilitator. HVO continued to make in-country arrangements for the team, including hotel accommodations and transportation. The second workshop was conducted exactly the same as the first, and several more projects were developed.

We enjoyed visiting the sites where the first sets of projects were being implemented. For example, as soon as the group approached Khe Tre Town, site of the immunization project, loudspeakers began telling the villagers that immunizations would be given that day and that there would also be classes on immunization for the parents (the government health personnel came to each village once a month to conduct immunization clinics, and the students coordinated teaching activities to coincide with these clinics). Posters created by the students were displayed with both words and pictures relating to the immunization of children. The students collected pre- and post-vaccination data by questionnaire and came up with some interesting figures that showed increased understanding by parents of the importance of vaccination, potential side effects associated with vaccination, and management of such side effects (Hue Medical College Faculty of Nursing, 2005, pp. 53–55).

When the facilitators group visited Village II of Thuy Phuong commune, the students showed their assessment plan, which included meetings with the village chief and interviews with 30 households. Implementation strategies included education about the dangers of garbage and how to dispose of garbage. A follow-up evaluation was also conducted and included interviews of the households and observation of garbage practices after the teaching sessions. Garbage was classified as "home garbage," "cattle feces," and "other." The evaluation results were outstanding in that the people had learned about the "evil" of garbage and no longer threw it outside or into the river, but instead buried it or burned it. Last, the students recommended that the villagers talk with local authorities about possible garbage collection (Hue Medical College Faculty of Nursing, 2005, pp. 11–17).

A project titled "Malnutrition of Children Under Five Years" was conducted in Thuong Nhat Commune, a village in the mountainous area inhabited by the Katu group, an ethnic minority. Students reported that "[t]he emerging health problem here is malnutrition in children younger than 5 years (47.3%) to compare with the average rate 36.8% of the whole district (according to the data of 2003)" (Hue Medical College Faculty of Nursing, 2005, p. 27). This was an ambitious project that included assessing the knowledge of the mothers, assessing food resources, preparing training material, holding teaching meetings with the mothers, and observing the mothers practice what they learned. The mothers' knowledge was evaluated at the end of the project, and most demonstrated a fundamental change in knowledge: a "good" grade. Many of the mothers were illiterate and did not speak the local dialect, so evaluation strategies had to be adapted. The most amazing part of the evaluation came at the end of the year when local authorities and health officers evaluated the rate of malnutrition and found it had decreased to 36%!

The students carried out the above projects over a 6-month period, facing obstacles such as difficult transportation to these distant villages, expense of transportation, illiterate trainees, and lack of enough funding for training materials. DHF funds were available, but had to be spread among all the projects—so no project could be fully funded.

Van, Hoat, and van Schie (2004) conducted a study to determine barriers to the use of maternal care and family planning services by two ethnic minority groups in the remote areas of Nam Dong. Their results give credence to the difficulties faced as the nursing students implemented their projects: difficulty of terrain, cost of treatment, difficulty communicating because of minority language, illiteracy, and lack of a modern communication system. These were the same barriers observed by the Hue students and faculty as they ventured into the mountainous areas. Those authors concluded that there was an urgent need to bring clinical and health-promotion activities to rural people in Vietnam (Van et al., 2004, pp. 1–2).

In addition to visiting the aforementioned projects, the visiting team of DHF facilitators and Temple nursing faculty conducted the second workshop for the next class. Hue University faculty exhibited their leadership as PSBH facilitators throughout the workshop. Transfer of ownership clearly began at this time in year 2. After working 1 year with the material, they were quite proficient in their knowledge of the DHF problem-solving methodology. A total of seven projects were developed in the second round. Some were extensions of the previous year's projects but at different locations. The new projects were conducted in the schools and included preventing worm infection of children, prenatal teaching, and dental education for school-age children. One project, directed at poor hygiene in young children, demonstrated good hand washing and rationale. It is interesting to note that 5 years later two Vietnamese public health researchers, using a similar but much larger sample, showed results that demonstrated a poor level of hand washing with soap. The study was conducted at six primary and secondary schools in rural villages. Recommendations included prioritizing hand washing education to children in school in these areas (Xuan & Hoat, 2013, pp. 1, 6).

In March of 2006, two Temple University nursing facilitators made the third and last formal visit. This was mainly to observe the results of the second set of projects and to watch as the Hue University faculty conducted another round with the next set of students. The objective was to give support, as the university was now self-directing the workshops. This time, a new faculty member from the university was present who had just graduated from the BSN program, had been a student in the first Dreyfus workshop, had graduated, and was now eligible to be a teacher.

Since the PSBH workshop was now a definite part of the curriculum and was being taught by Hue faculty, the long-range goal had been met. A visit by a facilitator would be made when possible, hopefully within 1 or 2 years, to check all projects and to verify that the university was maintaining the program.

PROJECT OWNERSHIP

Several partnership projects report limited success, although long-term data addressing projects in Vietnam are scarce or nonexistent (Barrett, Ladinsky, & Volk 2001; Crow & Thuc, 2011; Gien et al., 2007). "Designing the future requires a thorough understanding of where the Vietnam partners see their health care and educational systems evolving"

(Crow & Thuc, 2011, p. 11). Shediac, Rizkallah, and Bone (1998) discuss the indicators of sustainability. According to these authors, several factors need to be considered in order to determine sustainability. The first is the inclusion of sustainability planning in the initial project planning. Questions need to be asked about the institution sponsoring the project and the recipients of the project to find out whether sustainability is feasible. Strategies need to be considered that will support long-term maintenance. Although the article is from 1998, the discussion has bearing on sustainability of projects in the present day.

DHF plans for sustainability by providing seed money for the initial implementation of a project and gradually decreasing the seed money as the project continues. The foundation continues to stay involved with field visits to support the strategic growth of each country program, but the local teams drive the day-to-day activities. When DHF experienced funding constraints in 2008, it notified the national coordinators in each country to explain that field visits and even limited program support were not possible for the time being. Despite the funding constraints, many countries, including Vietnam, sustained their programs.

Derstine visited several of the nursing faculty at the university in 2011 and was informed that the DHF problem-solving method was still an integral part of the nursing curriculum. In order to cope with the budget cuts, the Hue University nursing faculty revised the program so that students no longer traveled to distant rural villages but instead conducted their PSBH project activities in local or nearby communities. Students used their bicycles to go to sites in Hue City and to villages that were within bicycling distance. The students in the third-year community health course continued to identify problems and implement their projects. The loss is to the far-reaching villages where perhaps the need is more pressing, but the positive aspect is that the students will continue to travel to needy communities, and engage the people to become part of the solution. The faculty remains very positive about the experiences of the students in the projects. Every graduate of the nursing program has participated, and it is anticipated this will encourage some of them to work in the rural communities or in other community settings. Hue University continues to seek resources to scale up the existing program and resume outreach to rural villages.

Lessons learned in this experience reflect the ability of three distinct organizations to work together to effect change. This was enabled by having a clear, distinguishable goal as well as a vested interest in education and improving health in a developing country. Another lesson is that although funding had been cut, the organization (school) realized the importance of these projects both to the students and the community and managed to maintain them as an important part of the curricula.

VIEWING THE SECOND-YEAR PROJECTS IN ACTION

In November 2006, 3 years after the original problem-solving workshop launch, we met in Hue to confer with the faculty of the department of nursing about the program. The entire nursing faculty was present to showcase a presentation summarizing each year of projects. The results documented were impressive for the first 2 years. The faculty then briefed us on the identified health problems for the upcoming workshop.

Very early the next morning, we were on our way to Nam Dong in the director's car with the nursing students following us in two vans. The trip into the highlands was certainly a challenge: It was pouring down rain, and the mountain roads were in less than desirable condition. We visited five schools, all in different villages, to observe students implementing their projects. The villages consisted of small shelters that housed family units. A health center was identified in each village, again a small building with a large room and several smaller rooms. The schools were open on all sides with sturdy roofs. The classrooms had rows of students sitting at long desks. Despite the torrential rain, and even though the schools had very little protection from the weather, we were able to observe high school students, several classes of primary students, and a kindergarten class where the mothers were present. The nursing students were very professional, using slides and other visual aids.

One project in particular, A Dental Health Education Program to Improve Oral Hygiene for Pupils 6 to 8 Years, had lasting effects for all children throughout the country. As we walked into the room eager to learn more about the project, we noticed teaching posters on the wall. Nursing students sat with the children on the floor and demonstrated tooth brushing with a large set of dentures. Some of the school children were using the big toothbrushes on the models.

The students asked the following question: Would a 1-year dental health education program including oral hygiene education, tooth brushing demonstrations, and suitable nutrition reduce the prevalence of dental diseases in children aged 6 to 8 at Thong Lo Primary School in Nam Dong district? They planned to use a questionnaire to assess the children's knowledge about oral hygiene.

The students made contact with health officials in the Nam Dong district health center, the primary health center, local authorities, and the school. They then went to Nam Dong to assess the knowledge of the children using their questionnaire. Three student researchers traveled to the school 2 days each month to tutor students on proper brushing, use of Listerine, oral diseases, and nutrition. Post-intervention questionnaires were used to reevaluate their knowledge. The authors observed some classroom teaching and nursing students teaching the young children how to brush their teeth using brushes and teeth models.

Results, tabulated in simple columns, showed marked improvement in all areas. All students used toothbrushes and toothpaste at the end of the project. The nursing students provided the toothbrushes and tooth crème using some of the DHF seed funding allotted to their project.

Recommendations included continuing community education on dental care by the use of loudspeakers, posters, and brochures, and directing dental education to the parents as well as the children, encouraging attendance at routine checkups when offered. These recommendations were taken seriously and helped to make the case for developing a formal oral health program in 2001 directed at school children that resulted in nearly 10 million children receiving dental care (www.saigon-gpdaily.com.vn/health/2011/11).

CONCLUSION

In summary, we believe that program ownership is a key goal that must be at the forefront of discussion during the project planning phase. Input from all partners, especially the local institutions or entities, is critical throughout the process, and will help to ensure program success and ownership.

REFLECTIVE QUESTIONS

1. What group dynamics do you think needed to be addressed as these organizations began their initial collaboration?
2. What additional long-term impacts could the projects have at the local, nursing school, and national levels?
3. Would the DHF Problem Solving for Better Health approach be useful in your context? Why or why not?
4. What would be some indicators of host country ownership? What steps could you take to achieve this?

REFERENCES

Barrett, B., Ladinsky, J., & Volk, N. (2001). Village-based primary health care in the central highlands of Vietnam. *Journal of Community Health, 26*(1), 51–71.

Crow. G., & Thuc, L. B. (2011). Leading an international nursing partnership: The Vietnam nurse project. *Nursing Administration Quarterly, 35*(3), 204–211.

Dreyfus Health Foundation. (n.d). *Problem Solving for Better Health™ (PSBH™): Participants' handbook.*

Gien, L., Taylor, S., Barter, K., Nguyen, T., Bui, X. M., & Nguyen, T. L. (2007). Poverty reduction by improving health and social services in Vietnam. *Nursing and Health Sciences, 9,* 304–307.

Health Volunteers Overseas. (2007). *A guide to volunteering overseas.* Washington, DC: Health Volunteers Overseas.

Hoyt-Hudson, P. (2007). An international approach to Problem Solving for Better Health Nursing™(PSBHN™). *International Nursing Review, 54,* 100–106.

Hue Medical College Faculty of Nursing. (2005). *Projects of Problem Solving for Better Health Program.* Unpublished report.

O'Toole, M., Melli, S., Moore, M., & Derstine, J. (1996). Global gladiators: A model for international nursing education. *Nurse Educator, 21,* 38–41.

Potempa, K., Phancharoenworakul, K., Glass, N., Chasombat, S., & Cody, B. (2009). Leveraging the role of public health nursing in managing HIV/AIDS in Thailand: A journey of international collaboration. *Collegian, 16,* 49–53.

Shediac-Rizkallah, K., & Bone, L. (1998). Planning for the sustainability of community-based health programs: Conceptual frameworks and future directions for research, practice and policy. *Health Education Research, 13*(1), 87–108.

Smith, B., Fitzpatrick, J., & Hoyt-Hudson, P. (2011). *Problem solving for better health: A global perspective.* New York NY: Springer Publishing Company.

Van, T. V., Hoat, L. N., & van Schie, T. J. (2004). Situation of the Kinh poor and minority women and their use of maternal care and family planning service in Nam Dong mountainous district, Thuathien-Hue Province, Vietnam. *Rural and Remote Health 4,* 1–18.

Wang, Y., Collins, C., Vergis, M., Gerein, N., & Macq , J. (2007). HIV/AIDS and TB: Contextual and policy choice in programme relationships. *Tropical Medicine and International Health, 12*(2), 183–194.

Weinstein, S. (2004). Strategic partnerships. *Journal of Infusion Nursing, 27*(5), 297–301.

Xuan, L. T. T., & Hoat, L. N. (2013). Handwashing among school children in an ethnically diverse population in northern rural Vietnam. *Global Health Action, 6,* 1–8. 18869-http://dx.doi.org/10.3402/gha.v610.18869.

Impact of International Volunteers on Nursing Education and Services at Angkor Hospital for Children and Cambodia

Manila Prak

CONTEXT: CAMBODIA

The Kingdom of Cambodia, formerly known as the Khmer Empire, is located in southeast Asia. The total landmass is 181,035 square kilometers, bordered by Thailand to the northwest, Laos to the northeast, Vietnam to the east, and the Gulf of Thailand to the southwest. Cambodia is the 70th most populous country in the world. The official religion is Buddhism, with 95% of the population active participants. Unfortunately, the Cambodian civil war allowed the Khmer Rouge to take power from 1975 to 1979. After the Khmer Rouge fell from power in 1979, Cambodia started from zero, at genocide from the combined result of political executions, starvation, and forced labor. Many health care professionals, including nurses, were killed during that time. Nursing education, albeit in a limited fashion, only revived in the 1980s. Health statistics reflect the ongoing impact of the civil war (see Table 13.1).

BACKGROUND OF ANGKOR HOSPITAL FOR CHILDREN AND PARTNERS

Angkor Hospital for Children (AHC), opened in February 1999, is a pediatric teaching hospital. A Japanese photographer, Kenro Izu, our founder, came to Cambodia in 1993 to take photos of our beautiful countryside and temples, especially Angkor Wat. At the same time

TABLE 13.1 Country Statistics of Cambodia

Total population	14,138,000
Gross national income per capita (PPP international $)	2,230
Life expectancy at birth m/f (years)	64/66
Probability of dying between 15 and 60 years of age m/f (per 1,000 population)	260/220
Probability of dying younger than age 5 (per 1,000 live births)	43
Total expenditure on health per capita (Intl $, 2011)	135
Total expenditure on health as % of GDP (2011)	5.7%

Source: WHO (2013).

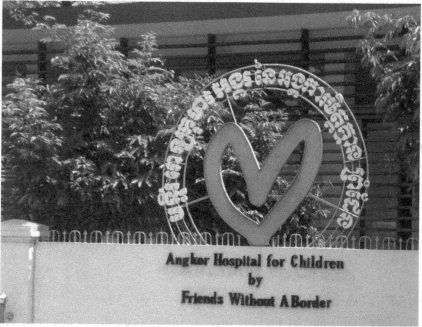

Front gate of the Angkor Hospital for Children.   *Credit*: M. Upvall

he saw many unhealthy and disabled children because of the previous civil war. However, those children were friendly and smiled at him. He remarked that the smile of those children touched his heart, and so he committed to raise money using his photos and come back to start a small hospital for those children.

As a nongovernmental and nonprofit hospital, AHC provides free high-quality treatment and compassionate care to children under 16 years old and their families from all over Cambodia, especially neighboring provinces. AHC is formally recognized as a teaching hospital by the Cambodian Ministry of Health (MOH). We work very closely with the MOH by playing roles as supporter and partners in order to fit with their strategic planning goal for 2008 to 2015: "to provide stewardship for the entire health sector and to ensure a supportive environment for increased demand and equitable access to quality health services in order that all the peoples of Cambodia are able to achieve the highest level of health and well-being" (Better Health Services Project, 2013).

With a strong support from the present executive director, Dr. William Housworth, the External Program Department (EPD) of AHC was started in February 2010. In the National Nursing and Midwifery Conference 2011, themed "Strengthening the Quality of Nursing and Midwifery Care Through Education and Professionalism," held in Phnom Penh, Cambodia, Dr. Housworth stated in his speech that "[t]he quality of care at AHC depends on three things. First, it depends on education. Without well-trained nurses, you cannot produce a quality health care system. Second, our quality depends on a culture of professionalism. Each nurse should have well-defined professional structure and guidelines that he or she follows. This instills a sense of obligation and pride in the nursing profession, which in turn results in quality. And third, and perhaps most importantly, the ideal nurse has a kind heart that seeks to help others regardless of the patient's wealth, social status, race, gender, or other potentially distracting factors. I actually believe that having such a kind heart is infectious. What I mean by this is that if one nurse works closely with another nurse with a kind heart, then this nurse, too, will develop a stronger sense of kindness and compassion over time. I have seen this at AHC and in Cambodia, and it is beautiful when it happens" (Housworth, 2011).

AHC was established and run in a system that was created by the ideas of people from different cultures around the world, making AHC a unique place. We believe that every child has the right to a healthy and loving life. Our vision is for Cambodian children to have access to quality medical care wherever they live, regardless of their ability to pay. AHC exists as a center for excellence in pediatric health care and training, fostering development and expansion of the public health care system.

The nursing process was used as a framework in delivering care to patients from the beginning of the hospital. With much support from the second director of AHC, Mr. Jon F. Morgan (2000–2007), nursing was viewed as a profession and incorporating the nursing process was initiated at that time. As a nurse with a master's degree in public health, Jon F. Morgan steered nursing at AHC in the right direction through strong leadership and management. He initially empowered nurses with education, leadership, and management roles. The three main organizations bringing nurse volunteers to AHC from the beginning were the United Nations Volunteers (UNV), Voluntary Services Overseas (VSO), and Health Volunteers Overseas (HVO). Nurse volunteers play crucial roles in making nursing at AHC stronger by encouraging autonomy in teaching, coaching, mentoring, and encouraging. These volunteers have been role models, increasing the knowledge, competencies, and skills of nurses at AHC as well as instilling the concept of lifelong learning.

Historical Perspective of Volunteers at AHC

I am grateful to Mr. Jon F. Morgan, the former director of AHC and the present director of Lake Clinic Cambodia, for his discussion of how nursing profession started at AHC and the history of volunteers. He was the one who empowered nurses at AHC to be strong, competent, and compassionate to rise to professional standards and level of care.

Volunteerism is a powerful means of engaging people in tackling development challenges, and it can transform the pace and nature of development. Volunteerism benefits both society at large and the individual volunteer by strengthening trust, solidarity, and reciprocity among citizens and by purposefully creating opportunities for participation (United Nations Volunteers, 2013). The second nursing director at AHC, Mieko Morgan, was such a volunteer from UNV. She, committed to promoting the nursing profession in Cambodia, initiated the idea of bringing Cambodian nursing students for clinical placement at AHC. Beginning in 2000, Mieko Morgan brought nurse volunteers from VSO for management roles and teaching Cambodian nurses.

VSO is an international nongovernmental organization linking the priorities of VSO and partners in achieving health targets, HIV and AIDS prevention, participation and governance, securing livelihoods, and promoting education. VSO is committed to gender equality in all work so that men and women have equal opportunities to realize their potential (VSO, 2013). From 2000 to 2002, VSO sent nurse volunteers to AHC to build the capacity and competency of Cambodian nurses. They worked alongside Cambodian nurses during both day and night duty, teaching Cambodian nurses pride in their profession. Eventually, Cambodian nurses grew stronger and gradually took ownership of teaching, coaching, managing, and leading the nursing department independently. VSO nurses also assisted to start up a nursing standard committee to develop the nursing procedures for the hospital. They also trained me, a Cambodian nurse on the job, to become a nursing education coordinator to coordinate all the nursing education for AHC nurses. Currently, I am the director of EPD, one of seven departments within the AHC, playing a significant role in supporting the MOH in improving the quality care for patients as well as strengthening the health care profession, mainly nursing. AHC signed the agreement with University Research Corporation (URC) for EPD to work with URC through various projects to improve the public health care system in Cambodia. URC requires both nursing and medical staff who have the expertise on clinical settings to teach and coach nurses and physicians in public hospitals, fostering interprofessional collaboration.

HVO, another important volunteer organization, is a network of health care professionals, organizations, corporations, and donors united in their common commitment to improving global health through education (HVO, 2013). HVO started work with AHC in 2002. Through HVO, we receive volunteers who have experience in clinical skills and education, and they are often advisors to nurses rather than working in a direct care role.

DEVELOPING LEARNERS INTO LEADERS

AHC nurses have learned much, and still continue to learn, from volunteers while taking ownership for management and leadership roles. Implementation of the nursing process is one of the successful projects within AHC nursing. In the past, volunteers taught the nursing process on an ongoing basis. Now, AHC nurses through EPD lead teaching of the nursing process and provide coaching roles to other nurses at public hospitals. Nurses play roles as advisor, educator, advocator, facilitator, and coach by working with nurses in the public hospitals. We are not just managing to make our new generations of nurses at AHC strong, competent, and professional, but we are also able to do so for nurses who work at the public health care settings in Cambodia as a whole through EPD.

Another project that was supported through volunteers was education of nursing students from nearby Battambang Nursing School. This project began 3 years after inception of AHC, when the nursing department started to receive the final-year nursing students from Battambang. The curriculum for these students was designed to supplement the nursing process, focusing on application of nursing process theory. Originally a pilot project, it was so successful that we continue to receive final-year students not only from Battabang, but also from all five nursing schools under the auspices of the MOH.

While providing supplement course focusing on the nursing process to students, we realized that the nursing instructors who accompanied students also have limited knowledge of the nursing process. In response in 2004, we designed a 2-week curriculum in cooperation with the Human Resources Department (HRD) of the MOH. The curriculum focuses on the application of the nursing process in clinical settings for instructors so that they have more knowledge and skills to help their students. Because of such initiatives, AHC is now well known for building a strong nursing profession in the country because of nursing process use. This resulted in HRD's supporting and assisting AHC toward its 2005 recognition by the MOH as a teaching hospital.

In 2011, the EPD of AHC and URC organized a workshop to "[e]stablish a nationwide consensus and commitment on how to uniformly implement the Nursing Process in practice and in theory" (Angkor Hospital for Children, URC Cambodia, & USAID, 2011). This event was greatly supported by the HRD and hospital services department of the MOH, presided by His Excellency Professor Thir Kruy, Secretary of State of the MOH, demonstrating the significance of the event. He was positively surprised by AHC nurses' professionalism and autonomy. Since the workshop, His Excellency continues to support the nursing process project for all nurses. Results of the workshop included a strategic planning process workshop on how to apply the nursing process, and in late 2012 the nursing process teaching material was developed, finalized, and approved for use by the MOH. In early 2013, the training of trainers and providers was started with follow-up and coaching at local hospitals. We selected 33 hospitals within 9 provinces to implement our project. EPD is now successfully making progress to in promoting quality and compassionate care nationwide, realizing the goals of the MOH.

Other significant events in 2011 in which EPD working with URC supported Cambodian nursing and midwifery of the MOH and Cambodian Nursing Council included the development of the code of ethics for Cambodian nurses. Holly Taylor, JD, a nurse volunteer, helped draft a code of ethics subsequent to discussion with and under guidance from Cambodian nurses. The code has been revised to fit the context of Cambodian nursing, and we have included the voices of nurses throughout the country for the final version. The new code of ethics now awaits approval from the MOH. However, to maintain momentum and to introduce the code to the general population of nurses, we presented the code in a workshop for all nursing leaders around the country. Two nurse volunteers from the University of Pittsburgh School of Nursing assisted in facilitating the workshop. These volunteers were advisors and supporters helping to establish understanding of the code. Finally, during the International Nurses Day May 9 event in Cambodia, the code of ethics for nurses was introduced with a case study application.

Nursing and midwifery protocols (nursing procedures) were also developed in 2011. Before this, no nursing procedures were written for the hospital setting. AHC nurses through EPD facilitated success of this project, supporting the Nursing and Midwifery Bureau of the MOH in both technical and financial support. A committee comprised of senior nurses from AHC/EPD, URC, VSO, and other nursing services and educational institutions under MOH developed 28 protocols that have been approved and published by the MOH. The process ended in late 2012 with distribution of the manuals of the national nursing and midwifery protocol to many hospitals throughout the country. Nurses and midwives use the 28 protocols in their daily work and teaching the nursing students at the clinical sites. The following is a list of the 28 nursing and midwifery protocols:

	Vital signs
1	Axillary Temperature
2	Oral Temperature
3	Rectal Temperature
4	Radial Pulse
5	Apical Pulse
6	Blood Pressure
7	Respiratory Rate
8	Oxygen Saturation
	Drug administration
9	General Drug Administration
10	Oral Drug Administration
11	Intramuscular Injection
12	Intravenous Injection
13	Intradermal Injection
14	Subcutaneous Injection
15	Eye Drug Administration
16	Ear Drug Administration
17	Nose Drug Administration
18	Nebulizer Therapy
19	Sublingual and Buccal Administration
20	Patch Administration
21	Topical Administration

(continued)

FACTORS ESSENTIAL IN BUILDING RELATIONSHIPS AMONG PARTNERS

Communication

AHC began with 40% expatriate staff, with no way to communicate in the Khmer language. It is now compulsory that all Cambodian staff study English. There are many benefits to maintaining English as the major communication vehicle for AHC. Without English, AHC nurses cannot work with volunteers, and without volunteers, we have no network. This networking with volunteers has promoted stronger nursing education and a higher level of professionalism. Nurses at AHC are proud to be part of promoting the nursing profession for the whole of Cambodia, and we have been empowered to lead projects and participate as policymakers and conference/workshop/training organizers.

Resources

Ongoing funding and coordination of volunteer activities will continue to promote the growth of nursing in Cambodia. Funding continues to be important to the MOH and public hospitals as they experience many financial constraints. The AHC–URC partnership with the MOH has helped, but funding of the AHC–URC partnership must continue.

Learning through volunteers continues at AHC and to promote continuity of projects, AHC hired a full-time volunteer coordinator in 2003. The main role of the coordinator is to link and work with volunteers prior to the arrival. Specific responsibilities include:

- Organize volunteer placement
- Collect necessary documentation from volunteer applicants
- Refer completed volunteer applicants to the appropriate supervisor
- Inform volunteer applicants of the AHC's decision
- Arrange logistics for volunteers' visit: accommodation, transportation, visa, supplies to bring
- Describe the application process to interested people
- Answer pre-arrival questions and problems
- Confirm logistics information prior to arrival
- Keep AHC and volunteers up to date
- Create weekly and monthly reports and send them to appropriate supervisors and volunteer organizations
- Pick up volunteers from the airport and introduce them to Siem Reap
- Provide a volunteer package and a hospital tour and introduce relevant staff
- Have the volunteers complete necessary paperwork on their arrival

- Be the volunteer's best friend. Initiate and maintain regular contact with volunteers during their stay at AHC. Answer any questions and respond to any problems
- Arrange a meeting with the executive director at the end of the volunteer's time
- Provide help desk support and hardware and software troubleshooting, and assist the IT manager as needed

CONCLUSION

Through ongoing support of volunteers and development of leaders within Cambodian nursing, we are raising standards for nurses across the country and promoting high-quality health care. The role of the volunteer has evolved from clinical care to project support, and, in turn, AHC supports volunteers through the coordinator role. Much work remains, but the past 2 decades have seen significant growth in the profession of nursing in Cambodia. Most important, it is the Cambodian nurses themselves who are actively seeking and making change.

REFLECTIVE QUESTIONS

1. What external events could influence the development of nursing in another country? What of the impact of war? Who is responsible for rebuilding?
2. At what point in the profession's development do volunteers become unnecessary? Can a transition be made?
3. What cultural factors could impact ongoing partnerships in Cambodia and elsewhere?

REFERENCES

Angkor Hospital for Children, URC, & USAID. (2011). Nursing Process Workshop, February 9–11, 2011, Phnom Penh, Cambodia.

Better Health Services Project. (2013). www.urccambodia.org/site/index.php

Health Volunteers Overseas. (2013). www.hvousa.org/whoWeAre/whywedo.shtml

Housworth, W. (2011, November 23). Introduction. Fifth Annual Nursing & Midwifery Conference, Phnom Penh, Cambodia.

United Nations Volunteers. (2013). www.unv.org/about-us.html

VSO. (2013). www.vso.org.uk/about/what-we-do

World Health Organization. (2013). Cambodia. www.who.int/countries/khm/en

Moving Forward for Global Health

Michele J. Upvall
Jeanne M. Leffers

The instructional content presented in the book chapters followed by the stories of global health nurses as told in the case studies illustrate multiple concepts of the model of partnership and sustainability (Leffers & Mitchell, 2011). Despite the separation of concepts and topics for global health nursing into distinct chapters, taken collectively and illustrated through the experiences shared in the case studies, there exists the important overlapping of partnership factors, processes, and factors influencing sustainability, including resources, leadership, and outcomes with the ultimate result of host country ownership. Incorporation of the strategies, assessment and evaluation tools, and insights from the case studies provide nurses who participate in global health projects ways to collaborate with partners to achieve improved health outcomes for people worldwide.

Nurses active in global health can no longer be content with providing direct service to the exclusion of the broader scope of global health. Issues such as poverty, access to clean water, and education—that is, social determinants of health—require reflection and action (Grootjans & Newman, 2013). These actions are grounded in the community with partnering to meeting the needs identified by the community, recognizing strengths and resources within the community (Anderko, 2010), not viewing the community through the prism of deficiency or as a community lacking resources. It will become increasingly important for global health nurses to take a more active role in shaping health policy, in collaboration with partners most affected by these health policies. Connections with ministries of health and other sectors of the government will be important as partners work together to seek and implement solutions that go beyond the provision of curative services in clinics and hospitals. Nurses can no longer work in isolation from other disciplines and as policymakers as funding sources change from government to private foundations.

Yes, partnerships are more important, indeed more critical, than at any time in the history of global health as we confront problems requiring solutions grounded in the acceptance of the nursing profession's accepting social responsibility for these problems. Solutions are important, but global health nurses must also be able to measure results of these efforts. Both quantitative and qualitative data will become increasingly important to demonstrate effectiveness of solutions and are also as a precursor to host country ownership of programs.

Throughout this book, we offer strategies to improve partnerships to develop sustainability and meet positive outcomes for global health. Each chapter offers specific strategies for partnership and sustainability, but taken collectively, they demonstrate the circular and recurring nature of components essential to global health work. Themes of collaboration, capacity building, cultural bridging, mutual respect, ongoing assessment, leadership, sustainable practices, and outcome evaluation cross all chapters and case studies.

For nurses beginning their global health work, the information shared in Chapters 1 through 5 provides guidance to facilitate nurses as they build and develop partnerships for global health. In particular, the need to ensure that the individual nurse partner explores his or her own motivations, cultural assumptions, readiness for global health work, match of skills and partner needs, and congruence between individual and organizational philosophy must occur prior to beginning a global partnership. The careful assessment of host partner factors and needs must precede mutual goal setting and planning activities. In addition, a careful assessment of resource requirements for the partnership is critically important to a successful partnership.

Chapter 8 offers examples of international organizations that foster both interprofessional collaboration across professions and cross-national collaboration of nurses to build the nursing profession. As nurses collaborate to solve global health problems through partnerships, capacity building, cultural bridging, and collaboration for leadership all contribute to successful outcomes. Chapters 6, 7, and 10 specifically address these essential components. Working collaboratively to advance the nursing profession with global nurse partners through the advancement of nursing education programs, the development and advancement of nursing associations and nursing councils, and the development of nurse practice acts will improve health outcomes across global settings. Leadership for global health partnerships and programs fosters sustainability beyond the actual program implementation.

Chapter 9 addresses the specific topic of global health nursing research, an area of growth and significance for building knowledge to solve global health problems and to advance capacity for nursing research across global settings. Global health nursing research requires particular attention to ethical concerns created by cultural, political, and economic factors.

Chapters 11, 12, and 13 offer solutions to the sustainability of partnerships and programs to achieve positive outcomes for health. With the advances in technology, our ability to communicate across miles has expanded opportunities to provide ongoing support by both partners to improve programs and maintain partnerships. The importance of building in sustainability planning at the outset of a program provides the scaffold necessary to promote sustainable outcomes. The ultimate goal of host country ownership of programs can be achieved through adequate planning, collaborative partnership, funding, leadership, and ongoing assessment for sustainability factors.

Practicing in the arena of global health nursing implies assimilation and expansion of multiple roles. For some nurses it may mean confronting postdisaster situations and helping to rebuild a country's health care and nursing education system. For others, global health nursing may require teaching best practices and learning how to adapt best practices in environments with limited or no resources. For global health nurses working in the public health sphere, there must be understanding of the mother walking more than 5 kilometers to the clinic with her children for immunizations and growth monitoring and, beyond understanding, the willingness to help the community confront problems of transportation. Global health nurses practicing in nursing education and capacity building may need to help students adapt study habits when there is no electricity or are no books available to study. But more than all these challenges, being a global health nurse requires a connection with our humanity and that of others, including those in our own communities, realizing that we do live in a global village and that we can find solutions from each other as we find our way home.

Initiatives developed during the past few years confirm that partnerships are the foremost goal for global health for nursing. Examples such as the Rwanda Human Resources for Health program and the Regis College Haiti Project, highlighted in our case studies, offer sustainable solutions to advance nursing education and ultimately improved patient outcomes in global settings. Most recently, the Global Health Service Partnership is a partnership between the Peace Corps, the President's Emergency Plan for AIDS Relief (PEPFAR), and SEED Global Health to improve clinical education, increase the number of nursing and medical educators, and build health care capacity. After more than a year of planning and recruitment, the inaugural team of nurses and physicians traveled to Uganda, Malawi, and Tanzania in July 2013 to begin 1 year of service in collaboration with schools of nursing and medicine (Peace Corps, 2013). SEED Global Health's mission is to "cultivate stronger, sustainable health systems by training a new generation of physicians and nurses" (SEED Global Health, 2013). Its resources include a library as well as the Global Health Service Partnership Hangout, accessible through its website.

Connections and collaboration have become much easier with recent advances in technology. Although we offer a chapter devoted to technology and how this impacts global health, the burgeoning online sources through listservs, online discussions, and web conferencing strongly support the need for nurses to learn from one another and from other health disciplines in order to improve health outcomes worldwide. One example is the online discussion source Global Health Delivery Online. Two expert panels were hosted by Global Health Delivery online (GHDonline) that included nurses and other health professionals for 1 week in September 2013. The first, hosted by the Global Health Nursing and Midwifery community, featured a panel of nursing experts from Botswana, the United Kingdom, and the United States to address nursing leadership to shape the future of global health. Discussants emphasized that while leadership is essential for successful global health programs, nurses must also consider strategies to collaborate to build nursing in global settings. The second panel was offered as a sitewide discussion and did not offer specific experts on the panel, but rather encouraged members of all communities to participate. In 1 week's time, health care professionals from 74 different countries and more than 130 organizations joined in the discussion (GHDonline, 2013). Through such connections nurses can learn from and collaborate with experts to build knowledge, partnerships, and shared strategies for solutions.

The Global Nursing Caucus, designed to build collaboration and disseminate information for the field of global health nursing, serves as a resource and discussion site for nurses in global health. Through their online blog, global health nurses can learn from one another, share resources, and connect through global health nursing conferences (Global Nursing Caucus, 2013). Collaboration among global health nurses creates partnerships and builds knowledge, develops competencies, shares innovations, and connects nurses new to global health with global health leaders.

The growing field of global health nursing programs in academia requires guidance that can be developed as nurses partner with other nurses in the global health arena. This guidance must address competencies, ethics, service-learning, and coordination with university international programs and partnering organizations and is currently a topic addressed in some academic settings. The Consortium of Universities in Global Health (CUGH) is dedicated to the balance between the educational needs of students and the needs of those partners in low- and middle-income countries. Their current initiatives include the development of shared competencies and curricula, as well as criteria and conditions for student placements for global health programs (CUGH, 2013). As academic nurses who participate in global health projects build or continue programs that involve nursing students, they must consider two important issues. First, academic programs must be partnered with host organizations to achieve ethical, responsible, and culturally appropriate models for nursing education and service. Second, current nursing students will build future generations of global health nurses and must learn about global health nursing through models that demonstrate partnerships and collaboration.

Global health nurses have an ethical and moral responsibility to be concerned with the world's suffering, as we are connected first through our humanity and then our professional values and social responsibility as nurses. Partnership is paramount to responding in a socially responsible manner and is at the heart of achieving sustainable outcomes. As we live our global professional relationships in partnership, we must also accept that mistakes will be made; these should be considered learning opportunities for all in partnership, with kindness and forgiveness an outcome of cultural humility. Finally, being a global health nurse requires courage and adapting to ever-changing goals, accepting at times the ambiguity of outcomes, but also taking comfort in the richness of possibility that serendipity allows.

REFERENCES

Anderko. L. (2010). Achieving health equity on a global scale through a community-based, public health framework for action. *Journal of Law, Medicine & Ethics, 38*(3), 486–489.

Consortium of Universities for Global Health (CUGH). (2013). Consortium of Universities for Global Health: Making the university a transforming force in global health. www.cugh.org

Global Health Delivery Online (GHDonline). (2013). Communities for global collaboration. www.ghdonline.org

Global Nursing Caucus. (2013). Global Health Nursing Caucus: A forum for everyone interested in global nursing issues. http://blogs.bu.edu/globalnursingcaucus

Grootjans, J., & Newman, S. (2013). The relevance of globalization to nursing: A concept analysis. *International Nursing Review, 60*(1), 78–85. doi: 10.1111\j.1466-7657.2012.01022.x

Leffers, J., & Mitchell, E. (2011). Conceptual model for partnership and sustainability in global health. *Public Health Nursing, 28*(1), 91–102.

Peace Corps. (2013). Global health service partnership. www.peacecorps.gov/response/globalhealth

SEED Global Health. (2013). SEED: Global Health. www.peacecorps.gov/response/globalhealth

Index

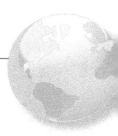